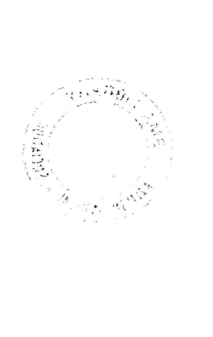

Rare Vascular Disorders

A practical guide for the vascular specialist

Created by Simon D Parvin

Edited by Jonothan J Earnshaw

A Joint Vascular Research Group book

tfm Publishing Limited
Castle Hill Barns
Harley
Shrewsbury
SY5 6LX
UK

Tel: +44 (0)1952 510061.
Fax: +44 (0)1952 510192
E-mail: nikki@tfmpublishing.com
Web site: www.tfmpublishing.com

Design & Typesetting: Nikki Bramhill

Cover photographs courtesy of:
Top right: Mr Geoffrey Gilling-Smith, Consultant Vascular Surgeon, Royal Liverpool University Hospital
Bottom right: Mr Simon D Parvin, Consultant Vascular Surgeon, Royal Bournemouth Hospital
Top left: Dr Bill Leen, Consultant Radiologist, James Cook University Hospital
Bottom left: Mr Mark Scriven, Consultant Vascular Surgeon, Birmingham Heartlands Hospital

First Edition © June 2005

ISBN 1 903378 32 X

Printed by Gutenberg Press Ltd., Gudja Road, Tarxien, PLA 19, Malta.

Tel: +356 21897037; Fax: +356 21800069.

Contents

Contributors

Mohan Adiseshiah MA MS FRCS FRCP Consultant Vascular & Endovascular Surgeon, University College Hospital, London, UK

Simon Ashley MS FRCS Consultant Vascular Surgeon, Derriford Hospital, Plymouth, UK

Ahmed Assar FRCS Specialist Registrar, Vascular Surgery, Queen's Medical Centre, Nottingham, UK

Roger N Baird ChM FRCS Consultant Vascular Surgeon, Bristol Royal Hospital for Children, Bristol, UK

Daryll M Baker PhD FRCS Consultant Vascular Surgeon, Royal Free Hospital, London, UK

Stephen Baxter FCS (SA) Consultant Vascular Surgeon, Southampton General Hospital, Southampton, UK

Jonathan D Beard MB BS BSc ChM FRCS Consultant Vascular Surgeon, Sheffield Vascular Institute, The Northern General Hospital, Sheffield, UK

Marcus J Brooks MD FRCS Specialist Registrar, Vascular Surgery, St. Mary's Hospital, London, UK

Bruce Campbell MS FRCP FRCS Professor and Consultant Surgeon, Royal Devon and Exeter Hospital and Peninsula Medical School, Exeter, UK

Nick JW Cheshire MD FRCS Professor of Vascular Surgery, Imperial College School of Medicine and St. Mary's Hospital, London, UK

Justin Cobb M Chir FRCS Consultant Orthopaedic Surgeon, London Bone Tumour Service, University College Hospital, London, UK

Philip Coleridge-Smith DM FRCS Consultant Vascular Surgeon, The Middlesex Hospital, London, UK

Simon G Darke MS FRCS Consultant Vascular Surgeon, Royal Bournemouth Hospital, Bournemouth, UK

Alun H Davies MA DM FRCS Reader in Surgery and Consultant Surgeon, Imperial College School of Medicine, Charing Cross Hospital, London, UK

Demosthenes Dellagrammaticas MB ChB MRCS Research Fellow, The General Infirmary at Leeds, Leeds, UK

Jonothan J Earnshaw DM FRCS Consultant Vascular Surgeon, Gloucestershire Royal Hospital, Gloucester, UK

Donna M Egbeare BSc MB BCh Senior House Officer, Vascular Surgery, Royal Bournemouth Hospital, Bournemouth, UK

Louis Fligelstone MD FRCS Consultant Vascular Surgeon, Morriston Hospital, Swansea NHS Trust, Swansea, UK

Peter A Gaines FRCP FRCR Consultant Vascular Radiologist, Sheffield Vascular Institute, Northern General Hospital, Sheffield, UK

Robert B Galland MD FRCS Consultant Vascular Surgeon, Royal Berkshire HospitaL, Reading, UK

Christopher P Gibbons MA DPhil MCh FRCS Consultant Surgeon, Morriston Hospital, Swansea, UK

Geoffrey Gilling-Smith MS FRCS Consultant Vascular Surgeon, Royal Liverpool University Hospital, Liverpool, UK

Michael J Gough ChM FRCS Consultant Vascular Surgeon, The General Infirmary at Leeds, Leeds, UK

Nandan Haldipur MB BS AFRCSI MRCS Ed Specialist Registrar, General Surgery, Sheffield Vascular Institute, The Northern General Hospital, Sheffield, UK

George Hamilton MD FRCS Professor of Vascular Surgery, Royal Free & University College School of Medicine, Royal Free Hospital Hampstead NHS Trust, London, UK

Denis W Harkin MD FRCS (Gen Surg) EBSQ-VASC Consultant Vascular Surgeon, Royal Victoria Hospital, Belfast, Northern Ireland

John Henderson MB ChB MRCP FRCR Consultant Interventional Radiologist, Birmingham Heartlands Hospital, Birmingham, UK

Michael Horrocks MS FRCS Professor of Surgery, Royal United Hospital, Bath, UK

Michael Jenkins BSc MS FRCS Consultant Vascular Surgeon, St. Mary's Hospital, London, UK

Ravul Jindal MS DNB FRCS Senior Registrar, Vascular Surgery, Imperial College School of Medicine and St. Mary's Hospital, London, UK

David Lambert MD FRCS Consultant Vascular Surgeon, Northern Vascular Centre, Freeman Hospital, Newcastle upon Tyne, UK

Peter Lamont MD FRCS Consultant Vascular Surgeon, Bristol Royal Infirmary, Bristol, UK

Peter Lewis MD FRCS Consultant Vascular Surgeon, South Devon Health Care Trust, Torquay, UK

Tom Loosemore MS FRCS Consultant Vascular Surgeon, St. George's Hospital, London, UK

Sumaira Macdonald MB ChB (Comm.) MRCP FRCR PhD Consultant Vascular Radiologist, Northern Vascular Institute, Freeman Hospital, Newcastle, UK

Shane MacSweeney MA MChir FRCS Consultant Vascular Surgeon, Queen's Medical Centre, Nottingham, UK

James Metcalfe MRCS Clinical Research Fellow, Vascular Surgery, Royal United Hospital, Bath, UK

Felicity Meyer MA FRCS Consultant Vascular Surgeon, Norfolk and Norwich University Hospital, Norwich, UK

Rob Morgan FRCR Consultant Vascular Radiologist, St. George's Hospital, London, UK

Graham Munneke FRCR Specialist Registrar, Vascular Radiology, St. George's Hospital, London, UK

A. Ross Naylor MD FRCS Professor of Vascular Surgery, Leicester Royal Infirmary, Leicester, UK

Ian Nichol MD FRCS (Gen) Specialist Registrar, Vascular Surgery, Northern Vascular Centre, Freeman Hospital, Newcastle upon Tyne, UK

Klaus Overbeck FRCS (Engl) Vascular and Endovascular Fellow, Northern Vascular Institute, Freeman Hospital, Newcastle, UK

Simon D Parvin MD FRCS Consultant Vascular Surgeon, Royal Bournemouth Hospital, Bournemouth, UK

David A Ratliff MD FRCP FRCS Consultant Vascular Surgeon, Northampton General Hospital, Northampton, UK

M Shafique Sajid FRCS Clinical Vascular Fellow, Royal Free Hospital, London, UK

Mark Scriven BSc (Hons) MB ChB MD FRCS Consultant Vascular Surgeon, Birmingham Heartlands Hospital, Birmingham, UK

Clifford Shearman BSc MS FRCS Professor of Vascular Surgery, Southampton General Hospital, Southampton, UK

Frank CT Smith BSc MD FRCS FRCS (Ed) FRCS (Glas) Consultant Senior Lecturer, Bristol Royal Infirmary, UK

Peter R Taylor MA MChir FRCS Consultant Vascular Surgeon, Guy's & St. Thomas' NHS Foundation Trust, London, UK

Rhys L Thomas BSc MB BS Senior House Officer in Surgery, Royal Surrey County Hospital, Guildford, UK

John F Thompson MS FRCS (Ed) FRCS Consultant Surgeon, Royal Devon and Exeter Hospitals, Exeter, UK

Matt Thompson MD FRCS Professor of Vascular Surgery, St. George's Hospital, London, UK

Dan R Titcomb MRCS Specialist Registrar, Vascular Surgery, Derriford Hospital, Plymouth, UK

Rao Vallabhaneni MD FRCS Endovascular Fellow, Malmö University Hospital, Malmö, Sweden

Anthony Watkinson FRCS FRCR Consultant Radiologist, Royal Devon and Exeter Hospital and Peninsula Medical School, Exeter, UK

Lasantha D Wijesinghe MA MD MB BChir FRCS Consultant Vascular Surgeon, Royal Bournemouth Hospital, Bournemouth, UK

John HN Wolfe MD FRCS Consultant Vascular Surgeon, St. Mary's Hospital, London, UK

Kenneth R Woodburn MD FRCSG (Gen) Consultant Vascular Surgeon & Honorary Clinical Lecturer, Peninsula Medical School & Royal Cornwall Hospitals Trust, Truro, Cornwall, UK

Michael G Wyatt MSc MD FRCS Consultant Vascular Surgeon, Northern Vascular Centre, Freeman Hospital, Newcastle upon Tyne, UK

Foreword

Vascular specialists confidently manage common conditions such as peripheral vascular disease and aneurysms, where the indications for treatment are agreed and interventions are justified by the results of large randomised research studies. This book is designed to be a practical help when an unfamiliar condition arises for which the clinician has no personal experience.

It was recognised some years ago that collating the details of unusual cases experienced by vascular colleagues would be a valuable resource. Simon Parvin and members of the Joint Vascular Research Group created the Rare Diagnosis and Operations Register (see Chapter 1). The aim was to analyse the investigation and treatment of uncommon conditions; this book is the outcome of the enterprise.

Some conditions identified in the Register and covered in this book are not all that rare; a patient with acute arm ischaemia may be seen by a vascular specialist every few weeks. Some conditions, however, may never be seen during a whole career - there is only one example of Moyamoya disease in the Register. All the disorders in the Register and in the book are characterised by a lack of scientific evidence in how best to investigate and manage them. The authors of this book have distilled all the available information to provide common sense advice.

This collection of rare disorders is the result of extensive collaboration between colleagues. A large number of vascular specialists were needed to provide all the cases described. The degree of co-operation is evidenced by the number of individual vignettes and loaned illustrations. The wealth of expertise found here will provide useful practical help.

The book's principal authors belong to a research collaborative of vascular specialists from the UK and Ireland: the Joint Vascular Research Group (see overleaf). The Group has collaborated in other textbooks, including *The Evidence for Vascular Surgery*, which examined common vascular conditions, and the scientific evidence for their optimal treatment. The present book should be seen as a companion.

This book also has significant contributions from others who are not members of the Joint Vascular Research Group. Thank you to all the clinicians who have been involved and given their time and experience. Thanks also to Mr. Michael Wyatt for his assistance in the preparation of the book and to Ms. Nikki Bramhill for her high quality publishing expertise.

Not everyone will agree on the conclusions about best treatment of some of these rare disorders. Ideally, this will spark further research and collaboration.

Jonothan J Earnshaw DM FRCS
Simon D Parvin MD FRCS
June 2005

The Joint Vascular Research Group

The Joint Vascular Research Group (JVRG) was born in March 1983 when 13 consultant surgeons met in Southampton and decided to collaborate in vascular research. From its inception, the prime objective of the Group has been to join together in designing and performing studies into the natural history of vascular disease and multicentre controlled trials of different vascular procedures. The members meet twice a year to propose new trials and to assess the results of current work. Each trial is the responsibility of one member of the Group. Over time the JVRG has been responsible for many communications at scientific meetings and its members have contributed widely to textbooks and surgical journals. A list of the original full papers produced by the JVRG appears on the facing page.

The JVRG is entirely self-supporting and relies on donations and profits from meetings, and ventures such as this volume. Once criticized for being an exclusive organisation, membership is now open and depends on a small annual subscription and contribution to JVRG studies. The Group has grown since 1983 and membership is now by centre rather than by individual; 22 geographic centres are current members, from 36 hospitals (see page xii). The driving force remains, however, very much the same as that which motivated the original Group 22 years ago.

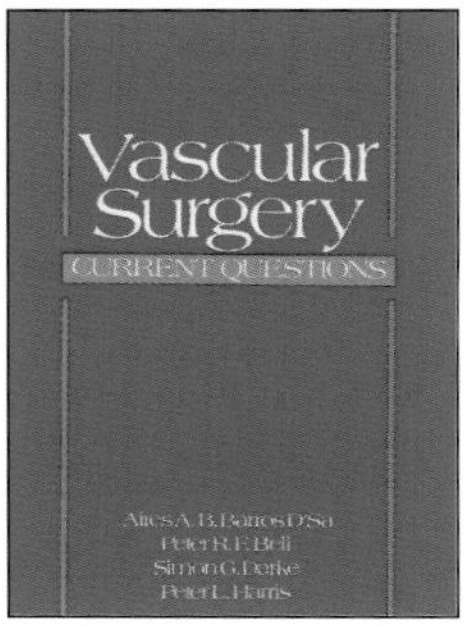

It has become obvious that many current vascular research projects require huge organisation and funding through central agencies and University departments. The JVRG specialises in clinical projects that require insubstantial funding, prospective audits and collaborative reviews. Whilst continuing to perform these studies, the Group has therefore changed its focus and expanded into education and training. The first JVRG book was published in 1991 (Vascular surgery - current questions, edited by Barros D'Sa, Bell, Darke and Harris).

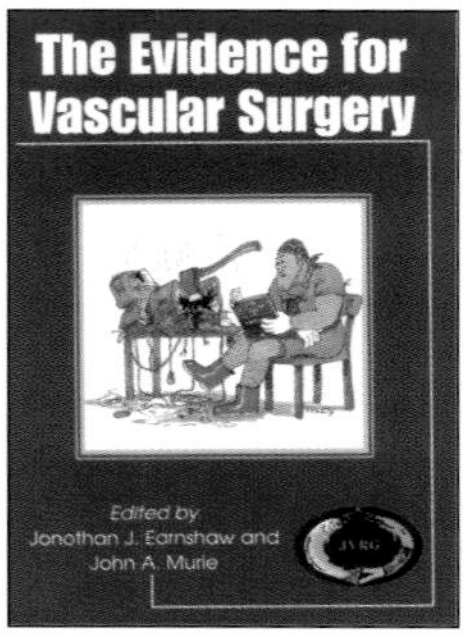

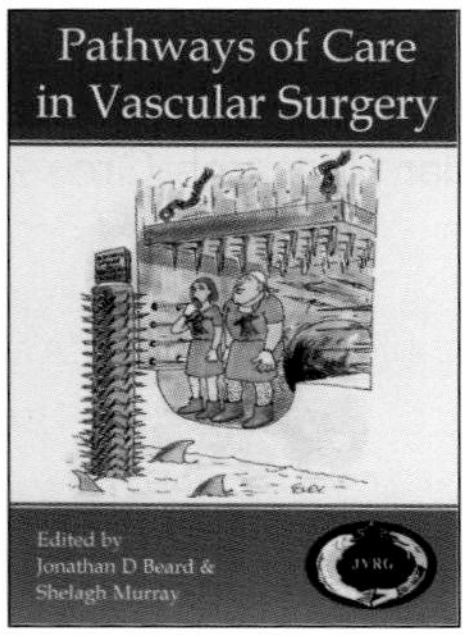

In recent years the Group has produced three more books (including this one) and promoted them through a series of conferences and courses. The Group has also recognised that vascular surgery is no longer the sole domain of the consultant surgeon, and has led the way into multidisciplinary teamworking. JVRG conferences are designed to appeal to surgeons, interventionists, specialist nurses and technologists; all of these share in the activities of the JVRG.

As older and sometimes less productive members have drifted away, they have been replaced by younger, more enthusiastic colleagues. In this way the JVRG remains a vibrant organisation with an exciting role to play in vascular surgery in the UK and Ireland. New challenges in the regulation of clinical research have been accepted and the Group is moving forward with confidence and an exciting portfolio of research activity.

Jonothan J Earnshaw DM FRCS
JVRG Chairman
Christine McGrath MSc BSc (Hons) RGN
JVRG Trials Co-ordinator

Original articles published by the JVRG

Darke SG, Lamont PM, Chant ADB, Barros D'Sa AAB, Clyne CAC, Harris PL, Ruckley CV, Bell PRF. Femoropopliteal versus femorodistal bypass grafting for limb salvage in patients with an isolated popliteal segment. *Eur J Vasc Surg* 1989; 3: 203-7.

Ruckley CV, Stonebridge PA, Prescott RJ, for the Joint Vascular Research Group. Skewflap versus long posterior flap in below-knee amputations: multicentre trial. *J Vasc Surg* 1991; 13: 423-7.

Tyrell MR, Wolfe JH. Critical leg ischaemia: an appraisal of clinical definitions. Joint Vascular Research Group. *Br J Surg* 1993; 80: 177-80.

Ranaboldo CJ, Barros D'Sa AA, Bell PRF, Chant AD, Perry PM. Randomised controlled trial of patch angioplasty for carotid endarterectomy. The Joint Vascular Research Group. *Br J Surg* 1993; 80: 1528-30.

Varga ZA, Locke-Edmunds JC, Baird RN, Joint Vascular Research Group. A multicentre study of popliteal aneurysms. *J Vasc Surg* 1994; 20: 171-7.

Thompson JF, Mullee MA, Bell PRF, Campbell WB, Chant AD, Darke SG, Jamieson CW, Murie JA, Parvin SD, Perry M, Ruckley CV, Wolfe JH, Clyne CA. Intra-operative heparinisation, blood loss and myocardial infarction during aortic aneurysm surgery: a Joint Vascular Research Group Study. *Eur J Vasc Endovasc Surg* 1996; 12: 86-90.

Stonebridge PA, Prescott RJ, Ruckley CV. Randomised trial comparing infra-inguinal polytetrafluoroethylene bypass grafting with, and without vein interposition cuff at the distal anastomosis. The Joint Vascular Research Group. *J Vasc Surg* 1997; 26: 543-50.

Galland RB, on behalf of the Joint Vascular Research Group. Mortality following elective infrarenal aortic reconstruction. *Br J Surg* 1998; 85: 633-6.

Lambert AW, Wilkins DC, on behalf of the Joint Vascular Research Group. Popliteal artery entrapment: collaborative experience. *Br J Surg* 1998; 85: 1367-8.

Braithwaite BD, Davies B, Heather BP, Earnshaw JJ, on behalf of the Joint Vascular Research Group. Early results of a randomised trial of rifampicin-bonded dacron grafts for extra-anatomic vascular reconstruction. *Br J Surg* 1998; 85: 1378-81.

Earnshaw JJ, Whitman B, Heather BP, on behalf of the Joint Vascular Research Group. Two-year results of a randomised controlled trial of rifampicin-bonded extra-anatomic dacron grafts. *Br J Surg* 2000; 87: 758-9.

Robinson J, Nawaz S, Beard JD, on behalf of the Joint Vascular Research Group. Randomised, multicentre, double-blind, placebo-controlled trial of the use of aprotinin in the repair of ruptured abdominal aortic aneurysm. *Br J Surg* 2000; 87: 754-7.

Naylor AR, Hayes PD, Darke S, on behalf of the Joint Vascular Research Group. A prospective audit of complex wound and graft infections in Great Britain and Ireland: the emergence of MRSA. *Eur J Vasc Endovasc Surg* 2001; 21: 289-94.

Pillay WR, Kan, YM, Crinnion JIN, Wolfe JHN, on behalf of the Joint Vascular Research Group. Prospective multicentre study of the natural history of atherosclerotic renal artery stenosis in patients with peripheral vascular disease. *Br J Surg* 2002; 89: 737-40.

Griffiths GD, Nagy J, Black D, Stonebridge PA, on behalf of the Joint Vascular Research Group. Randomised clinical trial of distal anastomotic interposition vein cuff in infrainguinal polytetrafluoroethylene bypass grafting. *Br J Surg* 2004; 91: 560-2.

Membership of the JVRG

Vascular specialists and their teams from the following Vascular Units currently contribute cases to JVRG studies:

Bath (Royal United Hospital)
Belfast (Royal Victoria Hospital)
Belfast (City Hospital)
Birmingham (Heartlands Hospital)
Bournemouth (Royal Bournemouth General Hospital)
Bristol (Bristol Royal Infirmary)
Dundee (Ninewells Hospital)
Edinburgh (Edinburgh Royal Infirmary)
Rotterdam (Erasmus University Hospital)
Exeter (Royal Devon and Exeter Hospital)
Gloucester/Cheltenham (Gloucestershire Royal and Cheltenham General Hospitals)
Cape Town (Groote Schuur Hospital)
Hull (Hull Royal Infirmary)
Leeds (Leeds General Infirmary and St. James' University Hospital)
Leicester (Leicester Royal Infirmary)
Liverpool (Royal Liverpool Hospital)
London (Charing Cross, Guy's, King's and St. Thomas', Royal Free, St. Georges, St. Mary's Hospital and, UCLH)
Newcastle (Freeman Hospital)
Norfolk and Norwich (University Hospital)
North Staffforshire (City General Hospital)
Northampton (Northampton General Hospital)
Nottingham (University Hospital)
Oxford (John Radcliffe Hospital)
Plymouth (Derriford Hospital)
Reading (Royal Berkshire Hospital)
Sheffield (Northern General Hospital)
South Tees (James Cook University Hospital)
Southampton (Southampton General Hospital)
Swansea (Morriston Hospital)
Torquay (Torbay Hospital)
Truro (Royal Cornwall Hospital)

Current projects (2005)

1. Register of rare diseases.
2. Scoring system to predict the outcome after bypass grafting to a single calf vessel.
3. Renal failure after arterial surgery.
4. Natural history of chronic mesenteric artery ischaemia.
5. Prospective study of outcome after short saphenous vein surgery.
6. Internal carotid artery subocclusion study.
7. Randomised trial of teicoplanin prophylaxis in amputation surgery.

Chapter 1

The Rare Diagnosis and Operations Register

Simon D Parvin MD FRCS, Consultant Vascular Surgeon
Royal Bournemouth Hospital, Bournemouth, UK

This book is born out of an idea conceived during a Joint Vascular Research Group meeting in the mid 1990s. At the time, the project was called the Rare Diagnosis and Operations Register.

The Rare Diagnosis and Operations Register is a collection of unusual vascular diagnoses and operations seen or performed by members of the Joint Vascular Research Group. Members contribute cases to the author who stores them in a database, which is then available to any member of the group. It was set up in May 1995 following the spring meeting of the Joint Vascular Research Group.

Aims

The database was set up with a number of aims in mind. These are as follows:

- To create a collection of unusual cases.
- To provide members with the opportunity of publishing, separately or jointly, collective reports of unusual vascular conditions.
- To allow expertise and advice to be disseminated between members for the management of unusual cases.
- To encourage contribution to the JVRG generally by promoting a competitive culture.

Method

From the outset, members were asked to contribute any cases they thought unusual. In order to encourage as many members to contribute as many cases as possible, no preconditions were set.

To facilitate data collection, a minimum of data were required on each case. These are summarised in Table 1. Latterly, hospital number has become the only patient identifier collected.

Each case submitted was entered in a database with the date of submission. At the beginning, there were a small number of categories that we particularly wanted to collect, though submissions were not confined to those groups. When more than three similar non-categorised cases were submitted, a new category was created.

Table 1. Data required on each case.

Surgeon data	Patient data
Name	Surname
Centre	First name
	Date of birth
	Hospital number
	Case details

Table 2. Categories of cases submitted.

Aortocaval fistula	Major vessel arteritis
Aorto-enteric fistula	Mesenteric ischaemia
Arm ischaemia	Mycotic aneurysm
Arteriovenous malformation	Other odd aneurysms
Brachial embolus	Paget Schroetter syndrome
Leg ulcer calcification	Popliteal entrapment
Carotid artery surgery	Profunda femoris aneurysms
Carotid body tumour	Right to left shunt or paradoxical embolism
Cystic degeneration	AAA with renal abnormality
Deep vein thrombosis	Subclavian steal syndrome
Radiotherapy arteritis	Thoracic outlet compression
Ehlers-Danlos syndrome	Vascular trauma
Klippel-Trenaunay syndrome	Visceral aneurysms
Systemic lupus erythematosus	Vena caval obstruction
Mid-aortic syndrome	Arterial disease in patients under 40 years

To start there were six categories. These included: popliteal entrapment, major vessel arteritis, carotid body tumour, mesenteric ischaemia, cystic degeneration and lupus. At the time of writing there are 30 categories and these are shown in Table 2.

The reports

Regular reports have been produced which are circulated to the membership. Reports are in several parts:

- A table of numbers submitted by category and by centre in total and since the last report.
- A list of all new cases showing contributing surgeon, category and details of case.
- A list of non-categorized cases with their details by centre.
- A newsletter.
- A proforma for subsequent case submissions.

Early on the cases were attributed to individual surgeons but as the size of the group has increased cases are now classified by referring centre. There are now 22 centres with approximately 30 contributing surgeons. Sent with the report are a newsletter and a proforma for completion during the next time interval. More recently, submissions directly by email have become possible.

The results

The Rare Diagnosis and Operations Register has been running for ten years. During that time 1322 cases have been submitted.

This book has chapter headings that reflect the categories in the Register. Chapter authors have been encouraged to contact other members of the group for material for their chapters as has previously been done for scientific publications [1,2]. The anonymised database is available on the JVRG website as a resource for members and others needing information and advice on how to manage that very unusual case, and to disseminate information.

References

1. Lambert AW, Wilkins DC. Popliteal artery entrapment syndrome: collaborative experience of the Joint Vascular Research Group. *Br J Surg* 1998; 85: 1367-8.
2. Varga ZA, Locke-Edmunds JC, Baird RN. A multicentre study of popliteal aneurysms. Joint Vascular Research Group. *J Vasc Surg* 1994; 20: 171-7.

Chapter 2

Anatomical variation for the vascular specialist

Klaus Overbeck FRCS (Engl), Vascular and Endovascular Fellow
Sumaira Macdonald MB ChB (Comm.) MRCP FRCR PhD, Consultant Vascular Radiologist
Northern Vascular Institute, Freeman Hospital, Newcastle, UK

Regional arterial variants

Aortic arch and carotid arterial anatomy

The derivation of a single aortic arch from six embryological arteries gives huge scope for the development of variant anatomy. Many such variants are relevant to endovascular procedures of the carotid or thoracic aortic territory. Those of the supracervical carotid segment are largely the concern of neuro-interventionists and neurosurgeons. Variants of the cervical carotid impact on vascular surgical practice when pathology presents fortuitously, or because the variant itself generates disease.

The bovine arch

A common origin of both common carotids and the right subclavian artery occurs in 10% of people. As five of six primary sources of cerebral perfusion arise from a single aortic branch, disease of this common trunk is a threatening disease pattern offering substantial surgical challenges; thankfully, it is uncommon. A large vascular unit accrued only six such patients over two decades [1]. Revascularisation strategies include: prosthetic bypass graft from the ascending aorta to the innominate or left common carotid arteries or both, or endarterectomy to include branch vessels. This small series reported two neurological complications, one fatal ischaemic stroke and one hyperperfusion syndrome, attesting to the threat posed by this pattern of disease. Furthermore, this pattern does not easily lend itself to a less invasive (endovascular) solution.

Variations in the position of the carotid bifurcation

The carotid bifurcation may lie higher than usual, at the level of the hyoid bone, or more rarely in a lower position than normal, level with the middle of the larynx or the lower border of the cricoid (Figure 1). Alternative patterns include absence of a recognisable bifurcation, when both internal (ICA) and external carotids (ECA) arise directly from the aortic arch, or failure of common carotid branching in the neck.

If the bifurcation is high, it may be difficult to expose a sufficient length of ICA to permit safe carotid endarterectomy (CEA). Adequate exposure may require division of the posterior belly of digastric and occasionally, disarticulation of the mandible. Endarterectomy in the setting of a high carotid bifurcation is associated with a greater incidence of

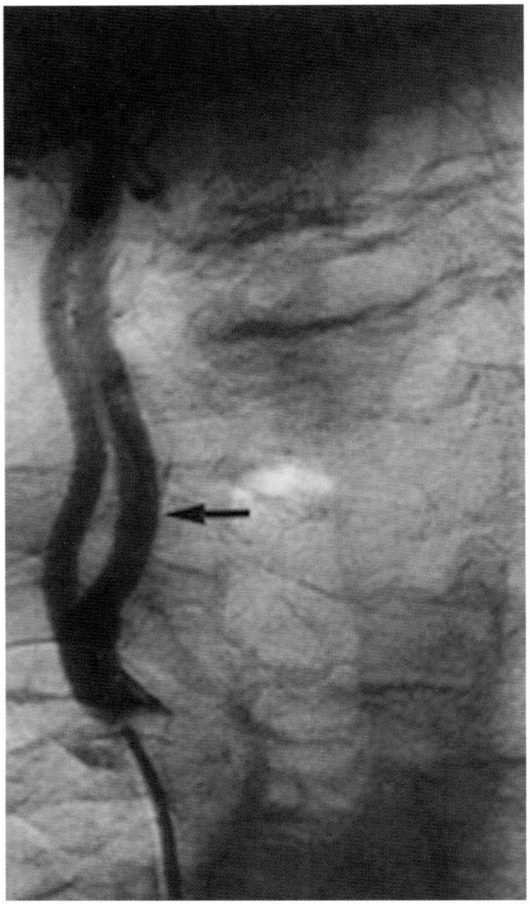

Figure 1. A low right carotid bifurcation demonstrated on selective catheter angiography (arrow).

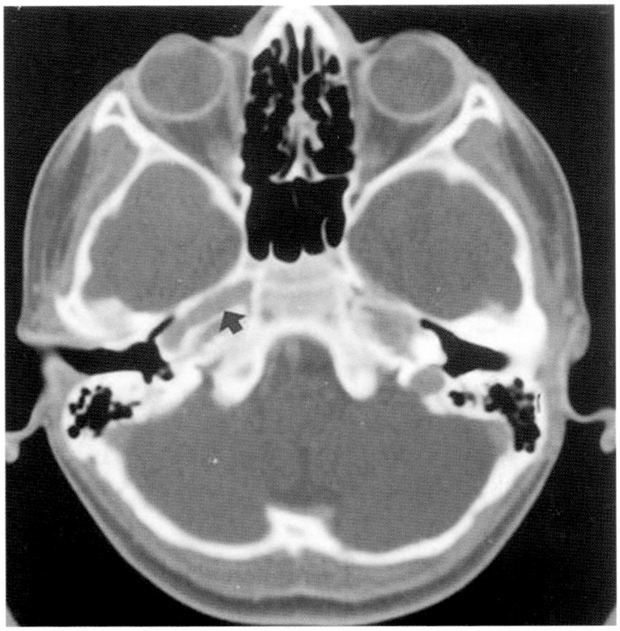

Figure 2. An unenhanced axial CT of the brain at the level of the carotid canals. The right carotid canal is highlighted (arrow). The left is absent, consistent with agenesis of the cervical portion of the left internal carotid artery.

nerve damage, although there is no increase in stroke rate. There is some suggestion that a low carotid bifurcation correlates with a longer extent of disease in the ICA [2].

To avoid the surgical pitfalls, pre-operative imaging should be accurate with a routine comment on the position of the carotid bifurcation.

Aplasia or agenesis of the cervical portion of the internal carotid artery (Figure 2)

This condition may be associated with subarachnoid haemorrhage (SAH), due to high-flow states in the collateral flow through the circle of Willis and resultant intracranial aneurysms. SAH occurs in 25% patients with bilateral ICA agenesis. SAH is

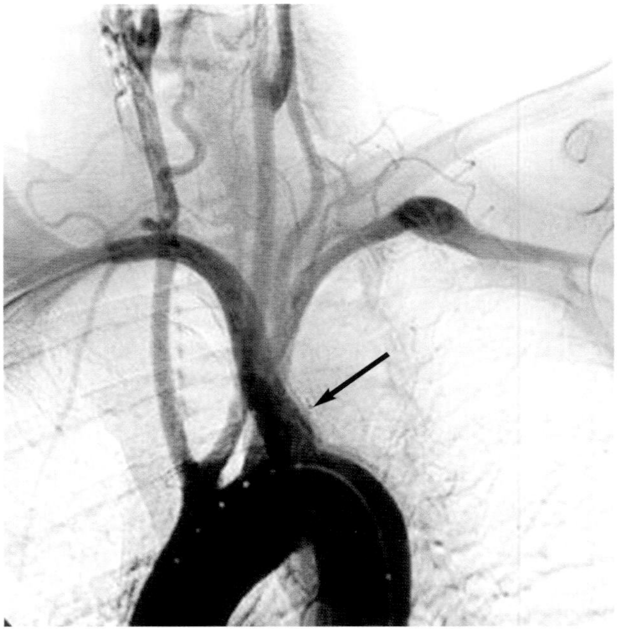

Figure 3. Catheter arch aortography demonstrating aneurysmal dilatation of an aberrant right subclavian (arrow), arising as the last branch of the aortic arch, in association with a common origin of the brachiocephalic trunk and the left common carotid artery (bovine-type arch).

more likely to present to a neurologist, but cerebrovascular ischaemia resulting from disease progression in the collateral pathways may present a clinical paradox to the vascular surgeon. The anterior cerebral circulation in these circumstances may be provided by the ordinarily, functionally remote vertebrobasilar and posterior communicating pathways. High-grade stenoses of the vertebral arteries may then manifest as carotid territory transient ischaemic attack (TIA).

The ECA may be ligated inadvertently in the mistaken belief that it is the thyroid artery during thyroid surgery when the carotid bulb is low. Head and neck surgery for cancer may be equally demanding when the ECA is ligated without recognising that there is agenesis of the ICA. Carotid imaging is not routine before these operations and the on-call vascular surgeon may be approached for technical expertise under these circumstances.

Aberrant right subclavian artery

Aberrant right subclavian artery occurs in 0.5% of the population and may be associated with a number of congenital heart diseases. This vessel may arise directly from the aortic arch at any point. When it arises as the last branch, it courses behind the trachea or both the trachea and oesophagus to reach the groove on the first rib. Resultant compression of the oesophagus by the right subclavian artery may cause dysphagia (dysphagia lusoria). The aberrant vessel and adjoining aorta are frequently subject to aneurysmal degeneration, which is commoner in the elderly. Figure 3 demonstrates an aneurysmal aberrant right subclavian and a bovine type arch, a frequent association. Aneurysms appear to be atherosclerotic in origin, but may also be caused by arteritis. The deviant vessel is commonly dilated at the arch origin (Kommerell's diverticulum). Rupture may be fatal in this setting and appears unrelated to aneurysm size. One fifth may have an associated abdominal aortic aneurysm (AAA).

Surgical treatment of such lesions is recommended because of the potential for rupture. Repair may be accomplished via a right or left posterolateral thoracotomy, or a median sternotomy. The subclavian artery is reconstructed by an interposition arterial prosthesis anastomosed proximally to the ascending arch of the aorta. Alternatively, a left posterolateral thoracotomy for proximal resection of the aneurysm coupled with a right supraclavicular incision for reconstruction of the subclavian artery by end-to-side anastomosis to the right common carotid artery has been described. A staged approach with right carotid to subclavian bypass or transposition (end-subclavian to side-carotid) preceding left thoracotomy and aneurysm resection with oversewing of the origin from the aortic arch is attractive because the risk of cerebral and right arm embolisation is minimised. Extra-anatomic reconstruction of the right subclavian artery has also been described. When, in addition to the aneurysmal aberrant right subclavian artery, there is aneurysmal degeneration of the aortic arch and the descending aorta, concomitant surgical treatment can be complicated and may require a two-stage approach, to include an elephant trunk reconstruction [3]. An endovascular option has also recently been reported [4] (see Chapter 23, Aneurysm of an aberrant right subclavian artery).

Upper limb vascular variants

Vascular forearm entrapment syndrome (Figure 4)

Although not strictly a vascular variant, this can give rise to vascular complications. The syndrome is caused by compression of the brachial artery by the ligament of Struthers, found in 1% of the population, which arises from a bony spur of the humerus beneath which the vessel is entrapped. Ulnar artery compression by a pronator teres muscle and a fibrous arcade of the flexor digitorum superficialis muscle has also been reported.

Visceral and mesenteric vascular variants

Coeliac artery or median arcuate ligament entrapment

Again, this non-vascular variant gives rise to vascular complications. It is a cause of small bowel ischaemic symptoms with postprandial abdominal pain, anorexia, food fear and weight loss. Arcuate ligament compression in which the coeliac axis is compressed by the median arcuate ligament should

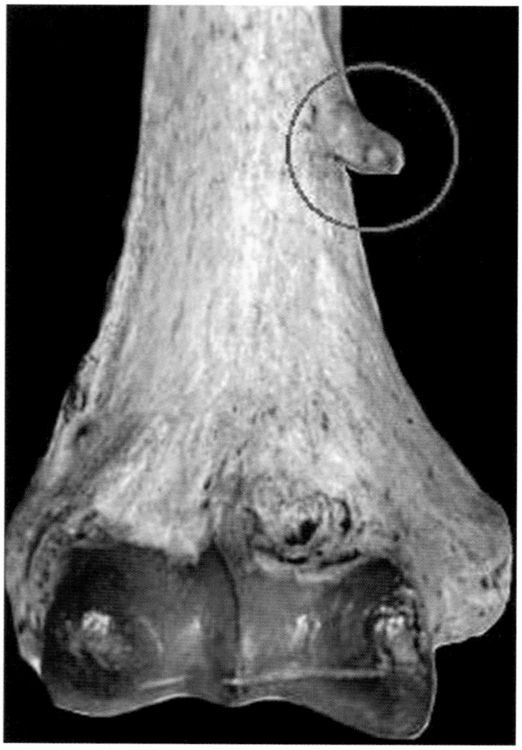

Figure 4. A case of brachial artery compression by a Struthers' ligament. Struthers' original dissection (Lancet 1873).

not be confused with stenotic disease of the coeliac axis ostium. An epigastric bruit is common and can be respiration-dependent. Duplex will elegantly display the characteristic features. Compression and raised velocities suggesting a stenosis are noted in the supine position and in expiration (Figure 5a). These changes revert to normality in the erect position and in inspiration (Figure 5b). A non-ostial asymmetric narrowing of the superior aspect of the coeliac artery is demonstrated. Symptoms may relate to compression of the adjacent symptomatic nerve plexuses. The treatment is surgical, involving resection of peri-arterial neural tissue only or division of the ligament either via open or, more recently, by a laparoscopic approach.

Renal and mesenteric arterial variant anatomy

Renal

Renal artery variations are very common and may be found in around 35% of individuals. This is due to the embryological ascent of the kidney from the pelvis to the lumbar region during which time it is vascularised by arteries originating from the aorta at continuously higher levels. The commonest variant, the so-called accessory artery occurs in around 28% of subjects. These are commoner above rather than

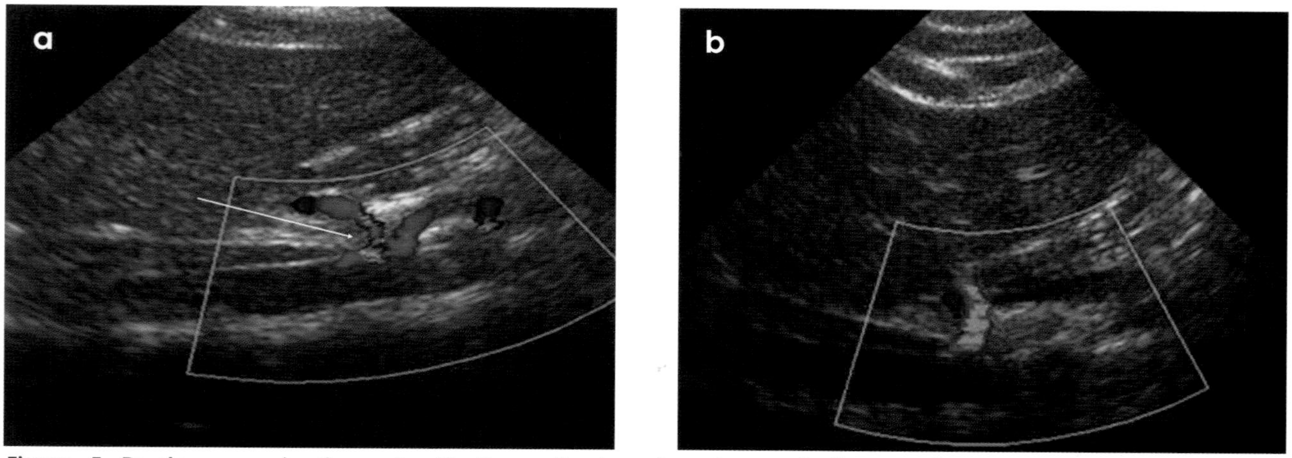

Figure 5. Duplex examination: a) with the patient supine demonstrating coeliac axis compression by the median arcuate ligament (arrow); b) with the patient erect demonstrating normal appearances of the coeliac axis.

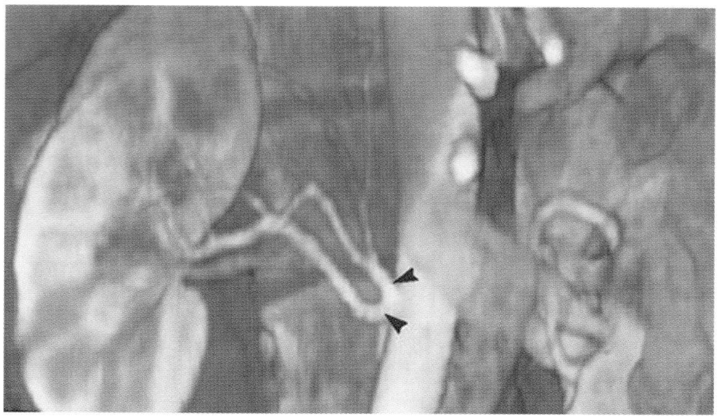

Figure 6. Early division of the main right renal artery on magnetic resonance angiography (arrows).

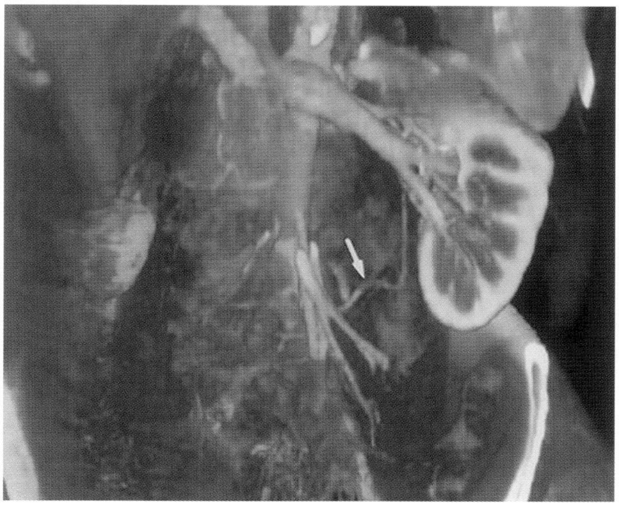

Figure 7. Prominent right renal arterial supply from the left common iliac artery on magnetic resonance angiography (arrow). The left renal venous return is prominently displayed on this image.

below the usual trunk and are more frequent on the left side. The term accessory is a misnomer as such vessels are not extra, but essential tissue-sustaining arteries and cannot be ligated without potential sequelae. The inferior phrenic is an inconstant branch and may arise from an aortic superior renal polar artery. As it is responsible for most or all of the blood supply of the adrenal, its identification is mandatory during renal pedicle surgery. Early division of the main renal artery may be misinterpreted as dual or multiple renal arteries (Figure 6).

Renal arterial variants may influence surgical technique during AAA repair. Bypass of a sizeable right renal accessory vessel that originates from an aneurysmal portion of either the aorta or right iliac segment may require a right retroperitoneal approach, if other visceral vessels do not require reimplantation. If this variant anatomy is present when suprarenal control is required to repair a juxtarenal aneurysm, the surgeon must weigh up the pros and cons of a left retroperitoneal approach, against a transperitoneal or right retroperitoneal approach for optimal right renal reimplantation. Variant left renal vessels are better reimplanted via the left retroperitoneal approach. Small arterial branches arising from aneurysmal aorta can be ligated with few consequences; however, any vessel greater than 2mm in diameter should be preserved, if possible.

Kidneys with major arterial supply from the iliac segment require a tailored approach (Figure 7). Anterior transperitoneal access is preferred and the minimisation of renal ischaemia during aortic cross-clamping and the position of the aortic graft are the main issues. Loop diuretics or mannitol may be administered before suprarenal aortic clamping as a renoprotective measure, but renal ischaemia should be limited to 30 to 40 minutes and, therefore, this method is feasible only in those patients in whom aortic reconstruction is simple and straightforward. Temporary (Gott-type) shunts may be employed to provide renal perfusion whilst the aneurysm is isolated between clamps. Alternatively, a temporary axillofemoral bypass, allowing retrograde perfusion during aortic clamping may be considered, but requires additional operating time for adjunctive inguinal and axillary exposures. In complex cases, where renal protection is anticipated, cold Ringer's lactate can be infused in the anomalous branches. This method affords sufficient time to achieve aortic reconstruction (up to 90 minutes).

Horseshoe kidney

Horseshoe kidney gives rise to variant vasculature that is highly relevant during aortic surgery (see Chapter 24, Abdominal aortic aneurysm with horseshoe kidney).

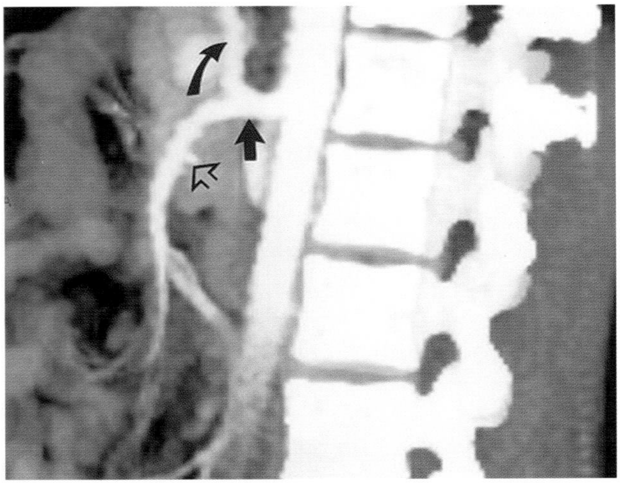

Figure 8. CT angiogram sagittal reconstruction demonstrating a common hepatic artery (curved arrow) arising directly from the superior mesenteric artery (open arrow). The short common trunk is highlighted (straight arrow).

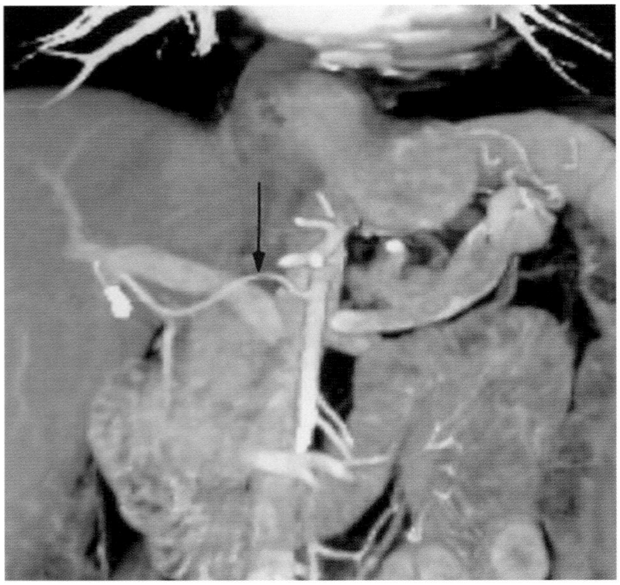

Figure 9. Magnetic resonance angiography (coronal reconstruction) demonstrating a replaced right hepatic artery arising from the superior mesenteric artery (arrow).

Mesenteric

These variants are common. The common hepatic artery may arise directly from the superior mesenteric artery (SMA) (Figure 8) or the aorta. The coeliac axis and SMA may have a common origin. An accessory left hepatic artery arises most frequently from the left gastric, an accessory right most commonly from the SMA (Figure 9).

Variants may exist in conjunction with more conventional anatomy or may replace the normal vasculature. Ligation of the common hepatic artery proximal to the origin of the gastroduodenal artery is usually well tolerated due to extensive hepatic collaterals, but inadvertent ligation beyond the origin of the gastroduodenal may be complicated by hepatic necrosis, as the only collateral supply is then via small inferior phrenic arteries.

These variations may impact on aortic surgery. If the main mesenteric trunks originate directly from the aneurysmal aorta, reimplantation will be required. Anticipating this eventuality is useful in order to optimise the approach i.e a left retroperitoneal exposure may be more appropriate for visceral reimplantation than a transabdominal approach. Ordinarily, the most appropriate site for proximal control of a juxtarenal aneurysm may be the (less diseased) supracoeliac aorta than the (more diseased) infrarenal aorta between the renal arteries and the SMA. The scope for safe proximal control may be limited by variant coeliac and/or SMA anatomy.

The inferior mesenteric artery is stable and not subject to much variation. It occasionally arises from the left common iliac artery (CIA). If the left CIA is aneurysmal and therefore included in the aortic repair, the surgeon may encounter brisk back-bleeding at the iliac level and not appreciate its cause or consider reimplantation.

Contrast-enhanced abdominal CT allows reliable estimation of such variant anatomy before aortic surgery or endovascular repair. CT is not requested by all surgeons before aortic surgery, unless the patient has been recruited into one of the endovascular aneurysm trials or otherwise has an endovascular repair planned.

The safe surgical and endovascular management of aneurysms of the hepatic, splenic and mesenteric vessels ordinarily mandates a sound knowledge of which branch vessels can be sacrificed safely, and variant anatomy adds a further layer of complexity.

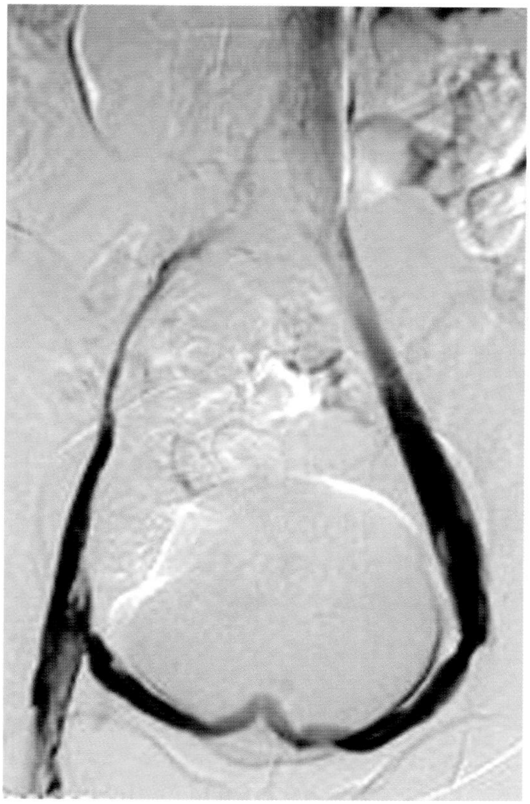

Figure 10. Ascending venogram with the patient prone demonstrating left common iliac vein compression by the right common iliac artery (May-Thurner syndrome). Note the cross pelvic collateral vein.

Pelvic vascular anatomy

May-Thurner syndrome (Cockett syndrome)

Chronic pulsatile compression of the left common iliac vein (CIV) between the overlying right common iliac artery (CIA) and the lowest lumbar vertebral body may induce focal intimal proliferation of the vein with venous web formation.

The syndrome was described first by McMurrich in 1908 and later by May and Thurner in 1957 and is also known as iliac vein compression syndrome (IVCS) (Figure 10). The syndrome may cause 5-30% of iliofemoral deep venous thromboses and may explain why symptoms and sequelae of venous disease may be more common in the left leg than the right. It is commoner in women (85% in one series), in the second to fourth decade of life. Some workers consider this entity to represent normal anatomy. Clearly, the syndrome is one end of a spectrum of normality in that in some individuals, arterial pressure is sufficient to cause venous trauma with time.

Although some clinicians suggest repair of any lesion discovered, reconstruction could reasonably be reserved for symptomatic patients, including those who had already had an episode of acute deep venous thrombosis.

Options include: decompression of the venous system with a Palma-Dale procedure (suprapubic crossed femorofemoral bypass with contralateral saphenous vein), direct exploration of the caval bifurcation with the use of a variety of techniques to release the iliac venous obstruction, transposition of the iliac artery behind the CIV or transposition of the right CIA to the left internal iliac artery to decompress the left CIV.

Endovascular stent placement provides effective symptomatic improvement of most patients. A recent retrospective analysis of 39 patients with IVCS treated by stent placement plus or minus thrombolytic therapy demonstrated a 91.6% 1-year patency for those presenting acutely and 93.3% for those with more chronic symptoms [5].

Lower limb variant anatomy

Persistent sciatic artery (Figure 11a)

The sciatic artery is a continuation of the internal iliac artery and is the primary blood supply to the lower limb bud during early foetal development. It normally involutes, but remnants persist as the popliteal and peroneal arteries after the superficial femoral artery (SFA) develops and establishes continuity with the popliteal artery. The sciatic artery may be complete from the internal iliac artery to the popliteal or may be incomplete, with small collaterals between it and the internal iliac artery or popliteal. An apparent paradox is created when the femoral pulse is absent yet distal pulses are full, being supplied by the persistent sciatic artery which enters the leg deeply through the sciatic notch (Figure 11b). This is known as Cowie's sign. The reported angiographic incidence of this anomaly varies from 0.025% to 0.06%. It is bilateral in 22% of

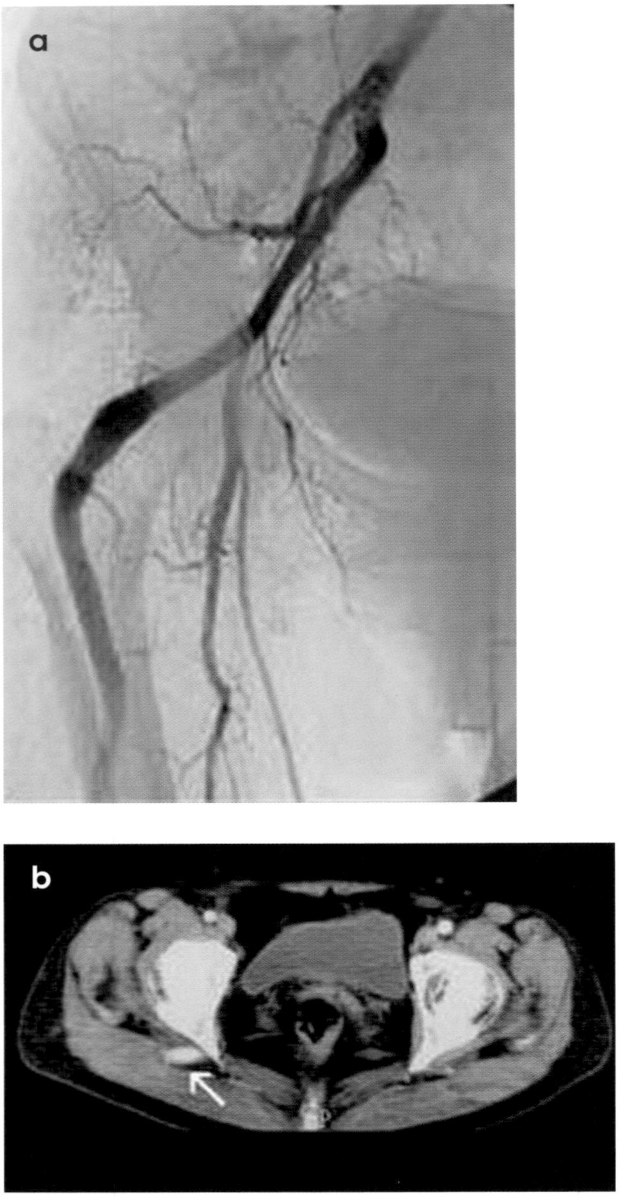

Figure 11. a) Femoral catheter angiography at the inguinal level demonstrating a persistent right sciatic artery arising from the right internal iliac artery. b) Contrast-enhanced axial CT demonstrating the path of a persistent right sciatic artery exiting the pelvis through the right sciatic notch (arrow).

subjects and is usually diagnosed in patients aged over 50 years, but may be noted throughout life.

Along with the presence of immature vascular elements, this condition causes early atherosclerotic changes and frequent aneurysmal degeneration (15-46% of subjects). This may cause critical leg ischaemia resulting from thrombosis or embolisation of aneurysm thrombus and may manifest as a soft-tissue pulsatile mass in the buttock that can compress the sciatic nerve with neurological sequelae.

If unrecognised, inappropriate bypass of apparent occlusive disease of the SFA may be undertaken. Acute lower leg ischaemia has been described in a child undergoing renal transplantation during which a persistent sciatic artery was ligated during anastomosis with the transplanted renal artery [6].

Options for vascular reconstruction for aneurysmal disease include interposition graft replacement and standard femoropopliteal bypass grafting if the common femoral artery is sufficiently developed to provide adequate inflow. As with other peripheral arterial aneurysms that cause thrombosis and distal arterial embolisation, intra-arterial thrombolytic therapy may be a useful adjunct in selected patients before definitive surgical revascularisation.

Short common femoral artery (CFA) with high profunda (PFA)/superficial femoral artery (SFA) bifurcation

This variant (Figure 12) is relevant to antegrade punctures made for infra-inguinal angioplasty. Accessing the short CFA may be prohibitively high i.e. above the inguinal ligament in this situation. In order to minimise haemorrhagic complications, ultrasound-guided direct proximal SFA puncture with small sheaths (4F) and sub-4F-shaft balloons and 0.018" wires may be advocated.

Variant popliteal anatomy and popliteal entrapment

Please see Chapter 38, Popliteal artery entrapment syndrome.

Crural arterial variants

The term trifurcation is a misnomer because the popliteal artery truly trifurcates in only 0.4% of individuals. A retrospective review of 1000 femoral arteriograms highlighted a normal branching of the

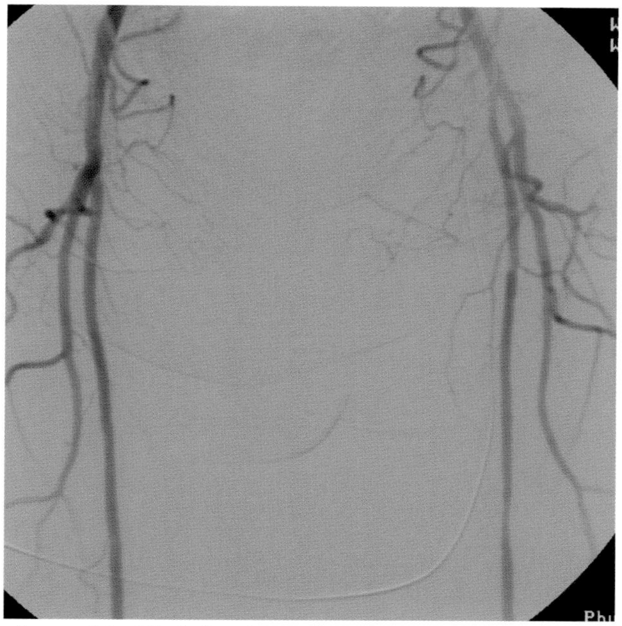

Figure 12. Digital subtraction angiography via the left common femoral artery demonstrating high left profunda/superficial femoral artery bifurcation.

popliteal artery in 92.2% [7]. Among the 7.8% incidence of variants, the majority (72%) were either high origin of the anterior tibial artery (AT) (Figure 13) or a true trifurcation pattern. Of variant patterns to the foot (5.6%), the most common was that the supply to the distal posterior tibial artery arose from the peroneal artery. This should be suspected when the infrapopliteal vessels show a hypoplastic or aplastic anterior or posterior tibial artery and compensatory hypertrophy of the peroneal artery.

Prior knowledge of these variants is important for planning of crural angioplasty and may influence the surgical approach and success of femorodistal bypass. For example, surgeons who routinely expose the proximal AT through a lateral incision with excision of the head of the fibula may be surprised that the AT is not where they expect it to be. This is likely to be avoided whilst comprehensive pre-operative arteriography remains the standard of care before femorodistal bypass procedures.

Venous variants relevant to abdominal vascular procedures

Spectrum of congenital anomalies of the inferior vena cava (IVC) and renal veins

The embryogenesis of the IVC is a complex process involving the formation of several anastomoses between three paired embryonic veins. The result is numerous variations in the basic venous plan of the abdomen and pelvis. There may be up to 14 theoretical variations in the anatomy of the infrarenal IVC. The commoner variants, their ontogeny and prevalence, where known, are given in Table 1. Diagrammatic representations of these variant anatomies are given in Figure 14. Knowledge of IVC anatomy is very important during aortic surgery when

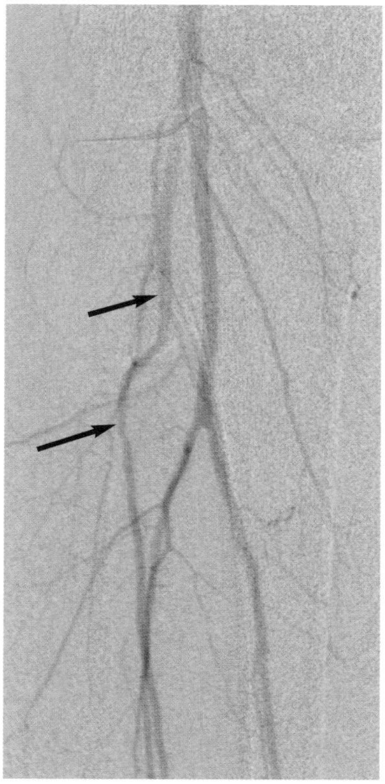

Figure 13. Digital subtraction angiogram demonstrating high take-off of the right anterior tibial artery (arrows).

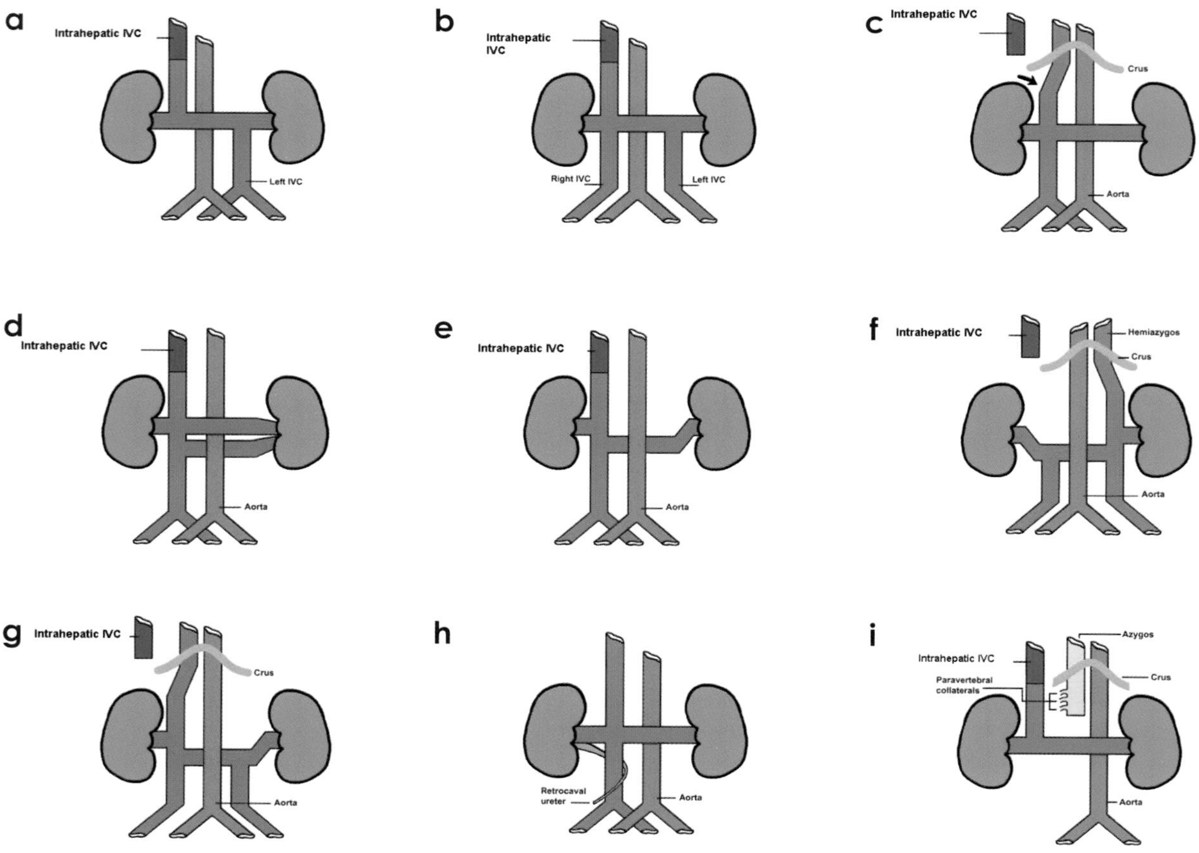

Figure 14. Diagrammatic representations of renal venous and caval variants. a) Left-sided IVC. b) Double IVC. c) Azygous continuation of the IVC. d) Circumaortic left renal vein. e) Retro-aortic left renal vein. f) Double IVC with retro-aortic right renal vein and hemi-azygous continuation of the IVC. g) Double IVC with retro-aortic left renal vein and azygous continuation of the IVC. h) Circumcaval ureter. i) Absent infrarenal IVC with preservation of the suprarenal segment.

the presence of a double IVC can lead to confusion (Figures 14b & 15a). One of the most dangerous variants is the retro-aortic left renal vein that can cause serious haemorrhage at aortic cross-clamping if not recognised (Figures 14e & 15b).

Lumbar venous variants

Great variation exists in the number and location of lumbar veins along the IVC. Most commonly, three lumbar veins enter on the left and two on the right. The left renal vein is entered in 43% of cases.

Failure to appreciate these anomalies may lead to inadvertent injury and major venous bleeding. These variants are likely to complicate left retroperitoneal approaches to juxtarenal or thoraco-abdominal aneurysms and occasionally to infrarenal AAA. A transperitoneal approach is preferable when the cava is left-sided. Pre-operative diagnosis can be made on CT, as is the case for renal arterial variants.

Table 1. Spectrum of congenital anomalies of the inferior vena cava.

Anomaly	Embryology	Prevalence
Left-sided IVC	Persistence of left supracardinal vein	0.2-0.5%
Double IVC	Persistence of both supracardinal veins	0.2-3%
Azygous continuation of the IVC	Failed right subcardial-hepatic anastomosis and atrophy of right subcardinal vein	0.6%
Circumaortic left renal vein	Persistent dorsal limb left renal vein and dorsal arch renal collar	8.7%
Retro-aortic left renal vein	Persistent dorsal arch of renal collar	2.1%
Double IVC with retro-aortic right renal vein and hemi-azygous continuation of the IVC	Persistent left lumbar and thoracic supracardinal vein and left suprasubcardinal anastomosis and failed right subcardinal-hepatic anastomosis	Rare
Double IVC with retro-aortic left renal vein and azygous continuation of the IVC	Persistent left supracardinal vein and dorsal limb of renal collar and regression of ventral limb and failed subcardinal-hepatic anastomosis	Rare
Circumcaval ureter	Failed right supracardinal system and persistent right posterior cardinal vein	Rare
Absent infrarenal IVC with preservation of the suprarenal segment	Absence of the infrarenal IVC implies failure of development of the posterior cardinal and supracardinal veins. ?True embryonic anomalies or the result of perinatal IVC thrombosis	Rare

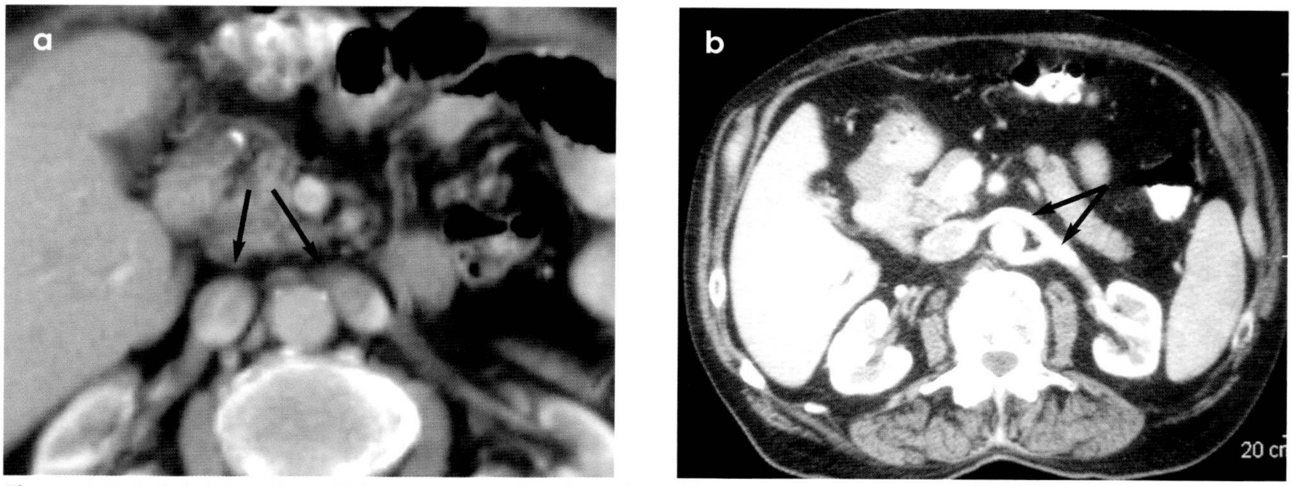

Figure 15. Axial CT and multiplanar reconstructions (MPR) of variant caval anatomy. a) Contrast-enhanced axial CT demonstrating a double IVC (arrows). b) Contrast-enhanced axial CT demonstrating a forked left renal vein, the posterior part lying behind the aorta (arrows).

Key points

- **Vascular specialists must be as aware of variant arterial and venous anatomy as normal anatomy.**
- **Pre-operative imaging often reveals variant anatomy that should be taken into account at the time of intervention.**
- **Modern imaging methods provide greater information and detail than has previously been available.**

References

1. Azakie A, McElhinney DB, Messina LM, *et al.* Common brachiocephalic trunk: strategies for revascularization. *Ann Thorac Surg* 1999; 67: 657-60.
2. Beiles CB. Effect of carotid bifurcation location on the length of internal carotid disease. *ANZ J Surg* 2003; 73: 909-11.
3. Frank MW, Blakeman BP. Two-stage elephant trunk reconstruction for aneurysm of an aberrant right subclavian artery in association with aneurysmal distal aortic arch and descending thoracic aorta. *Tex Heart Inst J* 2000; 27: 412-13.
4. Corral JS, Zuniga CG, Sanchez JB, *et al.* Treatment of aberrant right subclavian artery aneurysm with endovascular exclusion and adjunctive surgical bypass. *J Vasc Interv Radiol* 2003; 14: 789-92.
5. O'Sullivan GJ, Semba CP, Bittner CA, *et al.* Endovascular management of iliac vein compression (May-Thurner) syndrome. *J Vasc Interv Radiol* 2000; 11: 823-36.
6. Balachandra S, Singh A, Al-Ani, *et al.* Acute limb ischaemia after transplantation in a patient with persistent sciatic artery. *Transplantation* 1998; 66: 651-2.
7. Kim D, Orron DE, Skillman JJ. Surgical significance of popliteal aterial variants. A unified angiographic classification. *Ann Surg* 1989; 210: 776-81

Chapter 3

Paediatric arterial problems

Roger N Baird ChM FRCS, Consultant Vascular Surgeon
Bristol Royal Hospital for Children, Bristol, UK

Introduction

Vascular problems are rare in children, and present unusual challenges for the vascular surgeon [1]. There are distinct differences in the very young: the small size of the arteries, the need to accommodate growth and the absence of atherosclerosis in comparison with the usual middle-aged and elderly patients.

A major consideration is that an arterial bypass has to develop in size to accommodate the growth of the child. As adulthood approaches, additional procedures may be required to lengthen a hypoplastic extremity in conjunction with paediatric orthopaedic and plastic surgeons. The main problem is acute ischaemia following iatrogenic and external trauma of the arteries of the extremities; an aneurysm is occasionally encountered.

Acute arterial ischaemia

Iatrogenic injury following arterial catheterisation in the groin in infants is increasing in incidence [2]. Fortunately, the collateral circulation is good and intervention is seldom required in children under 2 years of age.

Following external injuries in older children, newly available investigations for suspected arterial damage include reconstructions of multislice CT with intravenous contrast. Images of excellent quality are provided without the need for arterial catheterisation, which may be difficult because of restlessness and the small size of a child's femoral arteries. General anaesthesia is usually required for CT or MRI.

Blunt and penetrating trauma

Trauma is a major cause of death in children; it has been estimated that each year, over 2 million children worldwide are disabled by injuries [3]. Some of these children have vascular injuries. Major arterial injuries in infants and small children always present difficult problems in diagnosis and management.

Blunt injuries to the aorta and iliac arteries are particularly rare in children. Examples include handlebar injuries that damage the iliac arteries and very severe abdominal injuries when, for example, an unrestrained child is projected from a car. The author's experience includes an aortic thrombosis, which was associated with a major dislocation of the lumbar spine causing paraplegia. For treatment, the lumbar spine was initially stabilised by the orthopaedic

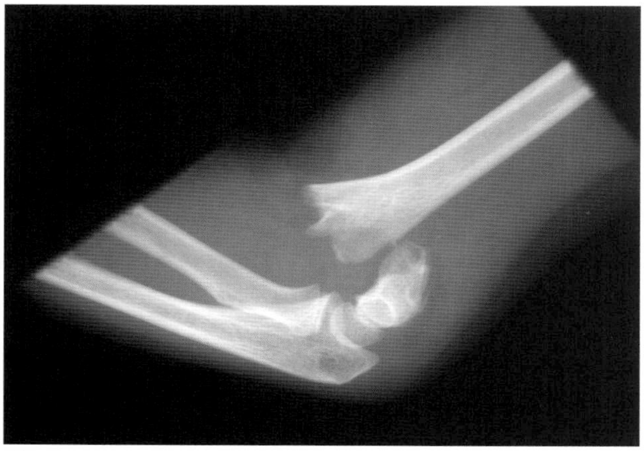

Figure 1. Badly displaced supracondylar fracture in an 8-year-old boy who fell from a quad bike. Arm ischaemia was unrelieved following reduction of the fracture.

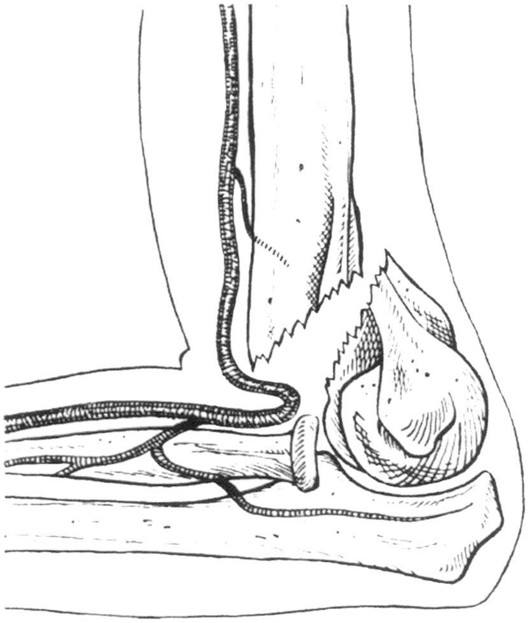

Figure 2. Mechanism of arterial injury in a supracondylar fracture.

surgeons. Thereafter, the disruption of the abdominal aorta was repaired using direct suture and a PTFE patch, with a good haemodynamic result, although the paraplegia was permanent.

In older children, blunt trauma can cause brachial arterial injury from supracondylar elbow fractures (Figure 1), and iliac and femoral artery injuries from bicycle handlebars [4]. If arterial ischaemia persists once a fracture is reduced (Figure 2), reconstructed multisliced CT with intravenous contrast can be used to localise intimal damage (Figure 3), leading to open repair by a longitudinal arteriotomy and vein patch closure.

Iatrogenic injury

Neonates are referred when umbilical or femoral artery catheterisation leads to complications. These include aortic and iliac artery thrombosis and arteriovenous fistula. Vigilance is required for the early

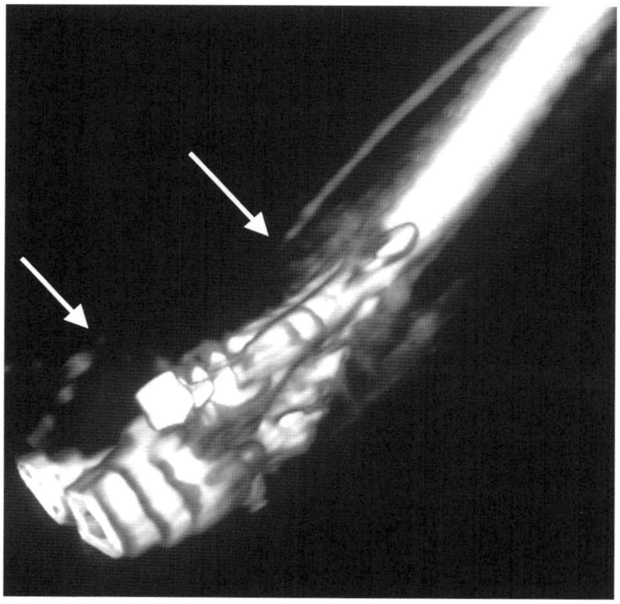

Figure 3. Reconstructed CT with arterial imaging using intravenous contrast. Arrows show the extent of the intimal flap damage to the brachial artery. This required open arterial repair of the intimal flap.

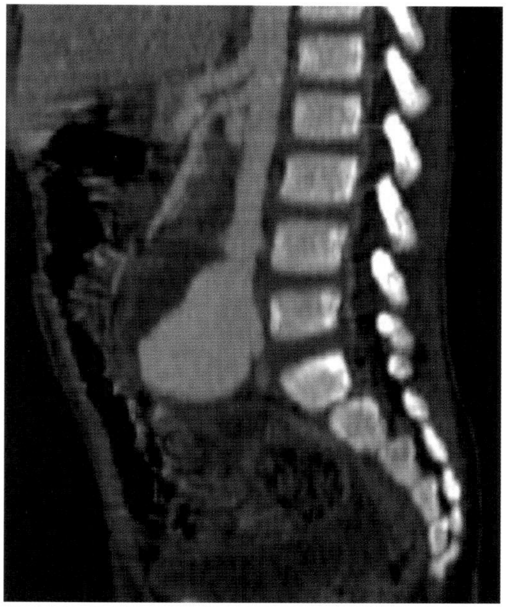

Figure 4. Sagittal CT reconstructive imaging with IV contrast of a saccular aortic aneurysm just above the aortic bifurcation in a 5-year-old boy. This was repaired with a PTFE patch.

detection of reperfusion injury and the compartment syndrome.

Remedial techniques include thrombolysis, embolectomy and fasciotomy. Revascularisation by saphenous vein bypass is usually deferred until the child is greater than 2 years of age. If very small arteries have to be reconstructed using microvascular techniques, the help of a plastic surgeon trained in microvascular repair may be required.

Ligation of the left subclavian artery in infants by cardiac surgeons undertaking repair of aortic coarctation and other cardiac operations can lead to left arm ischaemia of varying severity, ranging from impaired growth, to the acute compartment syndrome. Treatments include fasciotomy and carotid subclavian bypass using saphenous vein.

Profound digital ischaemia can occur in *purpura fulminans* complicating meningococcal septicaemia. There are no easy solutions, and skeletonisation of the digital arteries has been tried by paediatric plastic surgeons in an attempt to avoid multiple digital amputations.

Aneurysms - clinical experience

Aneurysms in children are rare and the causes are often unknown [5].

The author's personal experience includes the following.

Saccular aortic aneurysm (Figure 4)

Repair of a saccular aneurysm of the abdominal aorta in a 5-year-old child with a PTFE patch with a good long-term clinical result.

Ehlers-Danlos syndrome

Repair of carotid (Figure 5) and aortic aneurysms in a 12-year-old girl. Two years later, she died from a ruptured thoracic aneurysm caused by the underlying collagen disease.

Thoracic aneurysm in a 4-month-old baby

A congenital fibrosarcoma was successfully removed from a newborn baby. Subsequently, at the age of 4 months, a thoracic aneurysm was replaced by a 6mm PTFE tube, which was later replaced by a larger prosthesis when the child reached the age of 5 years.

Aneurysms - review of literature

Marfan's syndrome

The Marfan syndrome is an inherited autosomal dominant disorder of connective tissue with no sex or racial predilection. It is known after the Parisian physician, Marfan, who first described it in 1896 [6], and is said to occur in 1 in 10,000 of the general population.

The pathology is of disorders of collagen cross-linkage caused by mutations of Type 1 procollagen. Defects in elastin metabolism are also described.

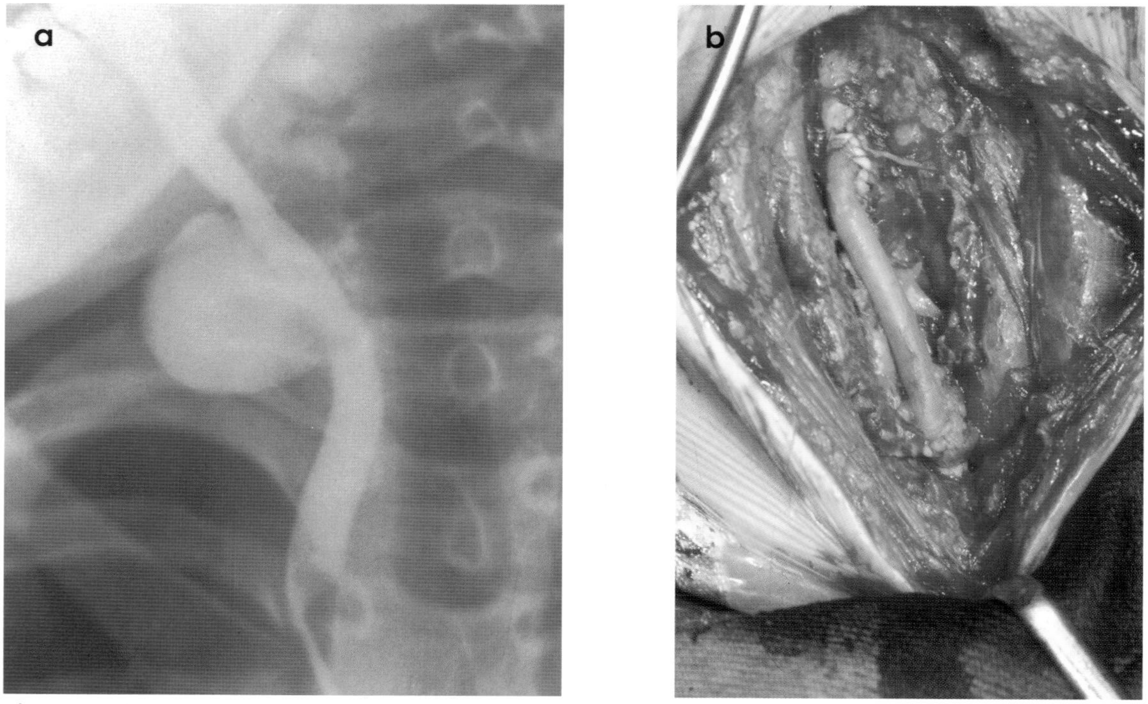

Figure 5. a) Arteriogram of a common carotid artery aneurysm in a 12-year-old girl with the Ehlers-Danlos syndrome. b) Following saphenous vein graft repair.

The clinical presentation is often with skeletal and occular abnormalities including short sightedness and other occular abnormalities. Patients with Marfan's syndrome are tall, thin individuals with long spindly fingers.

Cardiovascular abnormalities are an almost universal finding. Most commonly, there is dilation of the aortic root leading to aortic and mitral valve disease and predisposing to aortic dissection, beginning in childhood. Fusiform, saccular and dissecting aneurysms of the aortic arch follow. Histology reveals cystic medial necrosis with a striking disruption of elastin fibres. The average age of death in patients with cardiovascular involvement is 32 years. The causes of death include congestive heart failure, dissecting aortic arch aneurysms and valvular disease.

Ehlers-Danlos syndrome (see Chapter 7)

The clinical features of Ehlers-Danlos syndrome (EDS) were first described in 1682 by Job Van Meekeren [7]. He described a 23-year-old man who could stretch the skin of his right chest wall to his ear. Since then the term EDS has been used to describe patients with hyperextensible skin, hypermobile joints, bruising and abdominal scarring.

In 1960, Mories described a case of a 15-year-old boy with a fatal femoral artery rupture [8]. There have been numerous subsequent case reports and a few small series. Patients with EDS are at increased risk of vessel rupture in adolescence, during pregnancy and following operations. It is thought that increased collagenase activity leads to undue vessel fragility. Most patients die from vessel rupture before they are 30 years old.

Other aneurysms in childhood

There are case reports and small series of aneurysms in children arising following sepsis from umbilical catheterisation, inflammatory arteritis, Kawasaki's disease, and other uncommon conditions.

Acknowledgements

Good clinical results come from multidisciplinary surgical team working. I particularly acknowledge the contributions of my vascular surgical colleagues in Bristol and further afield: Peter Lamont, Frank Smith, Paul Lear, David Mitchell, Tony Baker, Euan Munro, George Hamilton and Simon Smith; in partnership with paediatric surgeons specialised in general paediatric surgery, orthopaedics, cardiac and plastics, including Richard Spicer, Eleri Cusick, Martin Gargan, Ash Pawade and Lisa Sacks.

Key points

- **Arterial disease in children presents special problems due to the size of the vessels and the need for any revascularisation procedure to accommodate growth.**
- **Good multidisciplinary teamworking is the key to good outcomes.**
- **Primary arterial disease is often part of a systemic disorder.**

References

1. Baird RN. Management of aneurysms and arterial ischaemia in children. *Vascular* 2004 S2; 12: S188-9.
2. Taylor LM, Troutman R, Felciano P, Menashe V, Sunderland C, Porter JM. Late complications after femoral artery catheterisation in children less than five years of age. *J Vasc Surg* 1990; 11: 297-306.
3. Perry MO. Arterial injuries in children. In: *Vascular injuries in surgical practice*. Bongard FS, Wilson SE, Perry MO, Eds. Prentice-Hall International; 1991: 327-30.
4. Sarfati MR, Galt SW, Treiman GS, Kraiss LW. Common femoral artery injury secondary to bicycle handlebar trauma. *J Vasc Surg* 2002: 35: 589-91.
5. Sterpetti AV, Hunter WJ, Schultz RD. Congenital abdominal aortic aneurysms in the young. Case report and review of the literature. *J Vasc Surg* 1988; 7: 763-9.
6. Marfan AB. Un cas de deformation congenitale des quatres membres, plus prononcée aux extremities, caracterisée par l'allongement des os avec un certain degree d'amincissement. *Bull Soc Chir Paris* 1896; 13: 220-5.
7. van Meekeren JA. De dilatabilitate extraordinaria cutis: observationes medicochirurgicae. Amsterdam 1682 Ch 32.
8. Mories A. Ehlers Danlos syndrome, with a report of a fatal case. *Scot Med J* 1960; 5: 269.

Case vignette

Ischaemic arm following reduction of supracondylar fracture of the humerus

Kenneth R Woodburn MD FRCSG (Gen), Consultant Vascular Surgeon & Honorary Clinical Lecturer
Peninsula Medical School & Royal Cornwall Hospitals Trust, Truro, Cornwall, UK

A 7-year-old girl fell from a horse, sustaining a severely displaced supracondylar fracture of the left humerus. Radial and ulnar pulses were impalpable before and after reduction of the fracture, which was stabilised by wires at the time of reduction. Despite a viable limb, with weak Doppler signals at the wrist, the brachial artery (arrowed) was found to be completely trapped within the suture line, requiring an interposition vein graft to restore normal circulation. If distal pulses do not return following reduction of supracondylar fractures in children, operative exploration should be undertaken, regardless of the viability of the arm, as limb development may otherwise be compromised.

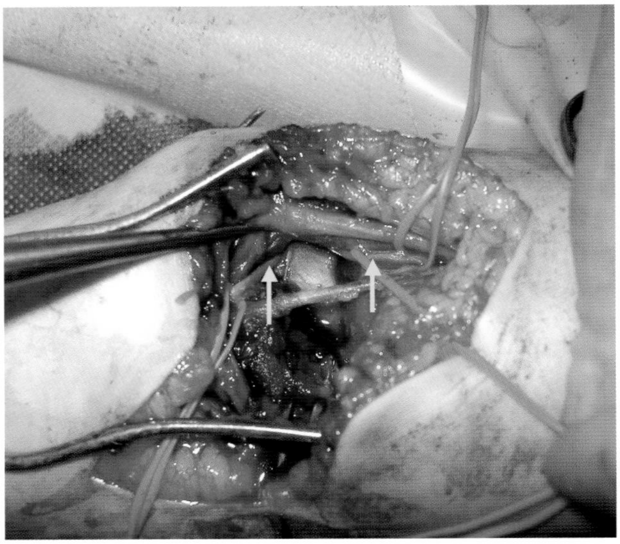

Chapter 4

Major vessel arteritis including lupus

Stephen Baxter FCS (SA), Consultant Vascular Surgeon
Clifford Shearman BSc MS FRCS, Professor of Vascular Surgery
Southampton General Hospital, Southampton, UK

Introduction

Vasculitis is a primary inflammatory disorder of blood vessels. Vessels of any type and size in any organ can be affected, resulting in a wide range of signs and symptoms. These may be self-limiting or potentially fatal, especially if associated with systemic inflammation. Although there are many different clinical syndromes or associations with other diseases, there are only a limited number of histological patterns which can make the diagnosis difficult to confirm [1]. Currently, the most widely used classification of vasculitis is based on blood vessel size (Table 1). This does appear to have clinical significance, although there may be considerable overlap. In smaller vessels, inflammation often leads to occlusion of the vessel and distal ischaemia such as skin ulceration. In larger vessels, damage to the vessel wall may result in aneurysm formation or dissection. Skin and visceral involvement are also less common in large vessel vasculitis.

In most cases no initiating factor can be identified. Drugs such as sulphonamides, infections including hepatitis C and B, HIV and malignancies can trigger the onset of vasculitis. Many patients report a non-specific malaise, night sweats, and weight loss prior to the onset of the vasculitis.

Patients with vasculitis are relatively uncommon in vascular practice, but it is essential to recognise them, as a missed diagnosis can be disastrous. This chapter will focus on vasculitis affecting the large and medium-sized vessels, which are those most likely to be encountered by a vascular specialist.

Large vessel disease

Large blood vessels are involved in two types of vasculitis. Takayasu's involves the vessels of the aortic arch (see Chapter 5, Takayasu's arteritis), while giant cell arteritis affects the extracranial, ophthalmic and aortic arch vessels.

Giant cell arteritis (GCA)

Also called cranial arteritis or temporal arteritis, GCA is the commonest form of vasculitis to affect adults. The aetiology is unknown, but it is rare under 50 years of age and most commonly found in those over 70. The ESR is markedly elevated in 90% of patients at presentation. Prevalence is greatest in those of Northern European descent and GCA is twice as common in women.

Table 1. Classification of vasculitis based on Chapel Hill Consensus Conference on the nomenclature of systemic vasculitis [8].

Large vessel	Medium vessel	Small vessel	Associated disease
Takayasu's arteritis	Polyarteritis nodosa	Wegner's granulomatosis	Systemic lupus erythematosus
Giant cell arteritis	Thrombo-angiitis obliterans	Henoch-Schönlein purpura	Rheumatoid arthritis
	Kawasaki disease	Microscopic angiitis	
	Mesenteric inflammatory veno-occlusive disease	Leukocytoclastic angiitis	

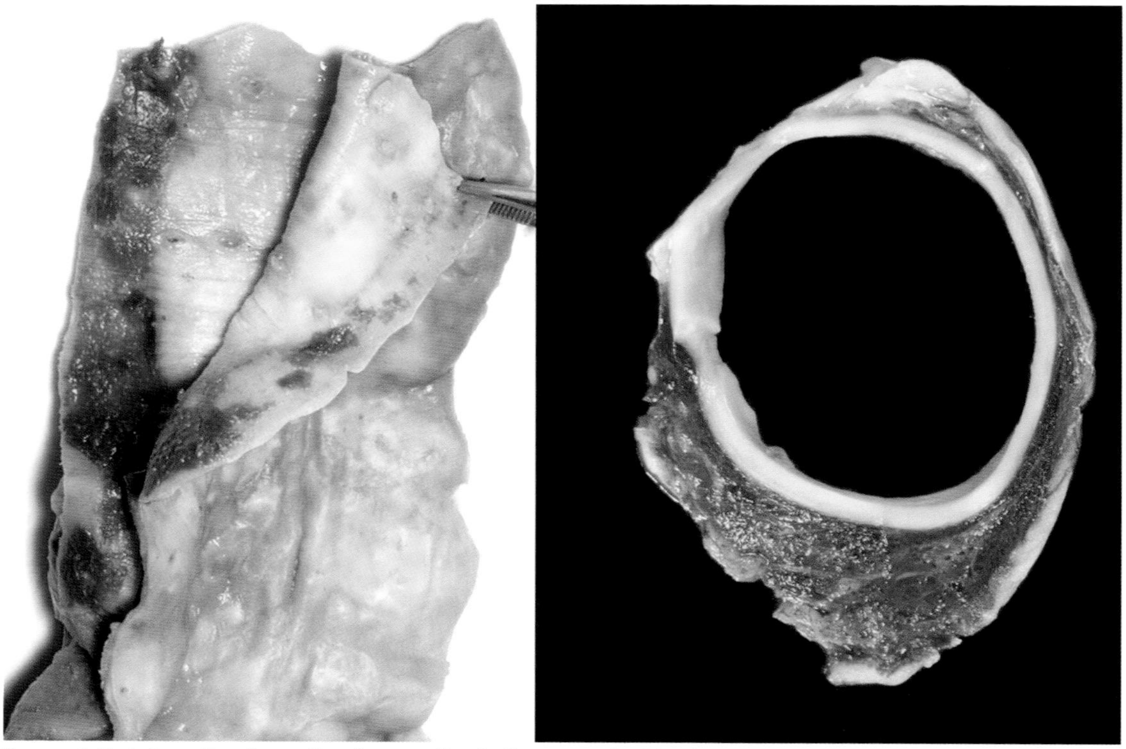

Figure 1. Fatal aortic dissection in a patient diagnosed with giant cell arteritis 18 months previously.

Giant cell arteritis results in transmural inflammation of the extracranial branches of the aorta, but spares the intracranial branches. In smaller vessels, this can lead to occlusion and end organ damage. In larger vessels, including the aorta, it causes damage to the vessel wall that can result in dissection or later aneurysm formation (Figure 1). The inflammation is most often segmental and histology demonstrates disruption of the internal elastic lamina. There is also a lymphocytic infiltration and giant cells can be identified in 50% of cases (Figure 2) [2].

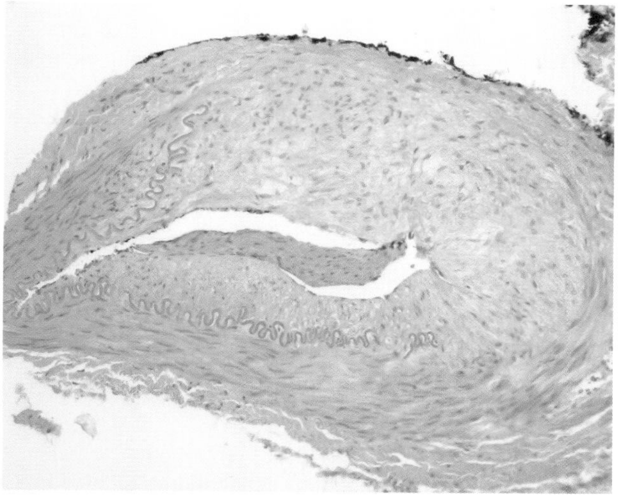

Figure 2. Temporal artery biopsy. There is transmural inflammation with disruption of the internal elastic lamina. Giant cells are visible at the junction between the intima and media.

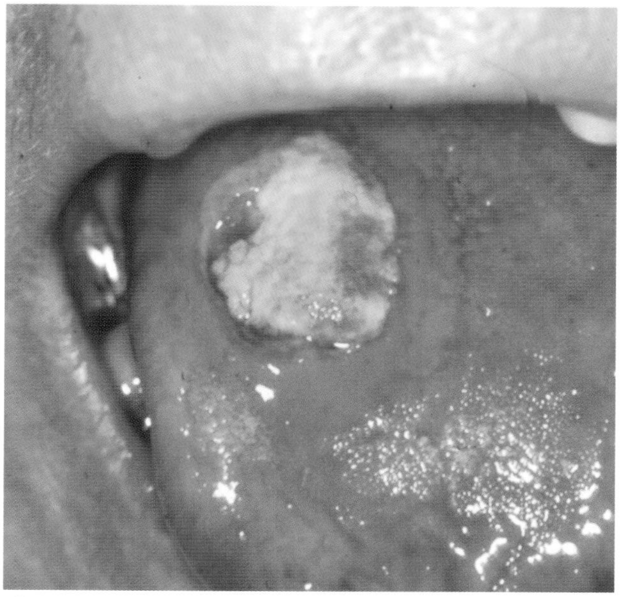

Figure 3. Ischaemic ulcer on the tongue of a patient with giant cell arteritis.

Headache and scalp tenderness are the commonest manifestations of GCA. Jaw claudication and tongue ischaemia may also occur (Figure 3). The onset is gradual in most patients and over half will have systemic symptoms of malaise, night sweats and low-grade pyrexia. Untreated, temporary or permanent visual loss occurs in up to 30% of patients due to retinal artery occlusion or optic nerve ischaemia. This can be bilateral in 30%. Peripheral neuropathy is also relatively common, especially affecting the arms. In 10-15% of patients, inflammation occurs in the larger branches of the aorta resulting in an audible bruit and may cause symptoms such as arm claudication. Thoracic aneurysms are significantly more common in patients with GCA supporting the suggestion that the aorta itself is often involved with the disease.

The diagnosis is usually made on the history and clinical signs supported by a high ESR and C reactive protein level. The superficial temporal artery is usually enlarged and tender and biopsy can confirm the diagnosis in 60% of cases. A negative biopsy does not exclude the disease and may be due to a delay in obtaining a biopsy after the commencement of steroids. It is also related to the patchy nature of the disease. Recently, the use of high resolution duplex ultrasound imaging has been shown to be superior to unselected surgical biopsy [3].

Treatment is based on immune suppression using high-dose steroids. This should be started immediately, before obtaining confirmation of the diagnosis. Very occasionally methotrexate may need to be added in those who do not respond. Low-dose aspirin has also been shown to be of help.

Medium vessel disease

Polyarteritis nodosa (PAN)

This condition was first described in 1866 by Kussmaul and Meier. PAN causes transmural necrotising inflammation of the blood vessels most commonly of the skin, joints, peripheral nerves, gastro-intestinal tract and kidney. This can result in gut infarction, heart failure or peripheral neuropathy. The damaged vessels are very prone to aneurysmal dilation (Figure 4). This typically occurs in the mesenteric vessels in up to 60% of patients. This can help with the diagnosis but may also cause retroperitoneal bleeding. PAN occurs most commonly in the 4th to 5th decades and is twice as common in men. An association with hepatitis B has been reported in a small number of patients. Patients usually have non-specific symptoms such as fever, malaise, weight loss and joint pains, and the kidney is

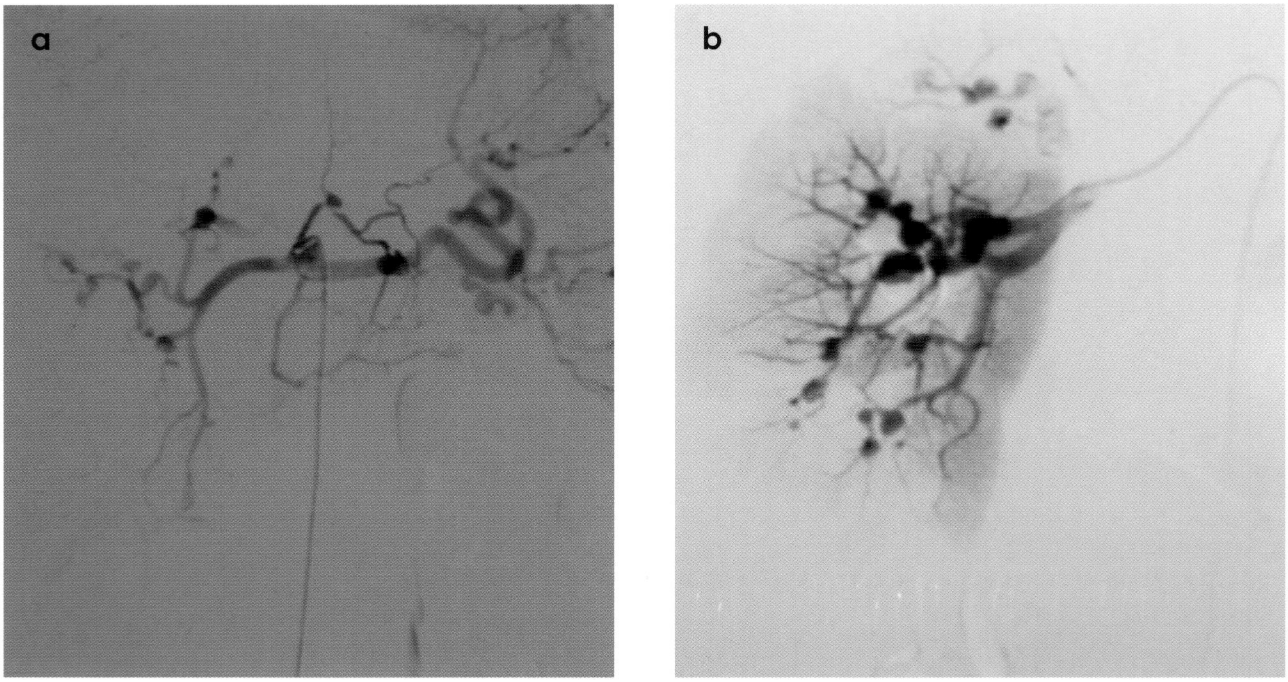

Figure 4. Selective angiography in a patient with polyarteritis nodosa. a) There are several mesenteric aneurysms visible; and b) multiple renal artery aneurysms.

involved in 60%, resulting in proteinuria. Skin abnormalities are very common and include nodules, ulcers and even gangrene of the digits. These changes are most common in the leg and are usually extremely painful.

The diagnosis is supported by elevated inflammatory markers. Mesenteric angiography may help but tissue biopsy is usually required. Treatment is with steroids.

Thrombo-angiitis obliterans (Buerger's disease, see also Chapter 41)

The aetiology of Buerger's disease is unknown, but the use of tobacco is inextricably linked with the disease and patients show hypersensitivity to the intradermal injections of tobacco extracts. Patients have been shown to have an increased prevalence of certain HLA types suggesting a genetic predisposition and anti-endothelial antibodies are usually elevated. It is three times more common in men than women.

The disease affects small and medium-sized arteries and veins of the arms and legs in a segmental pattern. Most patients present with pain and ischaemic ulceration of the toes, feet or fingers at a relatively young age, around 30-40 years (Figure 5). Thrombophlebitis is reported in 50% of patients. Progression leading to gangrene and tissue loss is usually associated with continued smoking, although the larger proximal vessels are rarely involved. On angiography the characteristic appearances are of segmental occlusion of the small vessels of the extremity with tortuous small collaterals (corkscrew collaterals) around the occluded vessel. The diagnosis can usually be made on the angiographic appearances, but similar appearances can be found in systemic lupus erythematosus, rheumatoid vasculitis and scleroderma. Histopathology of the blood vessels shows an inflammatory response with occlusive thrombi (Figure 6). The inflammation may spread to surrounding small vessels and nerves, but the elastic lamina of the vessel remains intact distinguishing it from atherosclerosis and other types of systemic vasculitis.

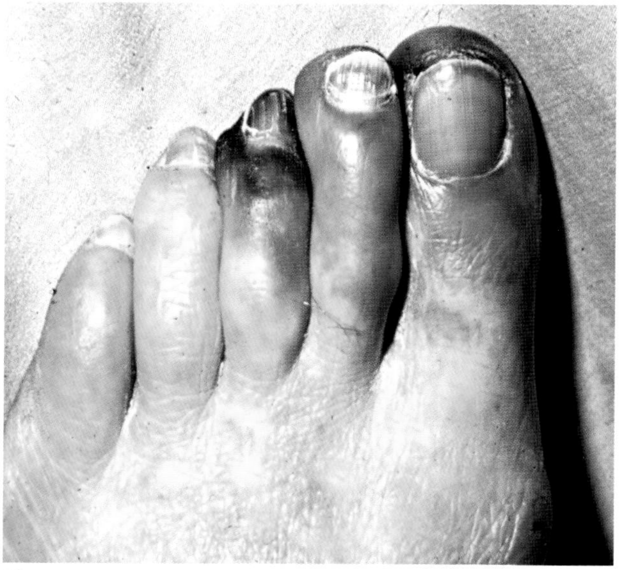

Figure 5. Gangrene of the toes in a patient with thrombo-angiitis obliterans (Buerger's disease).

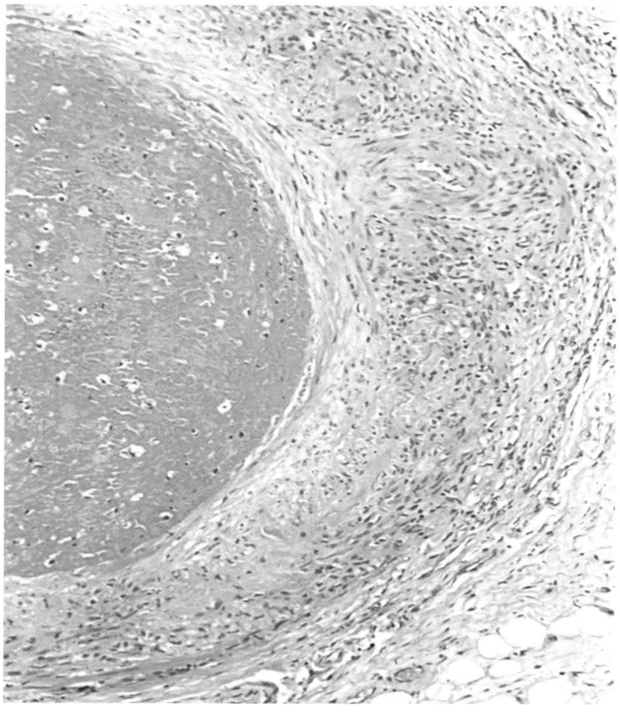

Figure 6. Small artery of patient with thrombo-angiitis obliterans. There is transmural lymphocytic infiltration and luminal thrombus. This patient was 32 and had undergone below knee amputation.

Kawasaki disease (KD)

KD (mucocutaneous lymph node syndrome) is an acute vasculitic syndrome affecting children, first described in 1967 by Tomisaku Kawasaki. Initially thought to be benign it was found that up to 25% of children develop cardiovascular complications including pericarditis, coronary artery ectasia and coronary artery aneurysms leading to thrombosis, myocardial infarction and sudden death. KD is seasonal, suggesting an infective element, but is also more common in those of Japanese descent and in males. The incidence has doubled in the UK in the last decade and is around 8.1/100,000 children under five. The peak prevalence is in children aged 18-24 months and 85% of children are under 5 years of age at presentation. The diagnosis is based on pyrexia of greater than 5 days duration, unresponsive to antibiotics, associated with conjunctivitis, cervical lymphadenopathy, a reddened oedematous mouth and tongue and erythema and desquamation of the skin of the hands and feet. The platelet count is usually very elevated. Treatment involves early administration of high-dose intravenous immunoglobulin and aspirin to suppress the inflammatory component and monitoring of the heart with echocardiography and, if necessary, cardiac catheterisation to identify coronary artery complications [4].

Mesenteric inflammatory veno-occlusive disease (MIVOD)

MIVOD was first described in 1994 as an isolated cause for acute intestinal ischaemia. MIVOD is a venulitis involving visceral organs and resulting in a thrombophlebitis. The majority of cases reported are between their 3rd and 5th decades with equal sex distribution. Clinical presentation is with abdominal pain and bowel infarction of variable extent. Resection of the affected bowel is usually curative, but recurrence has been reported at 15 months. The histological picture varies, but a predominantly lymphocytic venulitis is present in the majority of patients. There was no evidence of an underlying thrombophilia in the reported cases. Treatment is resection of non-viable bowel. At present there is no

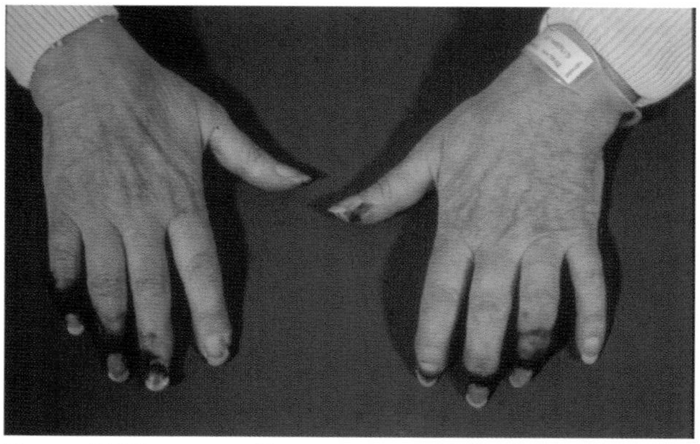

Figure 7. Woman with gangrene of the fingers due to fulminant SLE associated with antiphospholid syndrome. She was treated conservatively and after active medical treatment she only lost the tips of her fingers.

evidence that any prolonged medical treatment is effective.

Vasculitis associated with connective tissue disease

Vasculitis affecting small, medium or large vessels develops in up to 4% of patients with systemic lupus erythematosus or rheumatoid arthritis. The manifestations of this are described below but interestingly, both conditions are associated with an increased risk of atherosclerosis, perhaps related to inflammatory cytokines [5].

Systemic lupus erythematosus (SLE)

SLE was first described by Rogerius in the 13th Century and so named because it was thought that the cutaneous manifestations of the disease looked like a wolf bite. SLE is characterised by auto-antibodies; patients make antibodies against DNA, other nuclear antigens, ribosomes, platelets, erythrocytes and leucocytes. This results in immune complex formation which is deposited in vessel walls. SLE tends to affect women in their 3rd to 4th decades and the female to male ratio is 9:1. The characteristic skin lesion is a malar or butterfly rash.

Vasculitis occurs in nearly 30% of patients, usually involving the skin, but affecting the viscera in 15% [6]. Involvement of organs such as the lung, kidney, gut and eye is associated with an increased mortality risk. Skin lesions include palpable purpura, petechiae, papulonodular lesions, livedo reticularis, cutaneous infarctions and ulcers. Large vessel vasculitis is recognised, but it is unclear whether this is associated with subsequent aneurysm formation.

There is an association of SLE with antiphospholipid antibody syndrome (APS) which itself can be responsible for thrombosis and vascular disease. Patients with ulceration and tissue loss are more likely to have APS (Figure 7).

Steroids are the main line of treatment with the addition of immunosuppressive agents such as cyclophosphamide. It is also important to recognise that many of these patients with active vasculitis will be at risk of premature peripheral vascular disease and their risk factors should be addressed.

Rheumatoid arthritis (RA)

RA is a systemic inflammatory condition characterised by polyarthritis and extra-articular organ disease. Cutaneous vasculitis can cause skin ulceration which is difficult to distinguish from venous or arterial ulceration (Figure 8), peripheral gangrene, purpura or nail fold infarcts. It may also present as a neuropathy (either diffuse or mononeuritis multiplex). Biopsy may help, but often the findings are non-specific. To complicate matters the condition is usually multi-factorial with loss of calf muscle pump due to immobility [7]. Often the diagnosis cannot be confirmed and treatment is judged empirically based on the evidence of systemic activity of the RA balanced against the risks of immunosuppression on wound healing.

Conclusions

Vasculitis is relatively uncommon in vascular practice, but can present in a number of guises. The primary pathology is related to an abnormal immune response to an unknown stimulus which results in

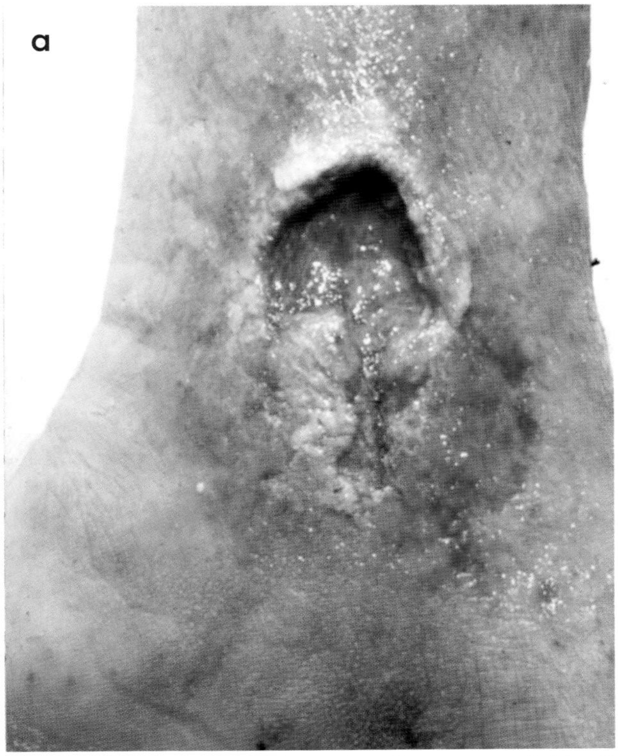

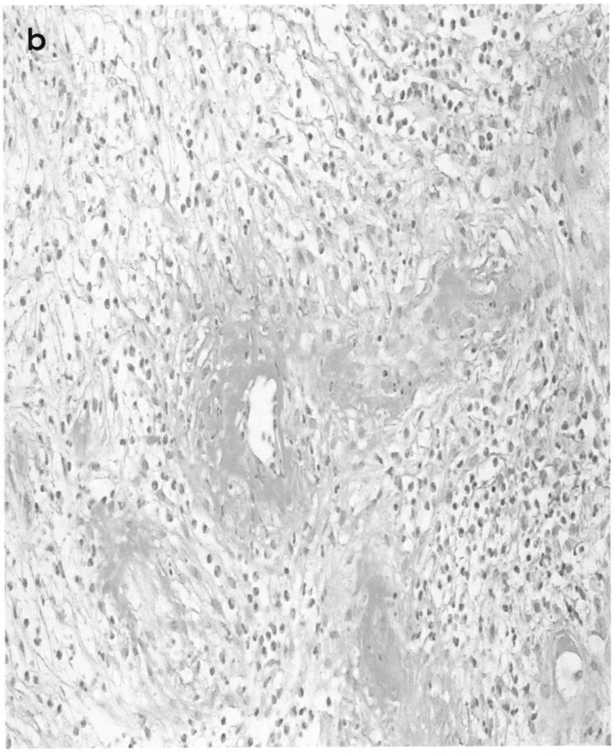

Figure 8. a) Patient with longstanding rheumatoid arthritis and a leg ulcer. b) Histology of a punch biopsy shows vasculitis of a small artery.

inflammation and necrosis of the walls of the blood vessels. Some of these conditions present with ischaemia, tissue loss and infection and so the vascular specialist will often become involved. Their main role is to be aware of the different conditions and to involve expert help expeditiously to diagnose and treat these complex diseases.

Acknowledgement

The authors would like to thank Dr. P Gallagher, Southampton General Hospital, for kindly providing Figures 1, 2, 3, 5, 6 and 8.

Key points

- Vasculitis can present with signs of leg or organ ischaemia.
- Systemic signs of inflammation (weight loss, night sweats, malaise, raised ESR or CRP) should suggest the diagnosis.
- Vasculitis can be fatal and diagnosis and treatment should be initiated urgently.
- Early involvement of an appropriate specialist (usually rheumatology) is essential.
- Following recovery the patient may have an increased risk of peripheral vascular disease, arterial aneurysms and dissection.

References

1. Jeannette JC, Falk RJ. Small-vessel vasculitis. *N Engl J Med* 1997; 337: 1512-23.
2. Salvarini C, Cantini F, Boiardi L, Hunder GG. Polymyalgia rheumatica and giant cell arteritis. *N Engl J Med* 2002; 347: 261-71.
3. LeSar CJ, Meier GH, DeMasi RJ, *et al.* The utility of colour duplex ultrasonography in the diagnosis of temporal arteritis. *J Vasc Surg* 2002; 36: 1154-60.
4. Burns JC, Glodé MP. Kawasaki syndrome. *Lancet* 2004; 364: 533-44.
5. Kaplan MJ, McCune WJ. New evidence for vascular disease in patients with early rheumatoid arthritis. *Lancet* 2003; 361: 1068-9.
6. Calmia KT, Balabanova M. Vasculitis in systemic lupus erythematosus. *Clin Dermatol* 2004; 22: 148-56.
7. Turesson C, Jacobsson LTH. Epidemiology of extra-articular manifestations in rheumatoid arthritis. *Scand J Rheumatol* 2004; 33: 65-72.
8. Jeanette JC, Falk RJ, Andrassy K, *et al.* Nomenclature of systemic vasculitides: proposal of an international consensus conference. *Arthritis Rheum* 1994; 37: 187-92.

Chapter 5

Takayasu's arteritis

Ian Nichol MD FRCS (Gen), Specialist Registrar, Vascular Surgery
David Lambert MD FRCS, Consultant Vascular Surgeon
Northern Vascular Centre, Freeman Hospital, Newcastle upon Tyne, UK

Introduction

Takayasu's arteritis (TA) is a chronic inflammatory disease of unknown aetiology that results in stenosis, occlusion or aneurysm formation in large arteries. The greatest incidence is in Asia, India and Latin American countries, although it has been reported worldwide. In the United States, Minnesota in Olmstead County has an incidence of TA of 2.6 per million per year [1]. The racial distribution is according to the population demographics, except in the Asian population who have a significantly higher prevalence. The spectrum of disease varies according to geographical region. Japanese patients are more likely to have ascending aortic aneurysms and aortic regurgitation due to aortic arch involvement, have more severe inflammation and be female. In Japan, 90% of all patients are young women. Indian patients, however, have higher rates of hypertension and left ventricular hypertrophy due to involvement of the thoracic and abdominal aorta, and are more likely to be men (37%). TA mainly affects the young, with a median age at onset of symptoms of 24 years, and at diagnosis of 28 years. About 80% of patients with TA are within the age range 11-30 years.

History of Takayasu's arteritis

The first description was published by Yamamoto in 1830. He described a 45-year-old man who presented with a high fever initially, and who later on developed an absent pulse in one arm and a weak pulse in the other [2]. Both carotid pulses subsequently became impalpable and the patient complained of dyspnoea and died suddenly, 11 years after the first presentation. The first scientific presentation of TA was given in 1905 at the 12th Annual Meeting of the Japanese Ophthalmology Society by the ophthalmologist, Mikito Takayasu. He presented the case of a 21-year-old woman with a retinal arteriovenous fistula in a wreath-like distribution around the optic disc, and micro-aneurysm formation. At this same meeting, two further patients were presented with absent radial pulses. The first pathological examination of a patient with TA was performed in 1920 by Ohta who described a panarteritis involving the intima, media and adventitia, and optic fundal changes resulting from ischaemia of the carotid vessels. In 1951, Shimizu and Sano described the features of TA under the title "pulseless disease". TA is also known by several other names including Onishi's disease, aortic arch syndrome, female arteritis and Martorell syndrome.

Aetiology

The arteries involved by TA are firm and thickened as a result of the chronic inflammatory process that affects all three layers of the vessel. When severe, the inflammatory process can involve adjacent structures in a manner similar to inflammatory aneurysms. Intimal lesions can be patchy with characteristic skipped areas. The microscopic appearance of the inflammatory process of TA features acute and chronic changes. The acute phase is represented by a panarteritis originating in the vasa vasorum with perivascular cuffing extending from the adventitia and an inflammatory infiltrate consisting of T-cells and dendritic cells. The media shows neovascularisation, elastic degeneration and lymphocyte infiltration. The intima is invaded by smooth muscle cells and fibroblasts. These processes lead to granulomatous nodules, acellular fibrosis and thickening of the media with gross kinking of the intima. These histological findings can also be found in patients with giant cell arteritis, when the clinical history and age assist in the differential diagnosis. The aetiology of the inflammatory process in TA has not been defined. Investigations of autoimmune markers have shown elevated levels of anti-endothelial cell, antinuclear antibody, anticardiolipin antibody, antimonocyte antibody, antineutrophil cytoplasmic antibody (ANCA) and anti-ß2GPI. Anti-endothelial cell antibodies have been reported to mediate complement-dependent cytotoxicity against endothelial cells and may therefore have a role in vascular injury. A further finding supporting an immune-mediated aetiology is an increase in CD-8 positive T-cell subsets and increased levels of IgG and IgM immunoglobulins. Infection has also been implicated in the development of TA. High rates of tuberculosis infection in patients with TA suggest that infection may have a role; however, mycobacteria have not been found in affected aortic tissue. Antituberculous treatment does not lead to improvement. The induction of TA-like lesions in animals infected with various viruses may point to a role for viral infection in the aetiology of TA. Genetic factors have been investigated following the report of TA in a set of twins. Japanese and Korean patients have an increased incidence of levels HLA-B52, A-10, B5, Bw52, B39, DR2 and DR4. Increased expression in TA is different in different geographical regions and correlates with a variation in clinical symptoms.

Clinical presentation

The clinical presentation of TA has three phases: an early prodromal pre-pulseless phase of a systemic illness with systemic symptoms; a second vascular phase, consisting of symptoms of stenosis, occlusion, or aneurysm formation; and a third remission phase of inactivity. Disease progression, however, rarely occurs in this manner because the early inflammatory phase often overlaps the later phases and remission may not occur in up to 25% of patients. The systemic symptoms include malaise, fever, weight loss, night sweats, myalgia, arthritis, skin rashes, headaches, dizziness and heart failure. Symptoms related to vascular lesions may occur months or years after diagnosis and are related to ischaemia of the end organ such as stroke, transient ischaemic attacks, visual disturbances due to ischaemic retinopathy, limb ischaemia, abdominal pain due to mesenteric ischaemia and fainting due to carotid sinus hyper-reflexia. The most frequent finding is a bruit in the carotid artery, usually on the left. Hypertension is common and correlates with the presence of renal artery stenosis. Takayasu's retinopathy occurs in a third of patients. TA generally has an indolent course with the most common causes of death being heart failure and stroke. The definitive diagnosis is made from biopsy, with identification of the histological changes of TA in vascular tissue. This is often impractical in the clinical setting and therefore, Sharma produced a set of diagnostic criteria consisting of three major and ten minor factors (Table 1) [3]. This diagnostic tool has been reported as having 93% sensitivity and 95% specificity.

Laboratory investigations reveal that 50% of patients have a normochromic normocytic anaemia, 15% have a positive rheumatoid factor, and antinuclear antibodies are usually absent. Attempts to assess disease activity have met with difficulty due to lack of a specific marker. C-reactive protein, ESR, tissue factor, von Willebrand factor, thrombomodulin, tissue plasminogen activator, ICAM-1, VCAM-1, E-selectin and PECAM-1 do not differentiate between healthy patients and those with active vasculitis. Interleukin-6 and RANTES (regulated on activation, normal T expressed and secreted) levels are elevated in patients with active disease and can mirror disease activity [4]. These cytokines correlated with ESR but not

Table 1. Modified Sharma diagnostic criteria for Takayasu's arteritis [3]. Two major, or one major and two minor, or four minor criteria indicate a high probability of Takayasu's arteritis.

Major criteria	Minor criteria
1. Left midsubclavian artery stenosis or occlusion	1. ESR >20 mm/hr
2. Right midsubclavian artery stenosis or occlusion	2. Carotid bruit
3. Signs and symptoms (>1 month duration)	3. Hypertension >140/90mmHg
a. Limb claudication	4. Aortic regurgitation
b. Absent pulses or >10 mmHg blood pressure differential in arms	5. Pulmonary artery stenosis or aneurysm
c. Exercise ischaemia	6. Left midcommon carotid artery stenosis or occlusion
d. Neck pain	7. Distal third innominate artery stenosis or occlusion
e. Fever	8. Descending thoracic aortic stenosis, occlusion or irregularity
f. Amaurosis fugax	9. Abdominal aortic narrowing, aneurysm or irregularity
g. Syncope	10. Angiographic evidence of coronary artery disease in a patient <30 years old without atherosclerotic risk factors
h. Dyspnoea	
i. Palpitations	
j. Blurred vision	

CRP levels. Antibodies to annexin V which is involved in inducing apoptosis of endothelial cells are increased in TA. These antibodies are associated with anti-endothelial antibodies and are related to disease activity.

Imaging

Angiography

Angiography, CT, MR and ultrasound imaging have all been used to evaluate patients with TA. Angiography is considered the gold standard (Figures 1 and 2). The Takayasu Conference in 1994 proposed a classification to describe the disease [5]. This consists of six disease patterns with the addition of a "C" or "P" to denote coronary or pulmonary involvement. The commonest pattern involves the entire aorta and primary branches above and below the diaphragm as represented by pattern V. The most frequently affected vessel is the subclavian (left greater than right) followed by the aorta, common carotid (left greater than right), renal, vertebral and innominate arteries. Indian patients are more prone to renal artery involvement and as such have a higher incidence of hypertension. The finding of a homogeneous circumferential thickening of an artery suggestive of an arteritis on ultrasound imaging may be useful in the early detection of TA, particularly in the subclavian and carotid arteries. Angiography is unreliable in diagnosing TA during

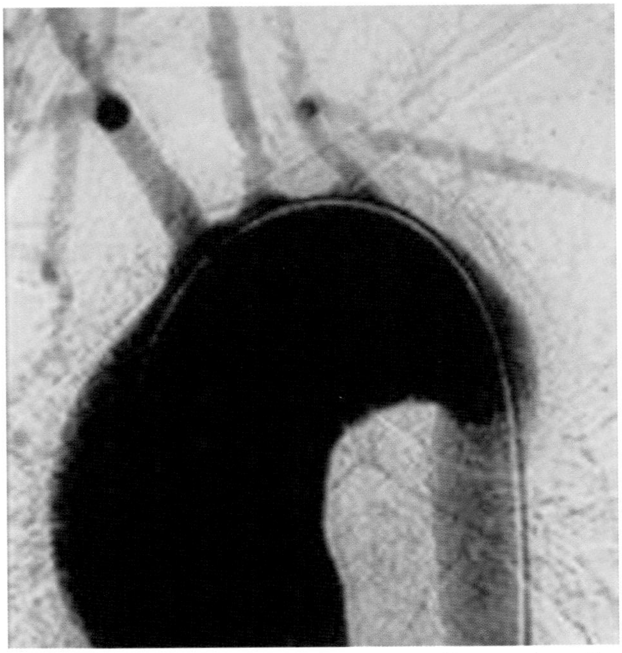

Figure 1. Angiogram showing ascending and aortic arch aneurysm, left carotid and post-vertebral left subclavian stenoses.

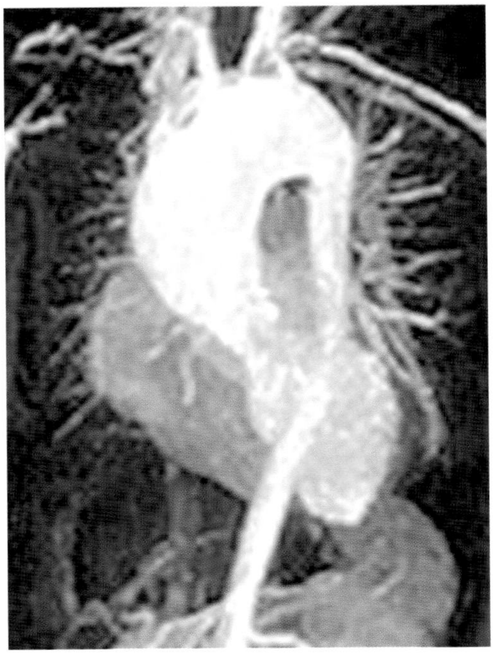

Figure 3. Magnetic resonance angiogram showing Takayasu's involvement of the subclavian arteries and a thoracic aneurysm with a distal aortic stenosis.

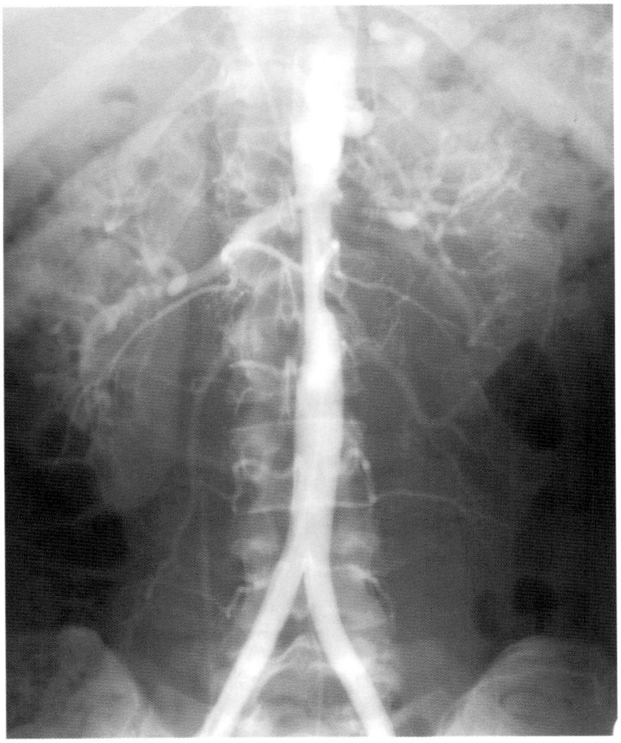

Figure 2. Angiogram showing an abdominal aortic stenosis in a young woman with Takayasu's arteritis.

the early inflammatory phase; it only identifies late fixed changes in the vessel lumen diameter.

Magnetic resonance angiography and positron emission tomography

Angiography is not able to provide information about the vessel wall or the inflammatory process. Magnetic resonance not only provides high resolution imaging of anatomical features such as luminal diameter and mucosal thickness, but is able to provide physiological information such as presence of oedema and mucosal enhancement (Figure 3) [6]. As MR is non-invasive it can be used to monitor response to treatment and does not involve the use of nephrotoxic agents in patients who often already have existing renal impairment. Positron emission tomography (PET) scanning has also been used to identify areas of arterial inflammation in patients who are in clinical and biochemical remission [6]. Fluoro-D-Glucose-PET scanning is a method of whole body screening for areas of arterial involvement and information about cellular activity within an inflamed arterial wall before morphological changes are apparent on other imaging studies.

Management

Pharmacological methods

The management of TA begins with controlling the acute arteritis to induce remission with pharmacological agents, followed by the treatment of fixed vascular lesions that are producing symptoms. Treatment begins with high-dose corticosteroids, starting with prednisolone for 1 to 3 months, with a gradual reduction and tapering of the dose once evidence of disease activity has disappeared and remission has been induced. If the patient does not enter remission or the inflammation recurs with reduced corticosteroid dosages, then cyclophosphamide, azathioprine or methotrexate can be added. Remission is reported to be achieved in 60% of patients, but half relapse with tapering of their steroids. In patients with steroid-resistant disease, methotrexate can induce remission in 50% of patients. In patients unable to tolerate the above cytotoxic agents, mycophenolate mofetil has been reported to be beneficial in three patients. Approximately one quarter of patients never achieve remission; this must be remembered when subjecting patients to long-term immunosuppression. Treatment with both azathioprine and prednisolone for 1 year has been evaluated using clinical, immunological and angiographic parameters, and found to be safe, well tolerated and effective in reducing systemic symptoms and levels of C-reactive protein and ESR. Lesions identified angiographically were halted but did not regress.

Surgery

The majority of patients present with TA after fixed vascular lesions have occurred; patients often have critical stenoses, ischaemia or enlarging aneurysms. The indications for intervention are the same as for patients without TA. As TA is rare, single centre cohorts tend to be small and data are limited concerning the durability of interventions to correct or stabilise fixed vascular lesions [7]. Before surgical intervention, the patient should be in remission, and any anastomosis should be performed in regions that are free from active disease. At the time of surgery, an arterial biopsy should be performed to establish that the anastomosis is to be performed in a non-involved region. There is a much higher incidence of anastomotic stricture or aneurysm formation when the anastomosis is done in an area of active disease. Due to the difficulty in establishing disease activity pre-operatively, some groups have advocated the use of routine peri-operative steroids to reduce the effects of subclinical disease. It has been suggested that if a trial of steroid therapy for 3-6 months is not beneficial, surgical intervention should be considered to limit end organ injury.

Cerebrovascular events in TA are usually the result of ischaemia, due to stenosis or occlusion rather than embolisation. As a result, in the carotid region, bypass is favoured in preference to local procedures such as endarterectomy or patch angioplasty. Crawford first described the durability of reconstruction as a means of treating occlusive arteritis in the aorta [8]. Bypass should originate from the ascending aorta as the great vessels are more likely to be involved in the disease process, and should extend beyond the site of active disease. Failure to adhere to this may result in premature graft failure, or result in anastomotic aneurysms, and postoperative haemorrhage. Perioperative steroids may reduce these risks, but the side effects of reduced healing and infection need to be balanced.

The treatment of renal artery and aortic disease are important in the management of hypertension which is a major cause of morbidity. Renal artery stenosis should be bypassed from uninvolved arteries such as the supracoeliac aorta or hepatic artery. Kidney autotransplantation has also been used. Both autologous vein and prosthetic grafts are acceptable, although the complication rate is lower using vein. Aneurysms are rare in TA and occur most commonly in the ascending, followed by the abdominal aorta. The rupture risk is said to be lower than for atherosclerotic aneurysms.

Angioplasty and stenting

Many stenoses and occlusions are relatively short and, therefore, amenable to endovascular management with balloon angioplasty and/or stenting. Stenting has been reported in the carotid artery by Sharma [9]. Five of six patients had a marked symptomatic improvement, but in one there was a procedure-related neurological event. In-stent restenosis occurred in two patients at 4-5 months, requiring further angioplasty.

Angioplasty has also been performed in the innominate and subclavian artery with a 96% success rate, though 6% had a transient ischaemic attack. Descending thoracic and abdominal aortic stenosis angioplasty has been reported in six patients, with a 67% patency rate at 21 months. Renal artery angioplasty and stenting appears to be effective in reducing hypertension. The restenosis rate is nevertheless very high, although the antihypertensive effect is often preserved.

The benefits of endovascular intervention can be short lived and there is a high failure rate compared to surgical bypass [10]. Nevertheless, bypass also has a significantly higher failure rate than in patients with atherosclerotic peripheral vascular disease, and can be complicated. In the absence of arterial biopsy, the endovascular procedure may be performed in a region of active TA disease. There are reports of endovascular biopsy using cutting balloons providing sufficient material to allow a histological diagnosis of TA in patients with early disease or uncharacteristic symptoms.

In patients with TA aortitis, 85% are improved or cured by endovascular intervention. The NIH study showed angioplasty of renal artery stenosis to be successful in only 43% of patients, with two thirds needing a subsequent bypass procedure. Thus, although endovascular therapy has a role in the management of the vascular disease of TA in the short term, long-term durability is less well defined. It should not be forgotten that the majority of patients are young and may require repeated procedures.

Key points

- Takayasu's arteritis occurs most often in young women.
- Initial management involves inducing remission of the acute disease by immunosuppression therapy, followed by treatment of any fixed arterial disease.
- The indications for intervention are similar to those with organ ischaemia or aneurysm formation without TA.
- Anastomoses should be performed to normal arteries in order to reduce postoperative bleeding, aneurysm formation and prolong graft survival.
- Endarterectomy and angioplasty are less durable than bypass procedures.

References

1. Hall S, Barr W, Lie JT. Takayasu arteritis. A study of 32 North American patients. *Medicine* 1985; 64: 89-99.
2. Numano F, Okawara M, Inomata H. Takayasu's arteritis. *Lancet* 2000; 356: 1023-5.
3. Sharma BK, Jain S, Suri S. Diagnostic criteria for Takayasu arteritis. *Int J Cardiol* 1996 (Suppl); 54: S127-133.
4. Norris M, Daina E, Gamba S. Interleukin-6 and RANTES in Takayasu arteritis. A guide for therapeutic decisions. *Circulation* 1999; 100: 55-60.
5. Moriwaki R, Noda M, Yajima M. Clinical manifestations of Takayasu arteritis in India and Japan - new classification of angiographic findings. *Angiology* 1997; 48: 369-79.
6. Andrews J, Al-Nahhas A, Pennell DJ. Non-invasive imaging in the diagnosis and management of Takayasu's arteritis. *Ann Rheum Dis* 2004; 63: 995-1000.
7. Valsakumar AK, Valappil UC, Jorapur V. Role of immunosuppressive therapy on clinical, immunological, and angiographic outcome in active Takayasu's arteritis. *J Rheumatol* 2003; 30: 1793-8.
8. Weaver FA, Yellin AE, Campen DH. Surgical procedures in the management of Takayasu's arteritis. *J Vasc Surg* 1990; 12: 429-39.
9. Sharma BK, Jain S, Bali HK, Jain A. A follow-up study of balloon angioplasty and *de novo* stenting in Takayasu arteritis. *Int J Cardiol* 2000; 75, Suppl 1: S147-52.
10. Liang P, Tan-Ong M, Hoffman GS. Takayasu's arteritis: vascular interventions and outcomes. *J Rheumatol* 2004; 31: 102-6.

Chapter 6

Behcet's disease

Ravul Jindal MS DNB FRCS, Senior Registrar, Vascular Surgery
Nick JW Cheshire MD FRCS, Professor of Vascular Surgery
Imperial College School of Medicine and St. Mary's Hospital, London, UK

Introduction

Behcet's disease (BD) is a multisystem vasculitis of unknown origin affecting all sizes of arteries and veins. It is seen worldwide, but occurs more commonly along the ancient Silk Road, extending from Far East Asia to Turkey. The prevalence in this area is one in 1000. It occurs less frequently in Northern Europe, North America, the UK and African-Americans, where the rate is one in 100,000. The clinical presentation of BD may vary across different geographic regions, which may result in underestimation of its true prevalence. System involvement is also different as central nervous system involvement is more common in Britain, France, and North America than in Iran, Turkey or Japan. A positive Pathergy test (hypersensitivity of the skin to simple trauma) is more common in countries where the incidence of BD is higher [1].

Definition

The symptom complex of recurrent oral and genital ulceration and chronic iridocyclitis was reported by a Turkish dermatologist, Hulusi Behcet in 1937 [2]. Behcet's disease is a chronic recurrent systemic inflammatory condition characterised by mucocutaneous ulceration along with a broad array of visceral organ involvement. It typically affects young adults with the most frequent age of onset in the third decade. Male gender and young age of onset are associated with more severe clinical manifestations such as retinal and central nervous system involvement.

The lack of a single diagnostic test makes the diagnosis of Behcet's disease difficult. The widely used criteria suggested by an international study group for Behcet's disease require recurrent oral ulceration at least three times in 1 year in all patients (Table 1). Only 3% of cases occur without oral ulceration [3]. It is a long-term cyclical disease and may start with just one or two small symptoms; other symptoms may gradually appear over the years.

Pathology

BD is a multisystem vasculitis affecting all size of arteries and veins. Viruses, streptococcal infections, environmental factors, racial and familial tendency, and auto-immunity have been implicated as causative factors, but none is proven. An increased incidence of HLA-B51 in these patients suggests a genetic component.

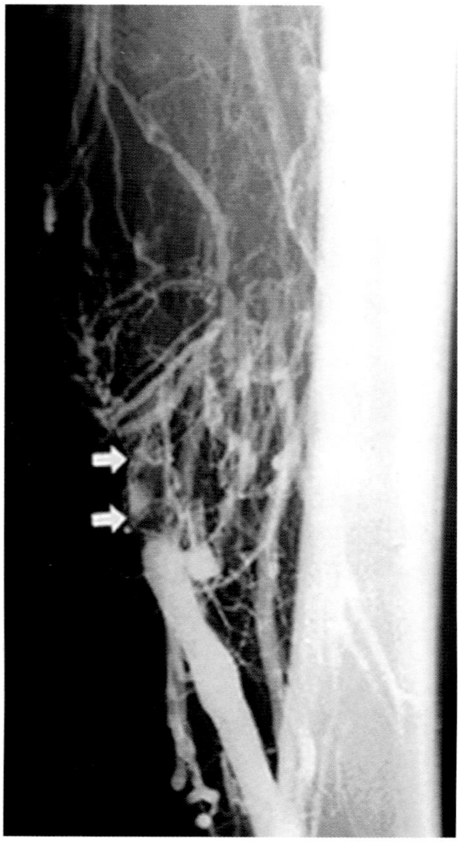

Figure 1. Ascending venogram in a young patient showing thrombus in the superficial femoral vein (arrow); one of the most common presentations of Behcet's disease.

The pathology of aneurysm formation is of inflammatory obliterative endarteritis of the vasa vasorum, probably caused by deposition of immune complexes, causing medial wall destruction and fibrosis. This results in weakness and aneurysm formation with subsequent rupture. The pathology of vessel occlusion has not been well documented but is thought to be due to endothelial cell dysfunction from immune-mediated vasculitis.

The underlying histopathology is of non-specific vasculitis. Tissue analysis shows adventitial thickening, fibrosis and perivascular lymphocytic infiltration, a decrease in elastic and muscular fibres in the media layer, and an increase in smooth muscle and fibroblastic cells in the intimal layer. The lesions are random and focal.

Anatomical variants

Vascular involvement affects 27% of patients with Behcet's disease, and almost 90% of these are venous (Figure 1). The most common vascular involvement is superficial and deep thrombophlebitis (12-25%). It mainly involves femoral and popliteal veins, but can involve inferior and superior venae cavae, mesenteric, iliac or renal veins. It also causes Budd Chiari syndrome due to involvement of the hepatic veins [1,4-6].

Table 1. The international study group criteria for diagnosis of Behcet's disease [3].

Diagnostic criteria	Definition
Recurrent oral ulceration:	minor/major aphthous ulceration on at least three occasions in 12 months
Plus two of:	
Recurrent genital ulceration:	aphthous ulceration or scarring
Eye lesions:	uveitis or retinal vasculitis
Skin lesions:	erythema nodosum or papulopustular lesions
Pathergy test: (hypersensitivity of the skin to simple trauma)	read in 24-48 hours

Note: Figures 1,2 and 3 are reproduced with permission from The British Institute of Radiology. Ko GY, Byun JY, Choi BG, Cho SH. The vascular manifestations of Behcet's disease: angiographic and CT findings. *Br J Radiol* 2000; 73: 1270-4.

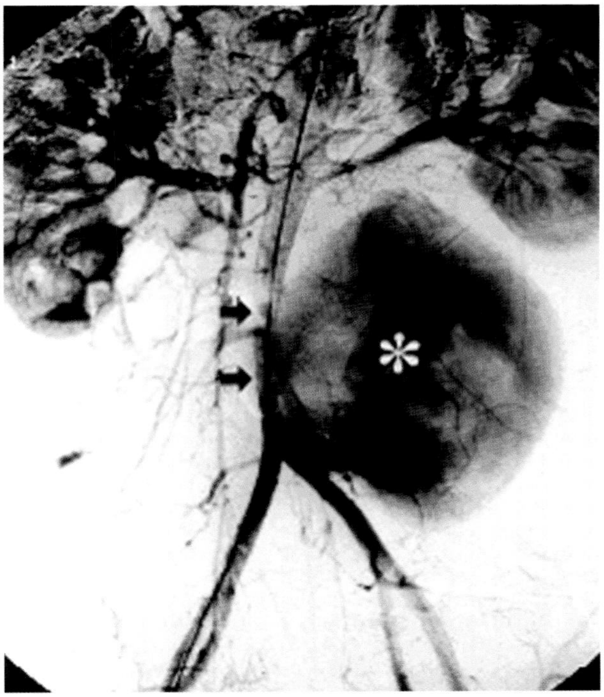

Figure 2. Angiogram showing infrarenal aortic aneurysm (star) in a patient with Behcet's disease.

Arterial involvement in Behcet's disease is rare and has a wide clinical spectrum. It is the most frequent cause of death in these patients. Arterial aneurysms are more common than occlusive disease. Unilateral and single aneurysms are common, the most frequent site being the aorta, followed by pulmonary, femoral, popliteal and visceral arteries (renal, coeliac or inferior mesenteric) [7]. The abdominal aorta is more frequently involved than thoracic aorta (Figure 2). These aneurysms often appear inflammatory, suggesting acute bacterial infection, although cultures are invariably negative.

Pulmonary involvement occurs in 5% of patients with BD and is the only systemic vasculitis associated with pulmonary artery aneurysms. It usually occurs at late stage of the disease and carries a poor prognosis. Aneurysms are multiple, bilateral, saccular and usually located at the origin of the lobar and segmental pulmonary arteries. Sixty percent of the aneurysms are complicated by rupture.

The most common location for arterial occlusion in BD is the pulmonary arteries followed by subclavian, radial and popliteal arteries (Figure 3).

The prevalence of cardiac lesions is 0.5%; these include myocardial infarction, coronary arteritis, endocarditis, myocarditis, valvular disease and arrhythmias. Approximately 50% patients have self-limiting arthritis, mainly affecting the knees. Nervous

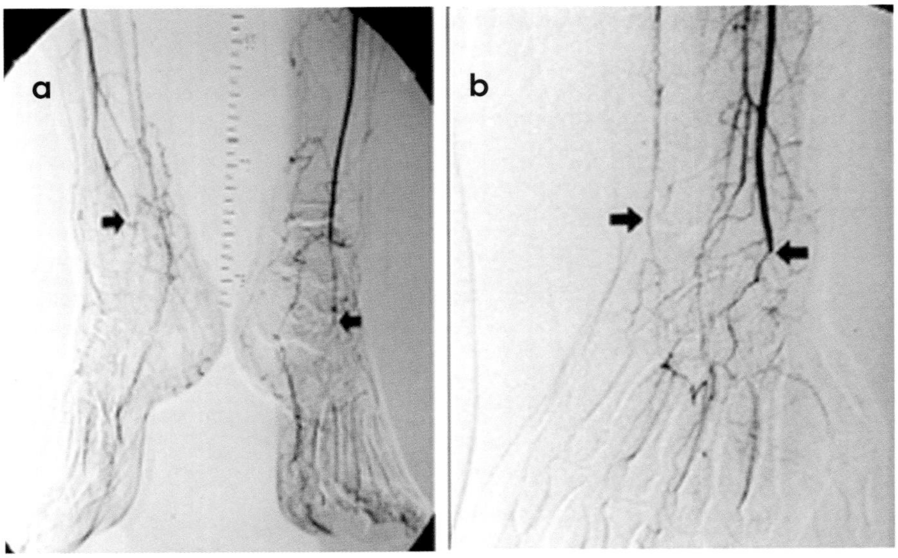

Figure 3. Multiple arterial occlusions are seen in: a) distal legs; and b) arm arteries.

system involvement carries a poor prognosis and is manifest by both motor and sensory neurological symptoms. Intestinal involvement is shown by multiple ulcers, mainly in the ileum and caecum; these frequently require surgery. Eye involvement is the most significant disease-associated morbidity and leads to loss of vision over approximately 5 years.

Diagnosis and treatment

The diagnosis should be considered if a young patient presents with unusual vascular symptoms, particularly with a history of oral and genital ulceration. Primary presentation with vascular symptoms is rare and it can be difficult to differentiate BD from Buerger's disease in areas where both diseases are common. Occlusive arterial involvement has a relatively more benign course than aneurysm disease. Aneurysms respond poorly to medical treatment and tend to enlarge and rupture.

Medical treatment

The main objective is to relieve symptoms, to suppress the inflammation and vasculitis, and to prevent recurrent ulceration and irreversible vascular and neurological damage. The choice of treatment is based on the severity of the systemic involvement, the clinical presentation and the site affected. No surgical or interventional therapy has a role in altering the course of the pathology; therefore, medical treatment is crucial to suppress the exacerbations.

The aim should be to bring the inflammatory markers under control before any surgical or endovascular intervention. Thrombophlebitis is treated with aspirin and dipyridamole (or clopidogrel). Cytotoxic agents, including cyclophosphamide and azathioprine, are given with corticosteroids in cases of arteritis and major venous thrombosis. Some clinicians prefer cyclosporin and colchicine because of the risk of infections with steroids. Others recommend combining low-dose steroids with low-dose cyclosporin in severe disease to prevent the nephrotoxicity of high-dose cyclosporin. After any surgery, medical treatment is continued postoperatively to control the disease activity for 3-6 months with close monitoring during follow-up [8].

Topical or systemic steroids are used for orogenital ulcers, eye symptoms and central nervous system symptoms; non-steroidal anti-inflammatory agents are used for joint involvement. High-dose corticosteroids alone can be used for isolated non-pulmonary arterial occlusive lesions. If pulmonary artery aneurysms are asymptomatic medical treatment should be started as they can disappear completely on follow-up. Colchicine is used as prophylaxis against disease flares. Thalidomide, tacrolimus, interferon-alpha and anti-tumour necrosis factor monoclonal antibodies are potential new therapeutic approaches, but no agent has predictably suppressed the disease completely. Results of treatment are difficult to interpret due to spontaneous remissions and the unpredictable course of BD.

Peri-operative management in Behcet's patients with vascular involvement

All these patients should be investigated extensively for multiple aneurysms and venous lesions. Non-invasive investigation is preferred because of the risk of aneurysm formation at puncture sites. For similar reasons, arterial punctures for angiography or arterial blood gas analysis should be restricted. Intravenous digital subtraction angiography can be employed, but is frequently complicated by puncture site thrombophlebitis. Magnetic resonance angiography (MRA) gives adequate information about aneurysm disease in these patients. Elective surgery should be avoided during an acute exacerbation of BD with flares of major symptom complexes and elevated C-reactive protein levels.

Anaesthesia

The presence of chronic oral ulceration, extensive scarring and adhesions can lead to difficult endotracheal intubation for general anaesthesia [9]. The anaesthetist should avoid any trauma to the scarred region. If emergency intubation is required, a fibre-optic laryngoscope, cricothyroidotomy needle, and a surgical set for tracheosotomy should be available.

Surgery

Surgical treatment of aneurysms is mandatory in Behcet's disease, as they are the major cause of

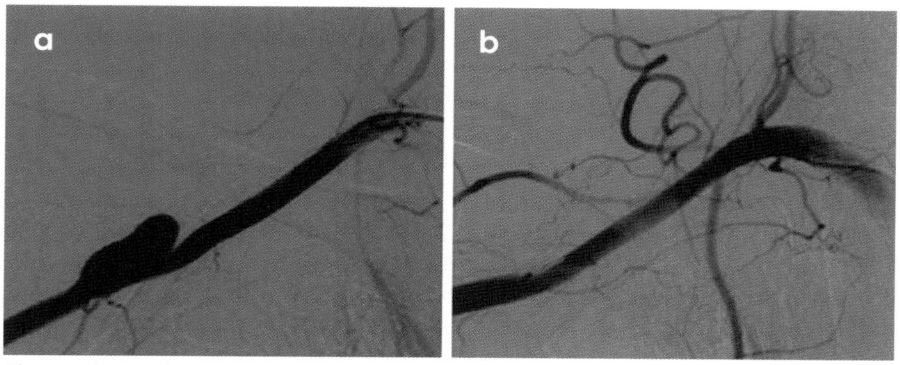

Figure 4. Angiogram showing a saccular aneurysm of the right subclavian artery a) before and b) after stenting. Reproduced with permission from The British Institute of Radiology. Hama *et al*, Endovascular management of multiple arterial aneurysms in Behcet's Disease. *Br J Radiol* 2004; 77: 615-9.

death due to rupture. Technical difficulties associated with the surgery are due to the nature of the histopathological changes in the vessel wall. During surgery the arterial wall has enough strength to hold sutures, but it may later become fragile due to arteritis, leading to anastomotic aneurysm formation. Recurrent false aneurysms occur after 30-50% of procedures. Anastomoses should be constructed in macroscopically disease-free segments of artery, and can be reinforced with Teflon felt. Alternative options include simple ligation of the aneurysmal vessel, where possible. Anastomotic aneurysms tend to grow and rupture and therefore require treatment. They still harbour the risk of recurrent aneurysm after every surgical repair. After infra-inguinal reconstruction, the mean delay to anastomotic aneurysm formation was 3.3 months and the average patency was 8.3 months [2,5,6,10].

The use of autologous or prosthetic grafts for arterial reconstruction is controversial. As veins are also affected in BD, some surgeons prefer to use a synthetic graft. The authors prefer vein if it is not involved macroscopically. A prosthetic graft is used if vein is not available or there is a complication from a previous vein graft such as thrombosis or aneurysm. Unfortunately, the use of interposition bypass grafts has a high rate of thrombosis, in addition to the risk of anastomotic aneurysms; long-term graft patency is the exception rather than the rule. Most of these patients, however, can tolerate graft occlusion without major ischaemia due to development of collaterals.

Endovascular

To avoid the complications and recurrence after surgical repair, endovascular methods have been used with good short-term results [4,11]. As patients are on immunosuppressive treatment, healing after open surgery is compromised. Endovascular treatment also has advantages of shorter hospital stay, less surgical trauma, avoidance of general anaesthesia, and thus decreased morbidity. Primary stenting is much easier in these patients as they are young and their arteries are not atherosclerotic. Good short-term results are available for aortic, coeliac and peripheral artery stenting (Figure 4). Patients continue on immunosuppressive treatment postoperatively, along with anticoagulation. Theoretical disadvantages of endovascular treatment include stent graft thrombosis and access site complications. Long-term results are awaited.

Pulmonary artery aneurysms are managed either by surgery or endovascular techniques. Percutaneous embolisation, either with coils or other embolic agents, requires a patent superior or inferior vena cava, which is not always the case in patients with BD. Pulmonary artery aneurysms may regress or may even completely disappear following medical treatment with immunosuppression. This response is believed to be a feature of false aneurysms and is due to repair of the arterial wall and lysis and absorption of extravascular haematoma.

Anticoagulation

Lifelong anticoagulation with warfarin is recommended in patients who develop venous thrombosis, but the role of prophylactic anticoagulation is uncertain in patients with arterial involvement. Anticoagulation should be avoided when there are pulmonary artery aneurysms because of the risk of rupture. In these patients, the presence of haemoptysis and deep vein thrombosis, with an abnormal ventilation perfusion scan, may erroneously lead to anticoagulation therapy for presumed pulmonary embolism. Anticoagulants and antiplatelet agents including warfarin, heparin and aspirin may be added to immunosuppressive therapy for large vessel arteritis, or after surgical intervention.

Prognosis and follow-up

Long-term follow-up is essential because of the relapsing nature of BD. The life expectancy is normal (mortality rate 3-4%) if not threatened by a ruptured aneurysm or major venous thrombosis. In Budd Chiari syndrome, the mortality rate reaches 60%. The course of inflammation is intermittent, but the disease stabilises in the majority of patients, becoming chronic in the affected organ system. The severity of symptoms and signs appears to diminish with time.

Prompt medical treatment and close follow-up should accompany the surgery to identify the potential complications of thrombosis and recurrent aneurysms. Because patients with BD are at high risk of angiographic complications, non-invasive monitoring is valuable for follow-up.

Key points

- **Behcet's disease should be considered in a young male patient with unusual vascular disease, particularly if accompanied by oral or genital ulceration.**
- **It affects both arterial and venous systems.**
- **Intervention should be avoided during an acute exacerbation.**
- **Long-term surgical results are poor because of graft thrombosis and anastomotic aneurysms.**
- **Endovascular treatment has good short-term results in selected patients.**
- **Long-term medical treatment and follow-up is required.**

References

1. Sakane T, Takeno M, Suzuki N, *et al.* Current concepts: Behcet's disease. *N Engl J Med* 1999; 341: 1284-91.
2. Ozeren M, Mavioglu I, Dogan OV, *et al.* Reoperation results of arterial involvement in Behcet's disease. *Eur J Vasc Endovasc Surg* 2000; 20: 512-6.
3. International study group for Behcet's disease: criteria for diagnosis of Behcet's Disease. *Lancet* 1990; 335: 1078-80.
4. Saba D, Saricaoglu H, Bayram AS, *et al.* Arterial lesions in Behcet's disease. *Vasa* 2003; 32: 75-81.
5. Sasaki SH, Yasuda K, Takigami K, *et al.* Surgical experiences with peripheral artery aneurysms due to Vasculo-Behcet's disease. *J Cardiovasc Surg* (Torino) 1998; 39: 147-50.
6. Ceyran H, Akcali Y, Kahraman C. Surgical treatment of Vasculo-Behcet's disease. A review of patients with concomitant multiple aneurysms and venous lesions. *Vasa* 2003; 32: 149-53.
7. Smith EJ, Abulafi M, Mcpherson GA, Allison DJ, Mansfield AO. False aneurysm of the abdominal aorta in Behcet's disease. *Eur J Vasc Surg* 1991; 5: 481-4.
8. Evereklioglu C. Managing the symptoms of Behcet's disease. *Expert Opin Pharmacother* 2004; 5: 317-28.
9. Turkoz A, Toprak H, Koroglu A, *et al.* Anaesthetic management and endovascular stent grafting of abdominal aortic aneurysm in a patient with Behcet's disease. *J Cardiothoracic Vasc Anaesthesia* 2002; 16: 468-70.
10. Schneider F, Gouny P, Van laere O, *et al.* Vascular complications after surgical repair of aneurysms in Behcet's disease. *J Cardiovasc Surg* (Torino) 2002; 43: 501-5.
11. Hernandez VB, Gutierrez F, Capel A, *et al.* Endovascular repair of concomitant celiac trunk and abdominal aortic aneurysms in a patient with Behcet's disease. *J Endovasc Ther* 2004; 11: 222-5.

Chapter 7

Ehlers-Danlos syndrome

Donna M Egbeare BSc MB BCh, Senior House Officer, Vascular Surgery
Lasantha D Wijesinghe MA MD MB BChir FRCS, Consultant Vascular Surgeon
Royal Bournemouth Hospital, Bournemouth, UK

Introduction

Ehlers-Danlos (ED) syndrome is one of the most frequently inherited connective tissue disorders. The syndrome is a collection of subtypes with various genotypes and phenotypes that have differing clinical presentations with the common feature of increased skin laxity. Subtypes I and especially IV should be of concern to the vascular surgeon as these patients are prone to present with catastrophic vascular problems [1,2].

The incidence of ED syndrome is 1 in 150,000, but this is probably an underestimate. Type IV is thought to represent about 4% of ED syndrome and its incidence is estimated to be between 1-10 per million. It affects men and women equally and its rarity means that it is less likely to be considered as a diagnosis when patients present.

Definition

ED syndrome is characterised by increased elasticity of the skin, hypermobility of joints, easy bruising and excessive gaping of wounds after minor trauma due to skin fragility. At present there are 10 distinct subtypes described (Table 1). They are due to various biochemical and genetic defects and have varying forms of inheritence. Spontaneous mutations have also been described [3].

Historical perspective and genetics

The syndrome was first described by a Dutch surgeon, van Meekeren, in the 17th Century. It was further characterised by Ehlers, a Dutch dermatologist, and Danlos, a French physician, at the turn of the 20th Century.

Type IV ED syndrome (also known as Sack-Barabas type) is autosomal dominant in inheritance (although there are incidences of recessive inheritance described) and characterised by mutation in the Type III collagen gene, COL3AI. There seems to be no correlation between mutation and type of complication [4]. Phenotypically it manifests as extreme fragility of blood vessels and hollow organs containing Type III collagen, resulting in spontaneous rupture of these tissues, often as the presenting feature. Multiple aneurysm formation and dissection of major vessels is common.

In 1975, Pope and his associates detected the Type III collagen defect that is responsible for the

Table 1. Main types and characteristics of ED syndrome subtypes.

Type	Name	Inheritance	Features
I	Gravis	Dominant	Most common form hyperextensible skin, easy bruising, varicose veins
II	Mitis	Dominant or recessive	Similar but less severe than Type I
III	Benign hypermobile	Dominant	Soft skin, marked large and small joint hypermobility, arthritis
IV	Arterial-ecchymotic or Sack-Barabas	Dominant or recessive	Thin skin, bruising, spontaneous arterial, bowel and uterine rupture
V	X linked	X linked	Similar to Type II
VI	Ocular	Recessive	Hyperextensible skin and joints, scoliosis, ocular fragility, keratoconus
VII	Types A, B and C	Recessive	Short stature, congenital hip dislocation, joint hypermobility and dislocation
VIII	Periodontitis	Dominant	Generalised periodontitis, skin similar to Type II
IX	X linked cutis laxa, occipital horn syndrome	X linked	Extensile lax skin, bladder diverticulae, limited pronation and supination, occipital horns, broad clavicles
X	Fibronectin defects	Recessive	Similar to Type II, but due to fibronectin defect

clinical manifestations and further subdivided Type IV ED syndrome into three types [5]:

- Classic type - complete Type III collagen defect.
- Long-lived type - incomplete Type III collagen defect.
- Atypical type.

Clinical presentation

The clinical diagnosis of Type IV ED syndrome is made on the presence of at least two of the following clinical criteria [6]:

- Easy bruising.
- Thin skin with visible veins.
- Characteristic facial features (wide-spaced eyes, lobeless ears).
- Rupture of arteries, uterus or intestines.

Patients often present with a vascular catastrophe and it is only later after the initial presentation has been dealt with that more information is gathered and a diagnosis of ED syndrome suggested. Often the diagnosis is made at post mortem. Many patients have relatives who have died suddenly of vessel rupture at a young age or relatives with hypermobile joints or lax skin who died suddenly from an unknown cause. Patients frequently suffer major complications, often fatal, in their twenties and thirties and survival beyond 50 is very unusual. In one review, 25% of patients suffered medical or surgical complications by the age of 20 and more than 80% by the age of 40 (see case report, Table 2). Approximately 85% of Type IV ED patients have skin symptoms, especially easy bruising and thin skin, and about 75% have lax joints.

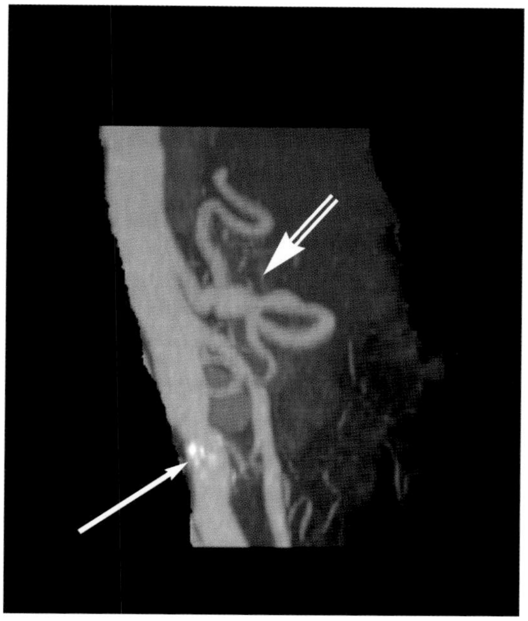

Figure 1. Postoperative surveillance CT in saggital plane showing dilatation of the coeliac axis (open arrow). High density areas at the site of the aortic repair are probably due to the pledgets used to effect aortic repair (closed arrow).

Vascular complications

The vascular complications of Type IV ED syndrome are often catastrophic and carry a high mortality [7]. Rupture of large arteries is the cause of death in 90% of these patients. Ruptures can be spontaneous, aneurysmal or following seemingly minor trauma. The most commonly affected arteries are the thoracic and abdominal aorta, followed by the head and neck vessels and the large vessels of the limbs (Figure 2a). Varicose veins, extensive bleeding after simple operative procedures, gross haematomas, false aneurysm and AV fistula formation are more common in patients with ED than in the general population. Patients have friable tissues and vessels.

Pathological examination of the arteries can show disorganised media, decreased or absent elastin and irregular hyperplasia of the media (Figure 2b). These findings are suggestive of connective tissue disorders, but are not specific to this disease or subtype. Diagnosis depends on the culture of a patient's fibroblasts to demonstrate the defect in Type III collagen synthesis or secretion.

Table 2. Case report.
A 41-year-old woman was admitted as an emergency with a 2-week history of a painful left leg. There was no relevant cardiovascular or family history. On examination the only abnormality was an absent left femoral pulse. An angiogram via a right femoral puncture showed a left external iliac artery occlusion. Under general anaesthetic a standard embolectomy was performed successfully. However, as the wound was being closed the patient became hypotensive and difficult to ventilate. The distal aorta and left iliac vessels were examined through a small iliac fossa incision. There was no haematoma or bleeding visible. Because the left side of the chest was not expanding, an intercostal drain was inserted which produced 6 litres of blood. A formal thoracotomy incision was made, but revealed no source for the haemorrhage. The incision was extended into the abdomen to expose the whole abdominal aorta. Just below the level of the renal arteries there was a small hole in the aortic wall that had probably been caused by passage of the embolectomy catheter. A short infrarenal section of aorta was replaced with a dacron tube graft sewn in with continuous 2.0 polypropylene sutures. The aortic wall was noted to be thin. On release of the aortic clamp there was catastrophic haemorrhage from the suture line. The anastomoses were redone using interrupted 5.0 sutures supported with dacron pledgets. On this occasion the aortic tissue held the sutures securely. The patient recovered without incident. The diagnosis of ED was suspected and confirmed by fibroblast culture. She has been followed-up by ultrasound surveillance and, more recently, CT (Figure 1), which shows a secure aortic repair and a small aneurysm of the coeliac axis.

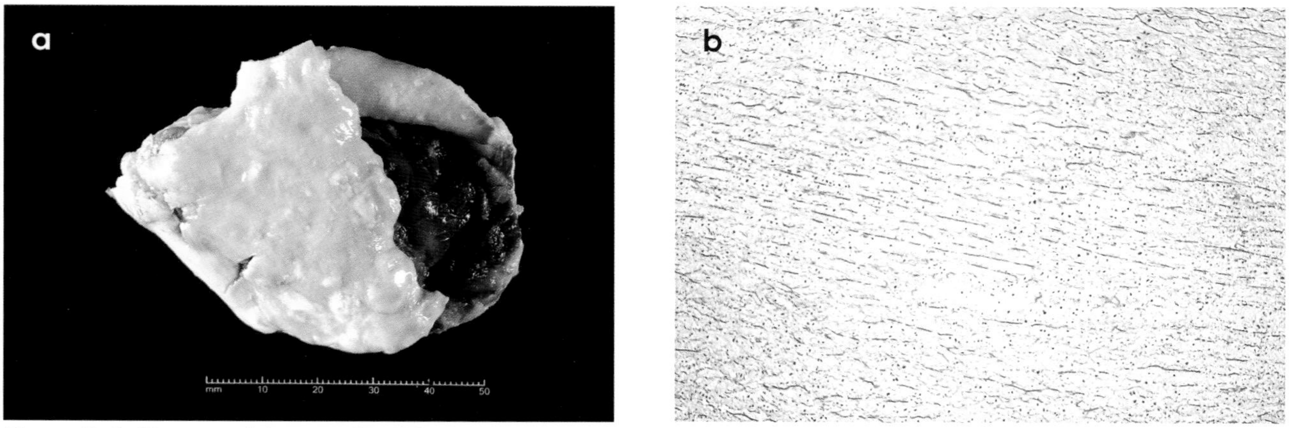

Figure 2. A 41-year-old man with Ehlers-Danlos syndrome died after thoracic aortic dissection. a) Macroscopic view of the intimal surface of the heart and ascending aorta. b) Microscopic view of the aortic media showing extensive fragmentation of the elastin fibres (stained pink) that is pathological in a person of this age. Courtesy of Dr. P Gallagher.

Clinical management

The outcome of arterial complications in Type IV ED syndrome is poor. There is no definite therapy or known cure. Patients should avoid unnecessary trauma, and know that pregnancy is high risk. Because of friable tissues and vessels, careful non-invasive surveillance is the preferred method of management. However, follow-up can induce both surveillance anxiety and false reassurance, since the arteries do not always become aneurysmal before rupture.

When investigating patients with ED syndrome, the method of choice is duplex ultrasound, magnetic resonance angiography (MRA) or CT. Arteriography is reported to have a complication rate in excess of 60% with a mortality rate of up to 17% and is relatively contra-indicated.

At the time of any surgery the use of soft clamps or intraluminal balloon occlusion catheters is advised to avoid damage to delicate vessels. Anastomoses should be made without tension using interrupted sutures. Teflon or dacron pledgets can be used to distribute pressure more evenly. Some surgeons recommend that skin closure should be done with steristrips, where possible. If sutures are used they should be kept in place for much longer than usual to mitigate the increased risk of dehiscence.

All patients diagnosed with ED syndrome should be referred for genetic counselling. This has two functions: to provide families with support, and to collate a knowledge base for clinicians.

The future

Pepin *et al* studied clinical records of 220 patients who had been confirmed as having ED [8]. They concluded that although no specific therapies delay the onset of complications in patients with ED syndrome Type IV, knowledge of the diagnosis influences their management including surgery, follow-up and pregnancy advice. Gene therapy may be useful in the future.

Acknowledgement

The authors would like to thank Dr. P Gallagher, Southampton General Hospital, for kindly providing Figure 2.

Key points

- Ehlers-Danlos syndrome should be suspected in a young patient with spontaneous vascular rupture.
- There are typical signs of the disease in the skin, eyes and joints, and the skin bruises easily. There is often a family history.
- Non-invasive investigations are advised.
- Fibroblast culture must be used to establish the diagnosis. Genetic analysis and family counselling have important roles to play in the management.

References

1. Cikrit DF, Miles JH, Silver D. Spontaneous arterial perforation: the Ehlers-Danlos spectre. *J Vasc Surg* 1987; 5: 248-55.
2. Habib K, Memon MA, Reid DA, *et al.* Spontaneous common iliac arteries rupture in Ehlers-Danlos syndrome Type IV: report of two cases and review of the literature. *Ann R Coll Surg Engl* 2001; 83: 96-104.
3. Beighton P, De Paepe A, Steinmann B, *et al.* Ehlers-Danlos syndromes: revised nosology. *Am J Med Genet* 1998; 77: 31-7.
4. Byers PH. Ehlers-Danlos syndrome: recent advances and current understanding of the clinical and genetic heterogenicity. *J Invest Dermatol* 1994; 103: 47-52S.
5. Pope FM, Martin GR, Lichenstein JR, *et al.* Patients with Ehlers-Danlos syndrome Type IV lack Type III collagen. *Proc Natl Acad Sci* 1975; 72: 1314-6.
6. Lauwers G, Nevelsteen A, Daenen G, *et al.* Ehlers-Danlos syndrome Type IV: a heterogeneous disease. *Ann Vasc Surg* 1997; 11: 178-82.
7. Bergqvist D. Ehlers-Danlos Type IV syndrome. A review from a vascular surgical point of view. *Eur J Surg* 1996; 162: 163-70.
8. Pepin M, Schwarze U, Superti-Furga A, *et al.* Clinical and genetic features of Ehlers-Danlos syndrome Type IV, the vascular type. *N Engl J Med* 2000; 342: 673-80.

Case vignette

Severe carotid ischaemia

Felicity Meyer MA FRCS, Consultant Vascular Surgeon, Norfolk and Norwich University Hospital, Norwich, UK

This 52-year-old heavy smoker was seen sitting in outpatients with his head in his hands (Figure 1). Removal of a dressing on the left side of his scalp revealed a large area of dry gangrene. Arch aortography showed occlusions of both vertebral, the right common carotid and left external carotid arteries (Figure 2). A full thickness skin graft was performed with a good result (Figure 3). Arterial reconstruction is awaited.

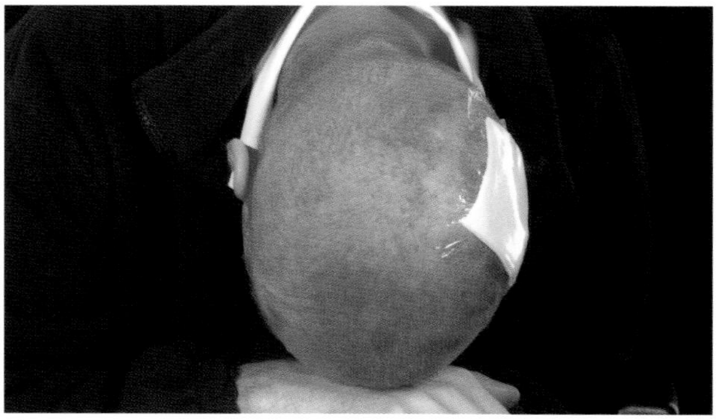

Figure 1.

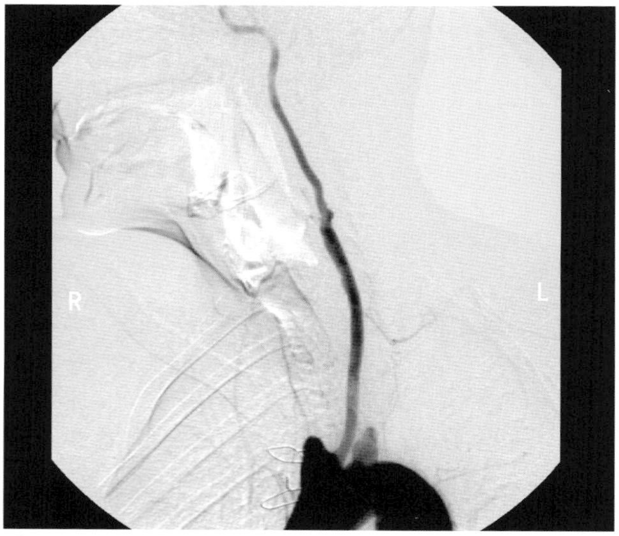

Figure 2.

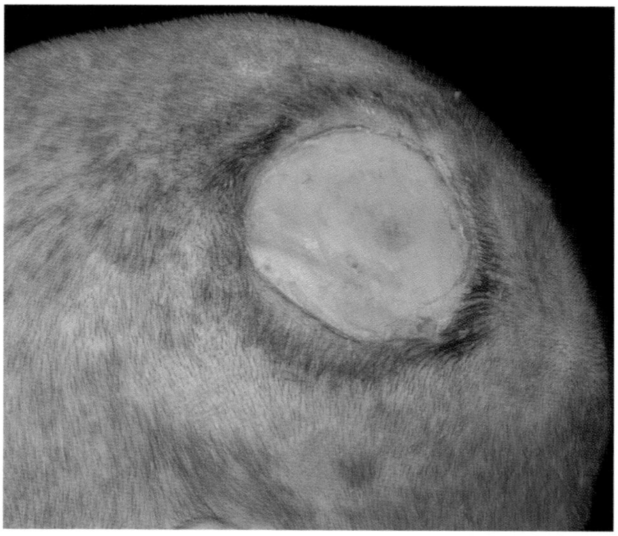

Figure 3.

Chapter 8

Moyamoya disease

Ian Nichol MD FRCS (Gen), Specialist Registrar, Vascular Surgery
Michael G Wyatt MSc MD FRCS, Consultant Vascular Surgeon
Northern Vascular Centre, Freeman Hospital, Newcastle upon Tyne, UK

Introduction

Moyamoya disease is a progressive occlusive cerebrovascular disease that affects the supraclinoid internal carotid arteries and proximal portions of the anterior and middle cerebral arteries with prominent collateral formation. The term Moyamoya means "wavering puff of smoke" which describes the abnormal vasculature found at the base of the brain on angiography.

History

Takeuchi and Shimizu reported the first case in 1957 as bilateral internal carotid artery hypoplasia. In 1968, Kudo described the spontaneous occlusion of the circle of Willis, and Nishimoto and Takeuchi reported a series of 96 patients in Japanese patients [1]. Moyamoya was the term coined by Suzuki and Takaku in 1969 to describe the abnormal vascular appearance on angiography [2]. Initially, Moyamoya was thought to be limited to Japan but it is now recognised across the world, especially in China and Korea. A recent report from Switzerland described a series of four patients with Moyamoya disease treated over 4 years. Moyamoya tends to affect children and young adults who present with neurological symptoms due to cerebral ischaemia or intracranial bleeding. It tends to affect males more than females with a ratio of 1:5 and has a higher incidence in individuals with Down's syndrome. A North American study reported an age range of 5 to 47 years and that 58% of patients were female.

Aetiology

The aetiology of Moyamoya remains unknown. Due to the increased incidence in Japan and Korea, and the familial clustering in both the Japanese, Caucasian, Innuit and North American Indian populations, a genetic aetiology is probable. Chromosome linkage studies suggest an association between the disease and markers at 3p24.2-26. The marker D6S441 on chromosome 6 where the human leukocyte antigen (HLA) gene is located also show possible linkage. HLA-B51 had a significant association with Moyamoya in a study of 32 Japanese patients. Several other studies have implicated HLA-B35. A role for Epstein-Barr virus (EBV) infection has been suggested based upon the finding of increased EBV DNA and antibody in patients with Moyamoya. Moyamoya-like changes occur in rats infected with propionobacterium acnes.

There are several factors that may play a role in the pathogenesis of Moyamoya disease [3]. Fibroblast growth factor and transforming growth factor ß-1 have been reported to be elevated in individuals with Moyamoya. Prostaglandins have also been investigated. It has been shown that arterial smooth muscle cells can activate the COX-2 enzyme in response to inflammatory mediators and produce excessive amounts of prostaglandin E, which is associated with increased endothelial permeability and vasodilatation. Analysis of cerebrospinal fluid (CSF) in patients with Moyamoya disease has shown high levels of cellular retinol A binding protein, the significance of which remains uncertain.

Pathology

Pathological studies have indicated that all lesions of Moyamoya disease are limited to the proximal parts of the circle of Willis and show stenosis and occlusion. Intimal thickening, luminal stenosis and occlusion are the result of the internal elastic lamina being very tortuous, winding and broken. The intima contains many smooth muscle cells of uncertain origin. The media is attenuated and atrophic with hyperplastic smooth muscle cells protruding inwards through the broken internal elastic lamina [4]. Immunohistochemical staining shows IgG and IgM immunoglobulin on the surface of the arterial wall, suggesting an immune-mediated aetiology. Patients with Moyamoya who present with ischaemic symptoms have less abnormal vessel proliferation and tend to present at a younger age compared to patients who present with haemorrhage. This suggests that the initial changes in Moyamoya are stenosis and occlusion of the main vessels of the circle of Willis. Ischaemia in early Moyamoya therefore results from an inadequate blood supply. This ischaemia induces compensatory vessel proliferation, leading to the formation of a network of thin-walled dilated vessels with the associated risk of intracranial bleeding. Miliary and saccular aneurysms may develop that can rupture and cause haemorrhage and stroke.

Clinical presentation

The highest incidence of Moyamoya disease is during the first decade of life, although it has a bimodal age distribution, with affected individuals in their fourth decade. Children typically present with recurrent episodes of sudden hemiplegia that may change sides as a result of transient ischaemic attacks or strokes. Fine involuntary choreiform movements of the limbs, seizures, headaches, speech disturbances and slowly progressive mental impairment are also features of Moyamoya. Motor symptoms are the most common mode of presentation, affecting 80%, whilst convulsions occur in 9-14%. Symptoms are frequently precipitated by episodes of hyperventilation, a rise in body temperature, crying, coughing or straining. Younger age (<3 years) is associated with a more severe and rapidly progressive Moyamoya. In addition, these children have more cerebral infarctions at presentation, resulting in poor outcomes. Adults more frequently present with symptoms resulting from intracerebral or subarachnoid bleeding from the fragile new vessels in the ventricles (30%), thalamus (15%), basal ganglia (40%) and subcortical regions (5%). Bleeding may occur in children, but more often symptoms are the result of progressive ischaemia. Hypertension and aneurysm formation contribute to the risk of haemorrhage. Blood pressure control may therefore reduce bleeding episodes, although these can occur years after the initial presentation. Females have an increased risk of haemorrhagic complications and there also appears to be racial variation; Korean children have a greater incidence of bleeding than Japanese children. Rebleeding is associated with increased mortality and after each rebleed the prognosis becomes poorer. Hypothalamic-pituitary and hypothyroidism have been associated with Moyamoya disease and children should be monitored for clinical symptoms. Arteriovenous malformations are rarely associated with Moyamoya disease.

Imaging

Angiography

Angiography reveals narrowing and occlusion of the supraclinoid parts of the internal carotid artery, the proximal portions of the anterior and middle cerebral artery, and abnormal collateral vessels (Figure 1) [5]. The ischaemic regions of the brain are supplied via

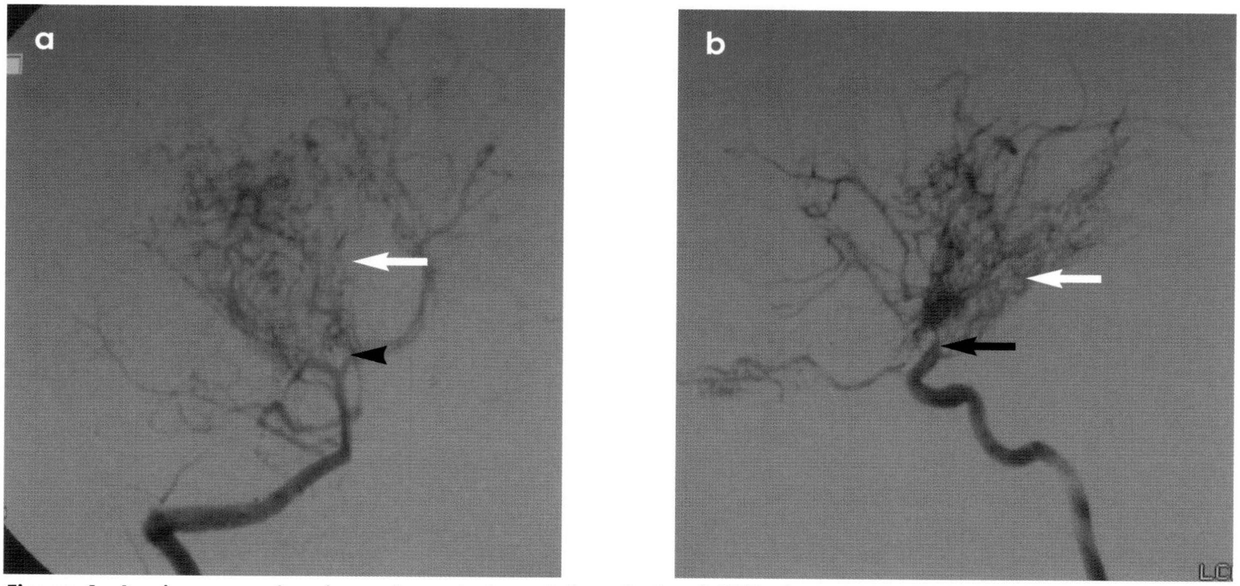

Figure 1. Angiograms showing: a) occlusion of the circle of Willis (arrow head); and b) occlusion of the supraclinoid internal carotid artery (black arrow) with abnormal collateral network (white arrows both images) in patients with Moyamoya disease.

Table 1. Angiographic stages of Moyamoya disease (Suzuki and Takaku [2]).

Stage I	Stenosis occurs bilaterally in the intracranial carotid artery
Stage II	Moyamoya vessels develop at the base of the brain as the carotid is narrowed
Stage III	Moyamoya vessels become prominent as the anterior circulation becomes stenosed and occluded
Stage IV	Moyamoya vessels increase to involve the posterior circulation
Stage V	Moyamoya vessels begin to reduce
Stage VI	Moyamoya vessels disappear and the brain receives blood through abnormal extracranial-intracranial anastomoses

large proliferating collaterals and transdiploic collaterals from the external carotid artery, giving rise to the Moyamoya network of abnormal vessels. These abnormal collaterals can originate from different feeding arteries. Those that form at the frontal base from the ophthalmic artery are termed ethmoidal Moyamoya. Posterior basal Moyamoya originates from perforating branches of the posterior cerebral artery. The development of extra and intracranial transdural leptomeningeal collaterals from pial vessels and branches of the external carotid artery is termed vault Moyamoya [5]. The angiographic appearance of Moyamoya has been classified into six stages according to Suzuki and Takaku (Table 1) [2]. The appearances are almost always bilateral; if found unilaterally, the diagnosis should be questioned. When the vessels of the circle of Willis, including the posterior cerebral arteries have occluded, the

Moyamoya network collaterals at the base of the brain begin to reduce and collaterals develop from the extracranial circulation. The "puff of smoke" appearance is not pathognomonic of Moyamoya disease, but can also be found in atherosclerosis, radiation arteritis, trauma, sickle cell anaemia and tuberculous meningitis.

Magnetic resonance angiography, computed tomography and positron emission tomography

Magnetic resonance angiography (MRA) and CT may reveal multiple dilated abnormal vessels, or narrowing and occlusions of the major arteries of the circle of Willis. Ischaemic infarctions or areas of intracerebral haemorrhage may also be identified (Figure 2). MRA has been used as a screening tool in Japan. In Moyamoya, reduced cerebral blood flow reflects the course of the disease. The limitation of standard MRA and CT techniques is that they are not able to assess cerebral perfusion and thus identify tissue at risk of infarction. Ultrafast Echo Planar MR imaging sequences can evaluate the passage of contrast through the intracranial vasculature. MR perfusion is performed before and after administration of a bolus of contrast such as gadolinium or dysprosium. A signal-intensity curve can then be plotted allowing conversion to cerebral blood volume. Areas of ischaemia show lower magnetic susceptibility-induced signal loss, or a delay in peak signal loss with perfusion imaging compared with normal tissue [6]. Positron emission tomography (PET) scanning with H(2)15O and acetazolamide has also been used to assess cerebral perfusion status. Xenon CT with acetazolamide challenge in children can be used to quantify regional cerebral blood flow and may allow assessment of stroke risk and response to surgical intervention earlier than conventional angiography [7]. Electroencephalographic (EEG) changes reported in Moyamoya disease are posterior slowing and centrotemporal slow activity, with sleep spindle depression. EEG has been used as a screening technique in the past, but has now generally been replaced by MR.

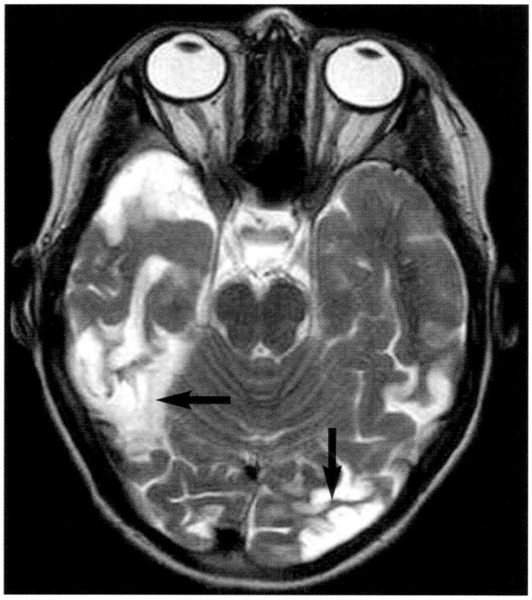

Figure 2. A CT scan of a patient with Moyamoya disease showing bilateral cerebral infarctions (arrows).

Management

Suzuki and Kodoma first described perivascular sympathectomy and superior cervical ganglionectomy to produce intracranial and extracranial vasodilatation in patients with Moyamoya in 1983. Krayenduhl proposed direct revascularisation using a superficial temporal artery to middle cerebral artery (STA-MCA) anastomosis to treat Moyamoya, although it can be difficult to identify suitable calibre vessels for inflow and outflow, especially in children with Moyamoya. Following revascularisation, rebleeding is the worst outcome and is greatest in patients aged 46-55 years. Therefore, patients must be followed-up throughout their lives, even if their neurological status is good. There are several other indirect revascularisation procedures described, the aim being to induce neovascularisation with arterial ingrowth directly into the cerebral surface and thus indirectly improve the blood supply. Encephalomyosynangiosis, described by Karasawa in 1977, involved suturing the temporalis muscle to surgically created dural defects in an attempt to place the muscle in contact with the surface of the brain. In 1981, Matsushima similarly described approximating the superficial temporal artery to the brain surface by suturing it along a longitudinal dural defect with the hope of developing vessel ingrowth [8]. In children, indirect revascularisation is preferred as it is easier and safer to perform than direct revascularisation. The best results are generally obtained in children in whom the main problem is one of ischaemia. In adults it is unlikely that revascularisation will prevent rebleeds as these patients have already formed an abnormal vessel network. Children who suffer frequent pre-operative transient ischaemic attacks are at greater risk of perioperative ischaemic complications, reflecting the instability of cerebral haemodynamics in these children. Goda recently reported a series of indirect revascularisation procedures in six children [9]. At follow-up of between 2 and 7 years, no child had developed further ischaemic complications. In five children the pre-operatively documented disease had advanced bilaterally. Angiography showed that collateral formation through the grafts was well developed. There was, however, no reduction in abnormal collateral formation from the posterior circulation which may indicate that these children are still at risk from haemorrhagic complications. Scott followed 126 patients after indirect revascularisation for 5 years and reported that only five suffered further neurological events. Indirect revascularisation and frequent transient ischaemia, reflecting more severe disease, were reported by Sakamoto to result in an increased incidence of postoperative ischaemic events. Follow-up angiography showed that indirect revascularisation procedures did not reduce collateral formation in the posterior circulation and therefore, the patients remained at risk of haemorrhage. In a further study of 52 patients, indirect surgery led to a poor intellectual outcome compared to combined indirect and direct revascularisation with STA-MCA bypass [10]. Previous stroke was also associated with poor outcome supporting early intervention to preserve intellectual function. Surgery is generally felt to be beneficial in comparison to the natural history of the untreated disease; however, there are no controlled series. Medical treatment with vasodilators, corticosteroids, and antiplatelet agents has been used, but without proven benefit.

Prognosis in Moyamoya disease

The prognosis in Moyamoya disease is different for children and adults. The overall mortality rate was reported in a large study of 518 patients to be 7.5%; 10% in adults and 4.3% in children. Bleeding was the cause of death in 55% of children and 63% of adults. Nishimoto described a good prognosis in 58% of 271 patients, including those who had undergone treatment. Many of the remaining patients were disabled. Patients with a transient ischaemic attack that do not receive surgical intervention suffer gradual deterioration in cognitive function despite resolution of their neurological symptoms. Yoshida reported that five of six patients with haemorrhagic Moyamoya died from rebleeding. The prognosis tends to be improved following surgical intervention, but in none of the studies has this reached statistical significance.

Key points

- Moyamoya disease occurs mainly in children who present with symptoms of cerebral ischaemia.
- Adults are more likely to suffer intracranial haemorrhage.
- MRI is non-invasive and can identify areas at risk of infarction.
- Treatment by both direct and indirect methods is successful in improving symptoms and prognosis.

References

1. Kudo T. Spontaneous occlusion of the circle of Willis: a disease apparently confined to Japanese. *Neurology* 1968; 18: 485-96.
2. Suzuki J, Takaku A. Cerebrovascular "Moyamoya" disease: disease showing abnormal net-like vessels in base of brain. *Arch Neurol* 1969; 20: 288-99.
3. Gosalakkal JA. Moyamoya disease: a review. *Neurology India* 2002; 50: 6-10.
4. Rao M, Zhang H, Liu Q. Clinical and experimental pathology of Moyamoya disease. *Chin Med J* 2003; 116: 1845-9.
5. Houkin K, Yoshimoto T, Kurodo S. Angiographic analysis of Moyamoya disease - how does Moyamoya disease progress? *Neurol Med Chir* 1996; 36: 783-7.
6. Khanna PC, Lath C, Gadewar SB. Role of magnetic resonance perfusion studies in Moyamoya disease. *Neurology India* 2004; 52: 238-40.
7. McAuley DJ, Poskitt K, Steinbok P. Predicting stroke in pediatric Moyamoya disease by xenon-enhanced computed tomography. *Neurosurgery* 2004; 55: 327-32.
8. Ueki K, Meyer FB, Mellinger JF. Moyamoya disease: the disorder and surgical treatment. *Mayo Clin Proc* 1994; 69: 749-57.
9. Goda M, Isono M, Ishii K. Long-term effects of indirect bypass surgery on collateral vessel formation in paediatric Moyamoya disease. *J Neurosurg Spine* 2004; 100: 156-62.
10. Kuroda S, Houkin K, Ishikawa T. Determinants of intellectual outcome after surgical revascularisation in paediatric Moyamoya disease: a multivariate analysis. *Childs Nerv Syst* 2004; 20: 302-8.

Chapter 9

Fibromuscular dysplasia

Louis Fligelstone MD FRCS, Consultant Vascular Surgeon
Morriston Hospital, Swansea NHS Trust, Swansea, UK

Introduction

Fibromuscular dysplasia (FMD) is a disease of unknown aetiology, defined as thickening of the arterial media by fibrosis and muscular hyperplasia, causing multifocal arterial stenosis. It was first described in 1938 by Leadbetter and Burkland [1]. Their initial description was of renal artery FMD associated with renovascular hypertension. The renal artery is most commonly affected, accounting for up to 80% of all cases. The internal carotid artery is the next most frequently affected artery, first described by Connett and Lansche in 1965 [2]. FMD is found in up to 1% of all carotid angiograms. Women are more commonly affected in a ratio of 3:1. The disease involves medium and small arteries; however, it has been described in almost every vessel. The renal and carotid arteries are both affected in up to 30% of patients; the vertebral arteries are affected in up to 10% of patients with carotid FMD. Fibromuscular dysplasia usually presents in the third to sixth decades.

The clinical presentation varies according to the vessel affected, but is similar to atherosclerotic disease: stenoses cause acute or chronic ischaemia, or distal embolisation.

Radiological findings

Fibromuscular dysplasia is often bilateral. In contrast to atherosclerosis, it is usually non-ostial and does not affect bifurcations. The classical angiographic finding is a string of beads; however, it is now accepted that there are three radiological types:

- Type I (80%) - series of stenoses alternating with areas of dilatation. On histology this is usually due to medial fibroplasia.
- Type II (15%) - unifocal or multifocal tubular stenosis. This is usually caused by intimal fibroplasia. It is more likely to result in dissection or vessel occlusion.
- Type III (5%) - one wall of the artery is affected with thinning that can result in true saccular aneurysm formation [3]. This is usually due to atypical fibromuscular dysplasia.

Pattern of disease

Ninety percent of FMD occurs in women. It usually involves the distal third of the renal artery extending into the segmental branches. Renal FMD causes hypertension due to the stenoses reducing renal perfusion. The kidney produces elevated levels of

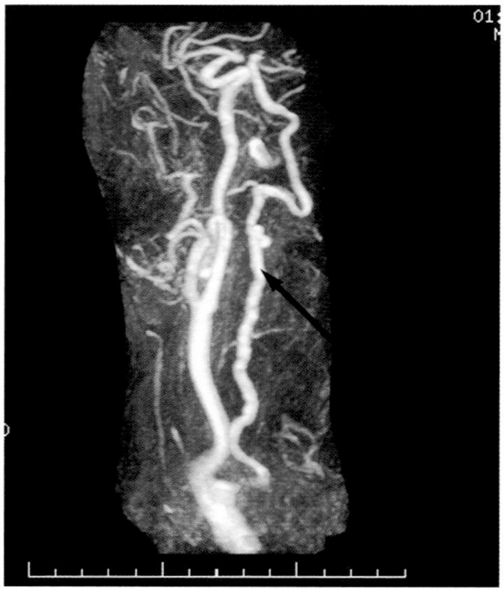

Figure 1. Magnetic resonance angiography showing normal carotid arteries, but typical beaded appearance of FMD in the vertebral artery with a series of mild stenoses and dilatation (arrow). The patient presented with vague symptoms of dizziness and headache. It was decided to treat the patient conservatively with antiplatelet therapy combined with warfarin; this controlled the symptoms.

renin and angiotensin, resulting in a raised systemic blood pressure and normalisation of renal perfusion. The patient is at risk of the side effects of uncontrolled hypertension, such as heart attack and stroke.

In the internal carotid artery, FMD is most often sited 3-4cm from the carotid bifurcation, though the disease usually ends outside the skull. Extracranial FMD can be asymptomatic, but can result in distal embolisation causing transient ischaemic attack or stroke. It may also be associated with a host of non-specific symptoms such as dizziness, headache, tinnitus, vertigo, visual disturbance or balance disorders (Figure 1). In contrast to renal FMD it can be associated with dissection of the internal carotid artery. Up to 50% of patients with extracranial FMD have associated intracranial aneurysm [4] and in up to two thirds these intracranial aneurysms are multiple. Likewise, patients with an intracranial aneurysm should be assessed for carotid and renal FMD.

Iliac artery FMD can cause intermittent claudication. A high index of suspicion is necessary when assessing young patients under 50 years of age, especially women with lower limb claudication. The differential diagnosis of FMD must be considered along with other rare causes of claudication, such as cystic adventitial disease, popliteal artery entrapment and vessel occlusion secondary to hypercoagulable states. Distal embolisation is unusual in FMD and is usually minor, causing patchy skin infarcts. It rarely causes acute leg ischaemia. Aneurysmal dilatation can occur, as can smooth focal stenoses; the latter can result in vessel occlusion.

Visceral artery FMD can cause both acute and chronic mesenteric ischaemia and can present with mesenteric angina, or segmental gut infarction.

Imaging

Duplex ultrasound imaging is useful in the carotid circulation and can identify beading distal to the carotid bifurcation due to stenoses and areas of dilatation. The distal internal carotid artery is most commonly affected and difficulty may be encountered with imaging the disease just below the skull base, resulting in a false negative report. In the presence of a good clinical history, CT or magnetic resonance angiography (MRA) may be useful to delineate the disease and confirm the diagnosis. Duplex imaging is also useful in the renal circulation, where renal resistive index can be calculated. This requires a transabdominal and lumbar approach to assess the renal vasculature. It has been shown to be valuable to monitor the outcome of percutaneous angioplasty for atherosclerotic renal artery stenosis, but to date, there are no studies in patients with FMD [5].

CT may be useful to diagnose intracranial aneurysms associated with carotid FMD. CT angiography may also pick up lesions suggestive of FMD. Nevertheless, resolution is limited and definitive diagnosis with formal digital subtraction angiography is recommended, and is carried out if any percutaneous intervention is planned.

MRI may also be used to diagnose intracranial aneurysms. MR angiography can identify lesions suggestive of FMD; resolution may be improved with gadolinium contrast. Movement artefact degrades the image and the motion of swallowing may create a string of beads appearance on reformatting. To avoid misdiagnosis, cross-sectional images should always be reviewed on the workstation.

Pathological classification

Histological classification of FMD is based on the layer of the arterial wall most affected. Originally classified as medial, intimal, peri-adventitial or peri-arterial, more recently, further subclassification includes medial fibroplasia, perimedial fibroplasia and medial hyperplasia.

The differential diagnosis of FMD includes, atherosclerotic disease, inflammatory arterial disease (e.g. Takayasu's disease), Mainis fibromuscular dysplasia, or vascular lesions of neurofibromatosis. Fibromuscular dysplasia is associated with other diseases including Ehlers-Danlos Type IV and alpha 1 antitrypsin deficiency.

Treatment

The earliest treatment of FMD was surgical. At open surgery, an arteriotomy was made and the stenoses dilated by the passage of graded dilators [6]. Renovascular hypertension associated with renal artery FMD was treated successfully by this method. Surgery, however, has a high risk of complications and is now reserved for failed angioplasty or when the disease extends into the hilar branches. Surgery remains the treatment of choice for associated aneurysmal dilatation. Contemporary surgical results are more than acceptable with success rates of up to 97%, and 77% improvement or cure of hypertension, but with a mortality rate of 0.5% at 6 months.

Renal fibromuscular dysplasia

Medical treatment is the first-line therapy for renal artery FMD causing hypertension. Treatment of hypertension should follow standard recommendations.

Indications for revascularisation include:

- failure to control blood pressure despite polypharmacy;
- recent onset of hypertension, where cure is likely;
- intolerance of antihypertensive drugs;
- falling renal size/volume despite treatment;
- non-compliant patients.

Most published data concern the outcome of interventional treatment for renal artery FMD. The best long-term outcomes are for endovascular treatment of FMD caused by medial fibroplasias, which is as effective as open surgery, but with lower morbidity. Percutaneous angioplasty is now the first-line treatment for renovascular hypertension due to fibromuscular dysplasia (Figure 2).

Immediate radiological success rates have been reported in 83-100% of patients [7-9]. Long-term patencies of 89% at 5 years, and 87% at 10 years have also been reported. Follow-up data are difficult to interpret due to differences in reporting. The most important clinical endpoint is effective reduction in systolic and diastolic blood pressure. Cure (restoration of normotension without need for antihypertensive medication) is achieved in between 14-59% of patients [10]. Percutaneous angioplasty is not without risk and reported complication rates vary from 0-28.5% [11], with an average complication rate of 11%, and mortality of 0.5%. The majority of the complications are minor, associated with puncture sites or segmental renal infarction. Arterial perforation, due to guidewire damage may occur, but complete vessel rupture is uncommon.

It can be technically challenging to quantify the result of angioplasty for renal artery stenosis with duplex imaging, but follow-up has suggested a recurrent stenosis rate of between 10-25%. Redo angioplasty is technically easier in FMD than primary angioplasty and is associated with a lower risk of vessel perforation or rupture. Stent placement in the renal artery is rarely required even for redo angioplasty, and currently, there is no place for primary stenting in renal FMD.

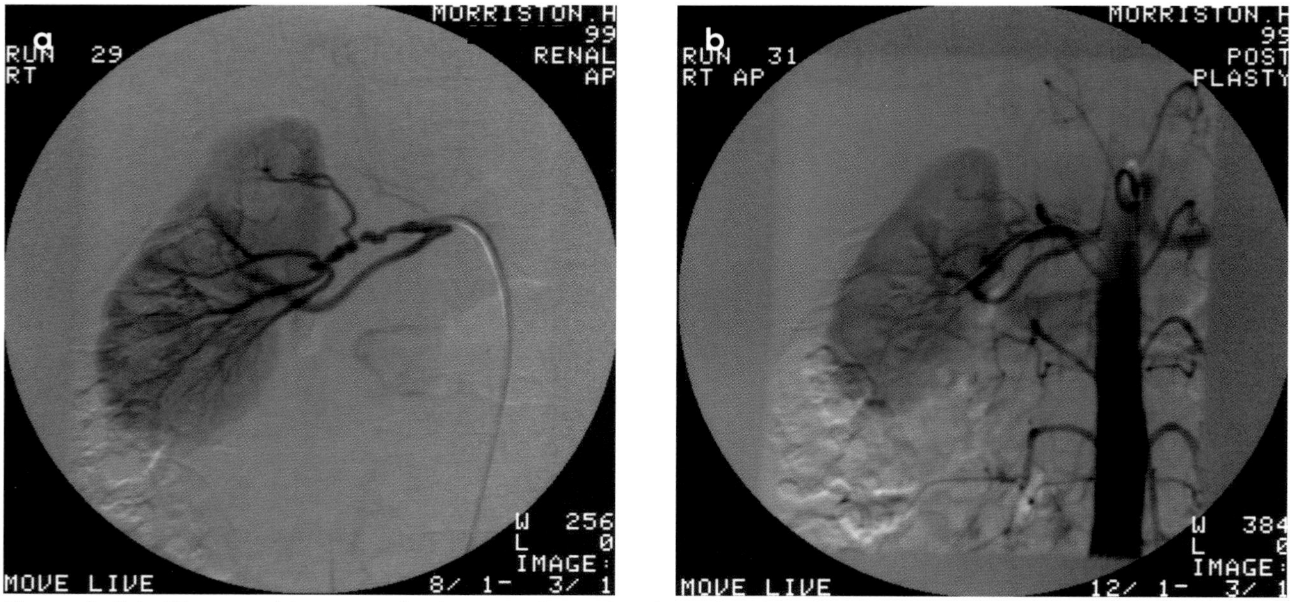

Figure 2. This 45-year-old woman had severe hypertension with deteriorating renal function. Renal ultrasound had shown a normal size kidney, but duplex imaging demonstrated an 80% non-ostial renal artery stenosis. a) Renal angiography confirmed renal artery stenosis, due to FMD, with a classical string of beads appearance. b) The patient underwent successful balloon angioplasty with good angiographic result. The patient became normotensive, without need for medication. Follow-up duplex imaging confirmed no recurrent stenosis.

FMD can cause hypertension in childhood. Treatment follows the same path as for adults, but the outcome of percutaneous transluminal angioplasty seems more favourable than other causes of renal artery stenosis, such as arteritis. The initial results depend on similar factors such as the length and complexity of the lesion. Restenosis occurs in up to 28.5%, a higher rate than in adults with renovascular FMD [12].

Carotid artery fibromuscular dysplasia

Carotid FMD was also previously treated by open carotid surgery, including patch angioplasty or autologous vein bypass. The lesions are usually 3-4cm from the carotid bifurcation and surgical access can be challenging. Due to these challenges, there is a clear attraction for percutaneous intervention which has also become the treatment of choice for symptomatic FMD of the internal carotid artery. Carotid lesions are at greater risk of dissection and therefore, it is more likely that a stent will be needed. The use of cerebral protection devices is a current focus of interest to reduce the small risk of stroke associated with this procedure.

Other areas affected

FMD can affect other sites in the arterial circulation and presents with the typical symptoms produced by atherosclerotic lesions. The age of presentation and the lack of the usual risk factors for atherosclerosis should increase the index of suspicion. Angiography provides definitive diagnosis and percutaneous angioplasty is usually the treatment of choice.

Acknowledgement

I would like to thank my radiological colleagues Dr. David Roberts and Dr. Sharon Evans for the images used in this chapter.

Key points

- Fibromuscular dysplasia most commonly affects the renal arteries where it may cause severe renovascular hypertension.
- In other arteries, fibromuscular dysplasia causes arterial stenoses (and occasionally aneurysms) that give rise to similar symptoms to peripheral vascular disease.
- In most areas the best treatment is balloon angioplasty for symptomatic lesions.
- The results of angioplasty for renovascular hypertension are particularly gratifying.

References

1. Leadbetter WF, Burkland CE. Hypertension in unilateral renal disease. *J Urol* 1938; 39: 611-26.
2. Connett MC, Lansche JM. Fibromuscular dysplasia of the internal carotid artery: report of a case. *Ann Surg* 1965; 162: 59-62.
3. Corrin LS, Sandok BA, Houser OW. Cerebral ischemic events in patients with carotid artery fibromuscular dysplasia. *Arch Neurol* 1981; 38: 616-8.
4. Luscher TF, Lie JT, Stanson AW, *et al.* Arterial fibromuscular dysplasia. *Mayo Clin Proc* 1987: 62: 931-52.
5. Radermacher J, Chavan A, Bleck J, *et al.* Use of Doppler ultrasonography to predict the outcome of therapy for renal artery stenosis. *N Engl J Med* 2001; 344: 410-17.
6. Starr DS, Lawrie GM, Morris GC Jr. Fibromuscular disease of the carotid arteries: long-term results of graduated internal dilatation. *Stroke* 1981; 12: 196-9.
7. Surowiec SM, Sivamurthy N, Rhodes JM, *et al.* Percutaneous therapy for renal artery fibromuscular dysplasia. *Ann Vasc Surg* 2003; 17: 650-5.
8. Tegtmeyer CJ, Selby JB, Harwell GD, Ayers C, Tegtmeyer V. Results and complications of angioplasty in fibromuscular disease. *Circulation* 1991; 83: Suppl I: I-155- I: I-161.
9. Davidson RA, Barri Y, Wilcox CS. Predictors of cure of hypertension in fibromuscular renal vascular disease. *Am J Kidney Dis* 1996; 28: 334-8.
10. de Fraissinette B, Garcier JM, Dieu V, *et al.* Percutaneous transluminal angioplasty of dysplastic stenoses of the renal artery: results on 70 adults. *Cardiovasc Intervent Radiol* 2003; 26: 46-51.
11. Birrer M, Do DD, Mahler F, Triller J, Baumgartner I. Treatment of renal artery fibromuscular dysplasia with balloon angioplasty: a prospective follow-up study. *Eur J Vasc Endovasc Surg* 2002; 23: 146-52.
12. Tyagi S, Kaul UA, Satsangi DK, Arora R. Percutaneous transluminal angioplasty for renovascular hypertension in children: initial and long-term results. *Pediatrics* 1997; 99: 44-9.

Chapter 10

Radiation-induced arterial disease

Peter R Taylor MA MChir FRCS, Consultant Vascular Surgeon
Guy's & St. Thomas' NHS Foundation Trust, London, UK

Introduction

Radiotherapy is a recognised and well accepted treatment for certain common and uncommon malignancies. Unfortunately, some incidental collateral damage to surrounding normal structures is inevitable. This chapter describes the effects of radiation on the arteries, a condition known as radiation arteritis.

Incidence

Radiation arteritis can affect any of the blood vessels adjacent to the common sites of malignancies sensitive to radiotherapy. The arteries commonly affected include the carotid arteries from radiotherapy for head and neck cancers, the subclavian and axillary arteries from treatment for breast cancer and lymphoma, the aorta and iliac arteries from treatment for lymphoma, and malignancies related to the gastro-intestinal tract, the urinary tract and the male and female genital tract. The effects of damage to the blood vessels can take many years to become apparent and they usually lead to ischaemia of the distal vascular territory.

Historical perspective

The effects of ionising radiation have been known for a long time. In 1899, Gassman described the effects of radiation on small vessels with swelling and proliferation of the endothelium of capillaries, venules and arterioles [1]. Windholz in 1937, also described endothelial cell proliferation, but noticed endothelial cell necrosis [2].

Pathophysiology

The acute effects of radiation on small vessels lead to cell death, luminal stenosis and ultimately, thrombosis. The endothelial cell seems to be very susceptible to the effects of radiation. The effect of radiation on the surrounding tissues limits the formation of collateral vessels; these are relatively rare compared with other causes of vessel occlusion such as atherosclerosis. Medium and large-sized arteries are also affected with endothelial cell damage associated with intimal fibrin deposition. After subsequent healing, the normal single layer of endothelial cells is replaced by conglomerations of irregular spindle-shaped cells. The acute injury seems to spare the media and adventitia. However, over the course of a few weeks, the media gradually increases in cellularity and starts to fibrose, which is attributed to damage to the vasa vasorum. This eventually leads to a stenosis of the arterial lumen, with subsequent thrombosis, occlusion or distal embolisation [3]. In the presence of other risk factors such as raised cholesterol, diabetes and hypertension, the irradiated artery may present after several years with the effects of premature atherosclerosis.

Clinical presentation

The clinical presentation is usually dependent upon the time interval following radiation [3]. Early lesions present within 5 years and are due to mural thrombus. Intermediate lesions occur within 10 years and relate to occlusion with poor collateral vessel formation. Late lesions take up to 25 years to develop and present as a peri-arterial fibrosis with accelerated atherosclerosis. There is always a history of radiotherapy to the affected vascular bed, and arteries are affected that are normally spared from atherosclerosis. Many patients have risk factors for atherosclerosis that can exacerbate the damaging effects of radiation. The most common vessels to be affected are the carotid, the subclavian/axillary and the aorto-iliac arteries.

Carotid

The carotid arteries are frequently irradiated during the treatment of common head and neck cancers. This usually affects the common carotid artery in the lower third of the neck, and more rarely the internal carotid artery (Figure 1). Patients are five times more likely to have duplex-detected haemodynamic stenoses following cervical irradiation than an age and risk factor-matched population. They are also 2-4 times more likely to have an audible carotid bruit, and to have double the incidence of neurological symptoms [4,5]. These usually occur 5-10 years after radiotherapy, but the range is from 2-17 years [5].

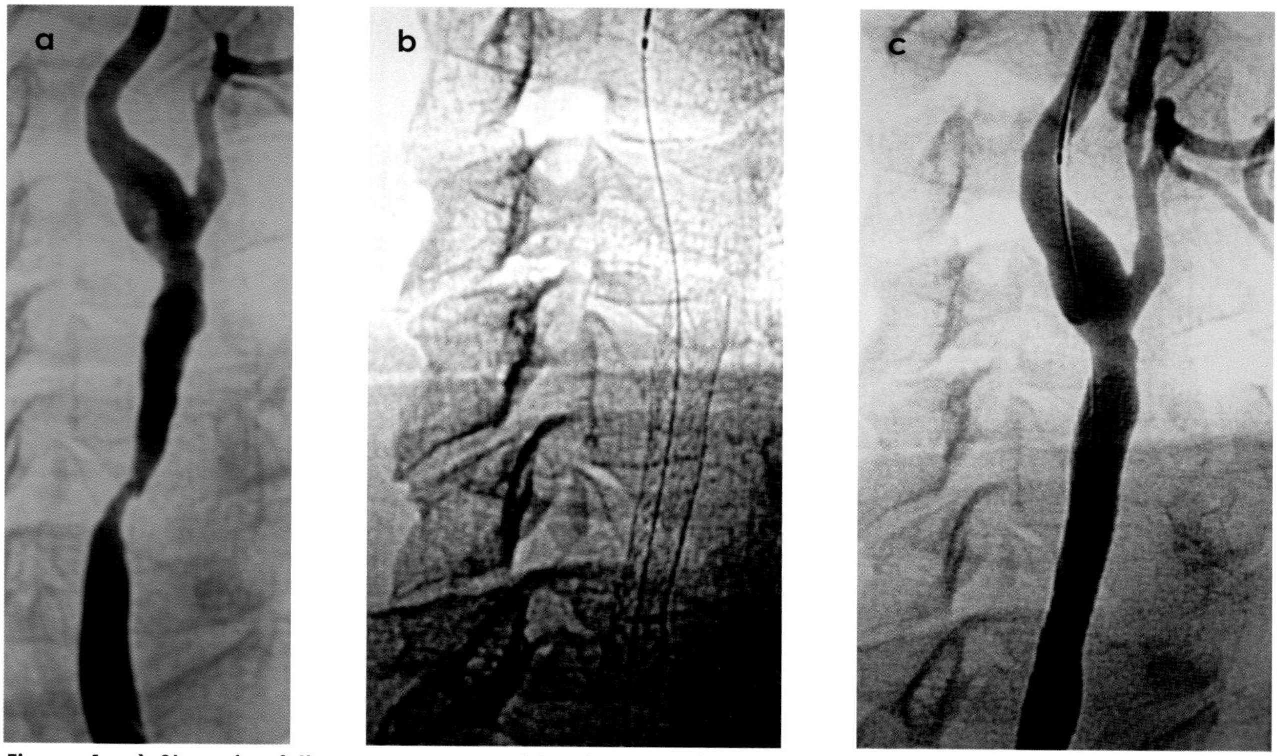

Figure 1. a) Stenosis of the common carotid artery causing transient ischaemic attacks of the ipsilateral hemisphere 15 years after radiotherapy for carcinoma of the larynx. b) A carotid stent used to treat the stenosis. c) Completion angiogram showing an excellent result.

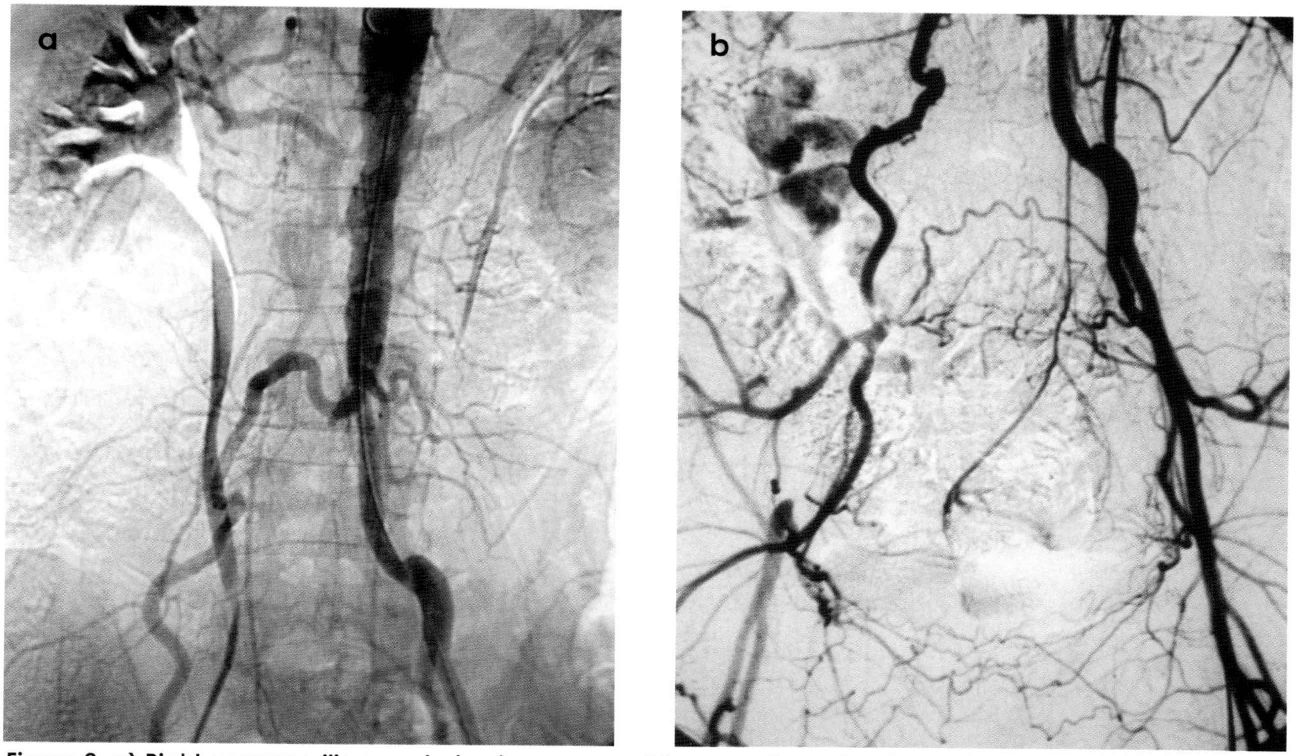

Figure 2. a) Right common iliac occlusion in a woman 12 years after extensive radiotherapy for carcinoma of the cervix. b) Reconstitution of the right common femoral artery via collaterals. This patient had a successful aortofemoral graft.

Investigation is primarily by duplex imaging, which shows a stenosis confined to the field of radiation. This is frequently the common carotid artery in the lower third of the neck, with relative sparing of the carotid bifurcation. Occasionally, there may be stenoses of the internal carotid artery with sparing of the other vessels. Rarely, this affects the whole of the extracranial internal carotid artery up to the base of the skull.

Subclavian/axillary

This may follow radiation for both breast cancer and lymphoma. Subclavian artery occlusion may follow 14-26 years after treatment and presents with ischaemia of the upper limb [6]. There may be exercise-induced muscle pain, but the ischaemia can be more severe with rest pain and tissue loss. Duplex imaging confirms long segment occlusion of the subclavian and axillary arteries and angiography may display a lack of collateral vessels [7].

Aorta/iliac

Stenosis and occlusion of these arteries usually follows at least 10 years after the radiotherapy for rectal, urological or genital tract malignancies. Patients usually present with lower limb ischaemia in the form of claudication, rest pain or tissue loss. Typically, the affected artery is in the radiation field and the arteries proximally and distally are spared in younger patients. In older patients the lesions cannot be distinguished from atherosclerosis (Figure 2). In this area, aneurysm formation caused by arterial disruption from the radiation has been reported. These are usually false or mycotic (infective) aneurysms.

Clinical management

Three factors impact on the treatment of radiation arteritis. The first is the patient's life expectancy. The treatment should not differ from that of patients presenting with atherosclerotic occlusive disease unless the prognosis from the underlying malignancy is very poor. Even then the quality of remaining life may be significantly improved by arterial reconstruction. The second consideration should be the patient's symptoms. Arterial reconstruction is mandatory in the presence of critical limb ischaemia. Exercise-induced pain may be treated conservatively, but unlike atherosclerosis, it is unlikely to improve with time, as the development of collaterals in the irradiated field is sparse. Usually, if a patient is concerned enough to present for an opinion, then they frequently request revascularisation. One advantage is that the vessels above and below the radiation field are likely to be normal, and therefore, the results of any interventions are relatively good. The third consideration is the patient's anatomy. Endovascular options may provide excellent results for short lesions. Bypass procedures may need to follow an extra-anatomical route to avoid the radiation field, and most authors recommend using an autologous conduit to avoid late graft infection which has been reported in irradiated fields [8].

Carotid

The stenoses caused by irradiation tend to cause neurological symptoms more often than atherosclerotic lesions. In addition, they are progressive and therefore warrant intervention. Sometimes the affected artery may be outside the normal field imaged by duplex, and therefore consideration should be given to other investigations such as angiography or magnetic resonance angiography to localise the full extent of the radiation-affected artery accurately. There may be additional lesions in the proximal common carotid arteries and distal internal carotid arteries that are outside the range of a routine duplex scan. Surgical endarterectomy is possible for lesions at the carotid bifurcation and in the distal common carotid artery, but the tissue planes are usually compromised and there is an increased incidence of cranial nerve damage. Patch angioplasty is usually performed to prevent restenosis. Occasionally, endarterectomy is impossible and the artery requires replacement with

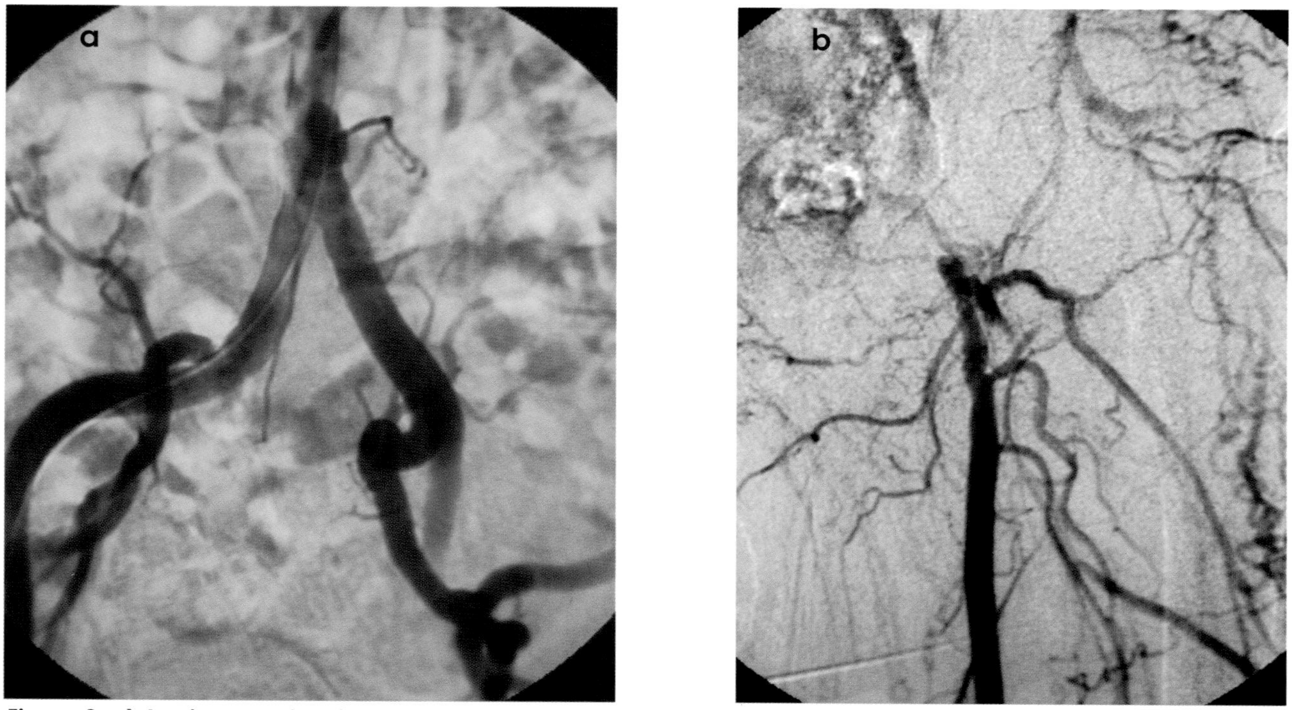

Figure 3. a) Angiogram showing occlusion of the proximal external iliac artery following radiotherapy of the left groin for metastatic carcinoma of the prostate 10 years previously. b) Reconstitution of the left common femoral artery via collaterals. The patient had a successful iliofemoral bypass.

an interposition graft. Autologous vein is preferred to prosthetic material in order to reduce the risk of late infection. Excellent results have been reported following surgery with regards to neurological outcome, but cranial nerve palsies have been reported after 23-28% of procedures [9]. The restenosis rate is not inconsiderable and is probably related to ongoing radiation damage to the arterial wall.

Carotid artery stenting has been used successfully in the treatment of radiation arteritis of the carotid arteries, particularly where it affects the proximal common carotid and distal internal carotid arteries [10]. The long-term outcome of carotid stenting for radiation-induced lesions has yet to be reported in adequate numbers.

Subclavian/axillary

Long segment occlusion of the arteries to the arm requires arterial bypass procedures using autologous vein. This is often placed in an extra-anatomical position to avoid radiation-damaged tissue. The danger is that the tissue may break down with the trauma of blunt dissection used to tunnel a graft into position. Sometimes the ipsilateral common carotid artery has to be used as the proximal inflow site if occlusion involves the proximal subclavian artery. Usually, the brachial artery and its run-off vessels are unaffected, and the outcome is excellent. Short lesions may be suitable for endovascular treatment and angioplasty with stenting has been reported with favourable outcomes in small series.

Aorta/iliac

Short lesions can be treated with angioplasty and stenting. The advantage is the avoidance of extensive dissection in the radiation field. Stent grafts or covered stents have been used to treat both occlusive lesions and false aneurysms. More extensive lesions are best treated by surgical bypass to and from arteries outside the radiation field (Figure 3). Extra-anatomic bypass (axillobifemoral graft) can be employed to stay outside the pelvis, thereby reducing the chances of infection, and the risk of damage to adjacent structures when tunnelling a graft.

Follow-up

Data are only available for the carotid artery, where an annual duplex scan is recommended to detect recurrent stenosis. Otherwise, routine scanning is probably not justified, unless the patient develops symptoms.

Key points

- Radiotherapy damage to the affected artery may present 10-20 years later.
- Duplex assessment may be inadequate and should be supplemented by angiography or magnetic resonance angiography, particularly in the carotid arteries.
- Bypass grafts should be performed using normal unaffected arteries proximal and distal to the radiation field.
- Prosthetic material should be avoided due to the risk of infection; autologous vein should be used, where possible.

References

1. Gassman A. Zur histology der roentgenulcere. *Fortschr Geb Rontgenstrahlen* 1899; 2: 199.
2. Windholz F. Zur kenntnis der Blutegefaessveraenderungen in rontgenbestrahlten Gebwe. *Strahlentherapic* 1937; 59: 662
3. Butler MJ, Lane RHS, Webster JHH. Irradiation injury to large arteries. *Br J Surg* 1980; 67: 341-3.
4. Moritz MW, Higgins RF, Jacobs JR. Duplex imaging and incidence of carotid radiation injury after high-dose radiotherapy for tumors of the head and neck. *Arch Surg* 1990; 125: 1181-3.
5. Carmody BJ, Arora S, Avena R, *et al.* Accelerated carotid artery disease after high-dose head and neck radiotherapy: is there a role for routine carotid duplex surveillance? *J Vasc Surg* 1999; 30: 1045-51.
6. Kretschmer G, Niederle B, Polterauer P, *et al.* Irradiation-induced changes in the subclavian and axillary arteries after radiotherapy for carcinoma of the breast. *Surgery* 1986; 99: 568-663.
7. Hashmonai M, Elami A, Kuten A, *et al.* Subclavian artery occlusion after radiotherapy for carcinoma of the breast. *Cancer* 1988; 61: 2115-8.
8. Phillips GR, Peer RM, Upson JF, *et al.* Late complications of revascularization for radiation-induced arterial disease. *J Vasc Surg* 1992; 16: 921-5.
9. Kashyap VS, Moore WS, Quinones-Baldrich WJ, *et al.* Carotid artery repair for radiation-associated atherosclerosis is a safe and durable procedure. *J Vasc Surg* 1999; 29: 90-9.
10. Branchereau AP, Berthet JP, Marty-Ane MH. Carotid artery stenting for stenosis following revascularisation for cervical irradiation. *J Endovasc Ther* 2002; 9: 14-9.

Chapter 11

Peripheral vascular anomalies

Peter A Gaines FRCP FRCR, Consultant Vascular Radiologist
Sheffield Vascular Institute, Northern General Hospital, Sheffield, UK

Introduction

Vascular anomalies are not uncommon and their management remains challenging. This review will focus on vascular anomalies affecting the peripheries, specifically excluding those affecting the lungs and central nervous system.

A basic understanding of the classification of vascular anomalies is required for the application of appropriate management. On the basis of clinical features, biological behaviour, and haemodynamics characteristics, Mulliken and colleagues classified vascular anomalies into haemangiomas and vascular malformations [1].

Haemangiomas, often referred to as a strawberry naevus, are characterised by endothelial hyperplasia, increased mast cell count and a multilaminated basement membrane. Characteristically, they are not present at birth, arise within the first 8 weeks and have a proliferative phase over the subsequent 3-9 months. They then regress at a rate of about 10% per annum. As a paediatric phenomenon, their diagnosis and treatment will not be considered further in this chapter.

Vascular malformations histologically do not show hyperplasia and have normal mast cells and basement membranes. They are an abnormality in development of one of the vascular components that is present at birth and persist throughout life. They are classified as either:

- high flow when they exhibit arteriovenous shunting; or
- low-flow vascular malformations which are sub-categorised according to their dominant vascular malformation (capillary, venous, lymphatic or mixed).

Although there have been advances in the field of vascular biology that provide some insight into the molecular basis of vascular malformations [2], to date this knowledge has had very little impact on the management of the condition.

Clinical presentation

When a vascular malformation has a cutaneous component, or is visible beneath the skin, then typically it is present at birth. The lesion grows proportionate to the overall growth of the child with occasional increase in size determined by hormonal factors (e.g. puberty or pregnancy), direct trauma (including medical intervention) or infection.

Often the initial presentation, particularly of low-flow lesions, is cosmetic. The impact on quality of life has had little attention in literature, but should not be underestimated. Occasionally the patients complain of pain. This is particularly true of venous malformations when they affect the muscles. More unusual presentations include mass effect, ulceration, bleeding, hyperhydrosis, pruritis, tissue overgrowth, high output cardiac failure or consumptive coagulopathy.

The basis of diagnosis is a good history and clinical examination. Clinical examination should be complemented by use of a hand-held Doppler, which is extremely valuable in confirming the clinical suspicion of a vascular malformation into low- and high-flow lesions. More extensive mapping by colour-flow Doppler is less helpful. The majority of lesions can be diagnosed successfully on the history and clinical examination without further investigation. Occasionally a mass lesion will defy clinical categorisation and biopsy is required. For patients who require active intervention, MRI examination is mandatory to determine the exact extent of the lesion and to help categorise lesions into low and high-flow malformations, to complement the hand-held Doppler examination. Only if Doppler examination and MRI indicate that a lesion is high flow will an arteriogram be required prior to intervention.

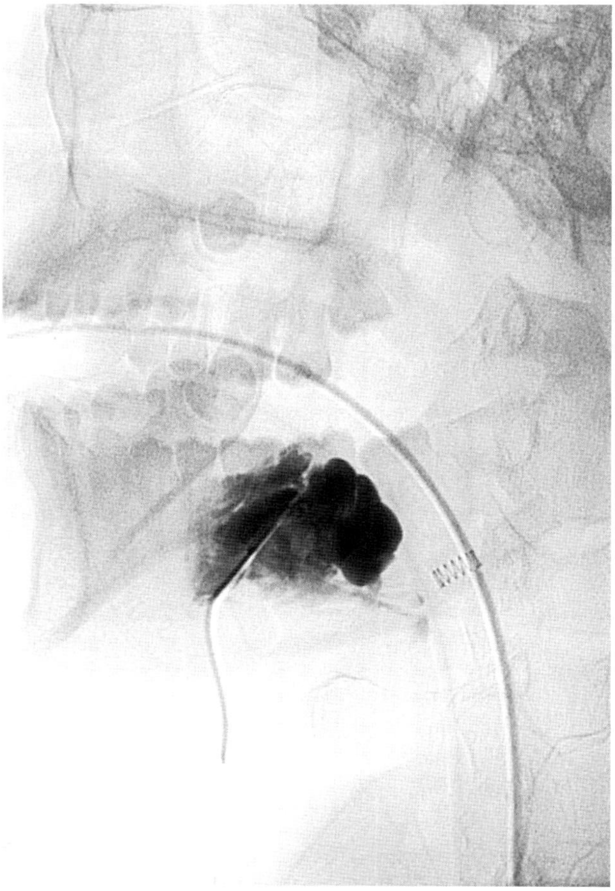

Figure 1. Direct puncture venogram of a low-flow venous malformation of the chin immediately before liquid embolisation. The venogram provides information on the volume of scerosant required and the anatomy of draining veins.

Treatment

A multidisciplinary approach is required for the management of vascular anomalies [3]. In Sheffield there is a team that includes plastic surgeons, vascular surgeons, interventional radiologists, a cosmetician and psychologist. It is important to recognise that current therapy largely offers palliation rather than cure, and that invasive therapy may require numerous attendances. In the majority, an explanation that this is a sporadic lesion without genetic transfer, is non-malignant and is never likely to be symptomatic, is all that is required to allay a patient's fears. If active treatment is required then, because of the high recurrence rate following surgery, embolisation is the therapy of choice. Surgery may be a first-line treatment where the malformation is focal and contains extensive stroma such that embolisation is unlikely to reduce its size, or as an adjunct to embolisation to debulk the lesion, provide a skin graft or to amputate an untreatable limb.

Low-flow capillary malformation

Although often occurring in isolation these are typically recognised as being part of the Sturge-Weber syndrome. In this condition the capillary malformation (port wine stain) involves the area of the first branch of the trigeminal nerve and includes ipsilateral vascular malformation of the leptomeninges and eye (coroidal angioma and glaucoma).

Cosmetic (camouflage) treatment is often successful at managing the capillary malformation. Laser therapy can be used when cosmetics have been unsuccessful.

Low-flow venous malformations

These lesions are often diagnosed as a cosmetic intrusion without major symptomatology and are then best managed by camouflage cosmetics.

If a lesion in the limb is painful, support hosiery may occasionally be of benefit. In lesions with significant symptomatology then the first-line treatment would be radiologically-guided percutaneous embolisation using a liquid sclerosant (Figure 1). Techniques to limit egress of the liquid are then required. Currently, for low-flow venous lesions, alcohol or sodium tetradecyl sulphate (STD) foam are favoured. Alcohol is highly effective but difficult to use because of potential damage to adjacent structures (nerves and skin) and the risk of circulatory collapse. Foam sclerotherapy has been popular in Europe, but is only now being used by vascular specialists in the UK. It is likely that expertise with foam will increase as it is used to treat patients with varicose veins.

Low-flow lymphatic malformations

These often cause a significant cosmetic problem with cutaneous vesicles. There is little experience with percutaneous embolisation and, where necessary, surgery is preferred.

High-flow malformations

Although the natural history of these vascular lesions is not well documented, the majority get treated because of the fear that they may eventually become symptomatic and the risk of high output cardiac failure in the long term.

It is important that treatment is directed to the nidus of the lesion. Particles (e.g. polyvinyl alcohol [PVA]) are difficult to use and not ideal because of the difficulty in choosing the correct size, the risk of paradoxical embolisation and the temporary nature of the occlusion. Similarly, in the majority of lesions, coils are not ideal because they only provide proximal embolisation and the subsequent ischaemia stimulates recruitment of new vessels to the nidus. To access and treat the nidus often requires microcatheters and a liquid embolisation agent (Figure 2). Again alcohol or cyanoacrylates are the agents of choice. When the malformation is complex, or has an extensive venous component, then embolisation of both the arterial and venous sides is often undertaken (Figure 3).

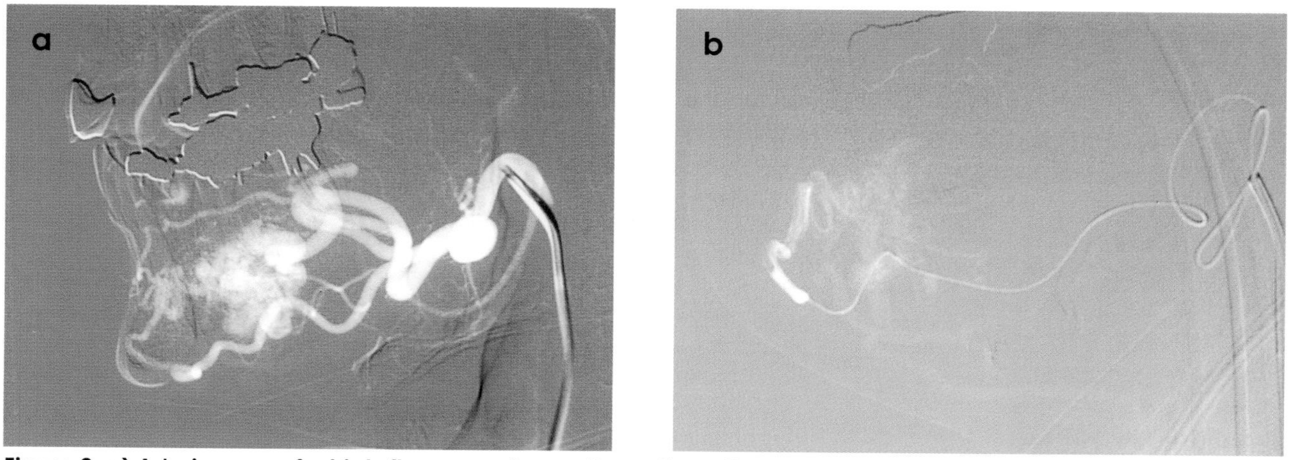

Figure 2. a) Arteriogram of a high-flow vascular malformation affecting the chin. b) A microcatheter is extended to the nidus in order to deliver cyanoacrylate.

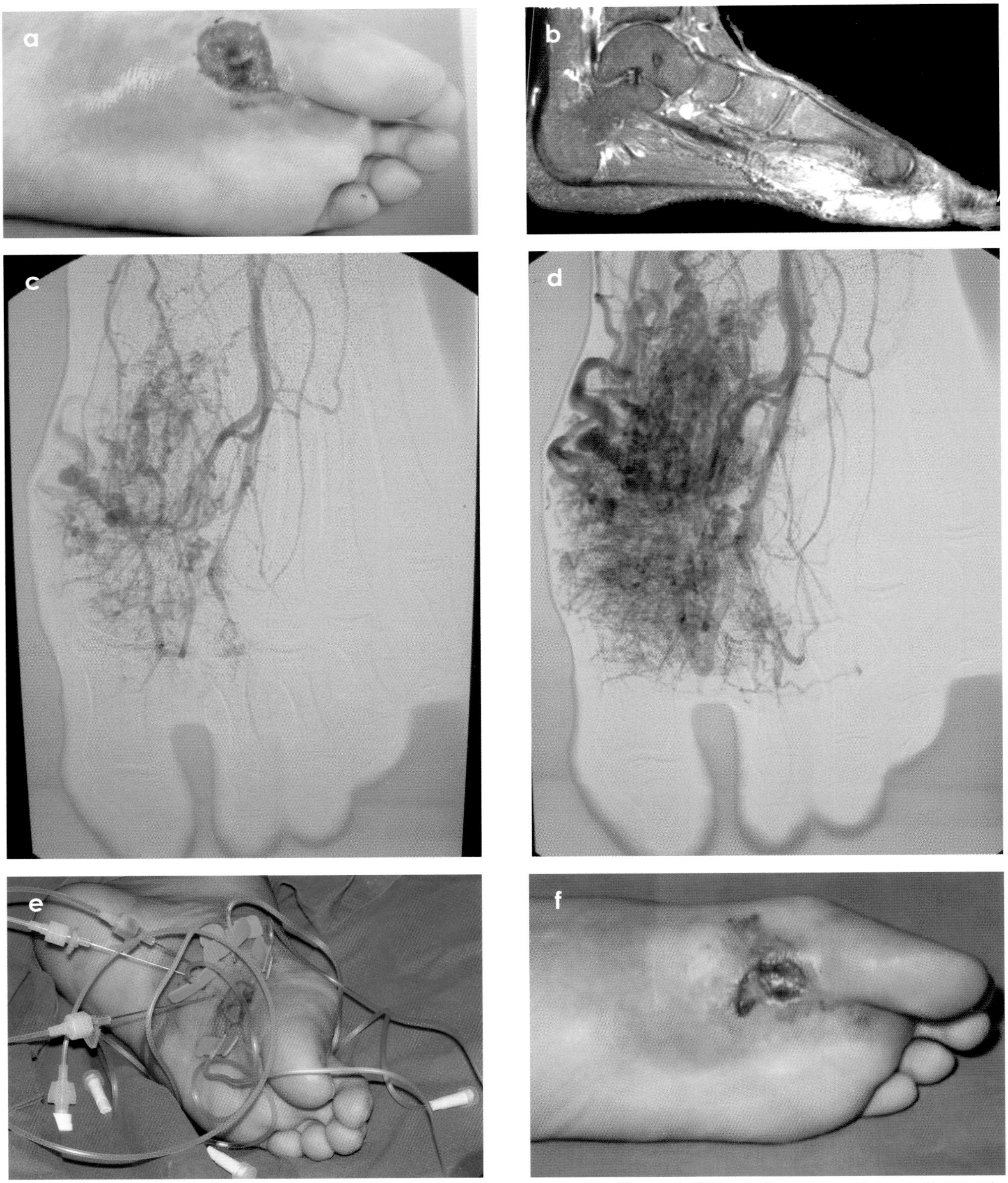

Figure 3. a) Ulcer of the foot due to a high-flow vascular malformation. b) MRI confirms the clinical diagnosis and delineates the extent of the lesion before treatment. c) Early phase angiogram demonstrates the arterial component of the lesion and shunting away from the toes. d) Late phase angiogram demonstrates the venous component of the lesion. e) To complement the arterial embolisation, venous embolisation is performed through numerous direct punctures to cover the whole lesion. f) Improvement in the ulcer before skin grafting.

Key points

- Peripheral vascular anomalies are clinically and therapeutically demanding and need an experienced multidisciplinary team.
- Choice of treatment is aided by accurate diagnosis and investigation.
- As expertise with ultrasound-guided foam sclerotherapy grows, it may become the treatment of choice for many vascular malformations.

References

1. Mulliken JB, Glowacki J. Hemangiomas and vascular malformations in infants and children: a classification based on endothelial characteristics. *Plast Reconstr Surg* 1982; 69: 412-22.
2. Vikkula M, Boon LM, Mulliken JB, Olsen BR. Molecular basis of vascular anomalies. *Trends Cardiovasc Med* 1998; 8: 281-92.
3. Oliva VL, Soulez G, Dubois J. Vascular malformations. In: *Comprehensive vascular and endovascular surgery.* Hallett JW, Mills JL, Earnshaw JJ, Reekers JA, Eds. Mosby 2005; 43: 665-74.

Case vignette

Transverse cervical arteriovenous malformation

Frank CT Smith BSc MD FRCS FRCS (Ed) FRCS (Glas), Consultant Senior Lecturer, Bristol Royal Infirmary, UK

This patient presented with a warm swelling in his left posterior triangle of the neck, which had been present for some years (Figure 1). On examination a thrill and bruit were detected. Angiography confirmed the presence of an arteriovenous malformation (Figure 2), which was managed conservatively in the absence of symptoms.

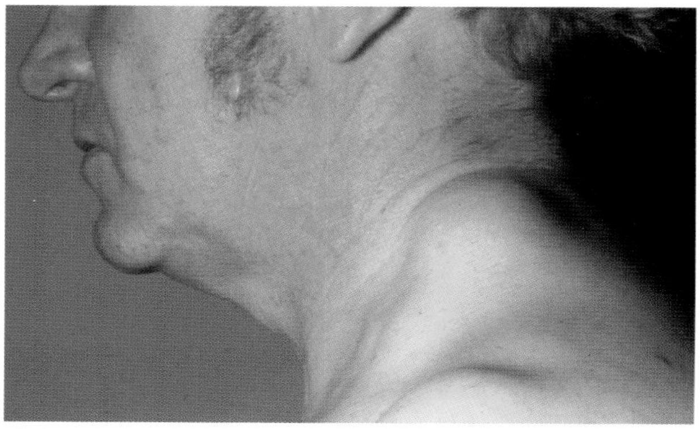

Figure 1.

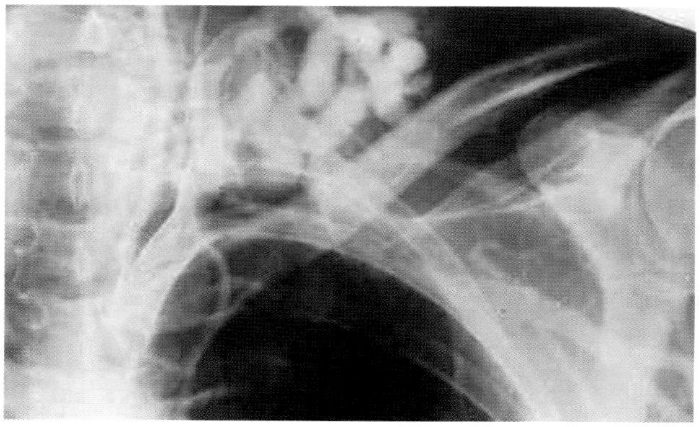

Figure 2.

Case vignette

Iatrogenic crural arteriovenous fistula

Frank CT Smith BSc MD FRCS FRCS (Ed) FRCS (Glas), Consultant Senior Lecturer, Bristol Royal Infirmary, UK

A 20-year-old man fractured his left tibia playing rugby. Initial orthopaedic intervention involved placement of an external fixator (Figure 1) during which the surgeon noticed bright red bleeding from a screw site wound. Examination at 4 weeks demonstrated persistent swelling of the calf with a palpable thrill and an audible bruit over the proximal anterior compartment. Angiography confirmed the presence of an anterior tibial arteriovenous fistula (Figure 2). The fistula was explored via a short vertical anterior compartment incision with venous ligation and vein patch angioplasty to repair the artery.

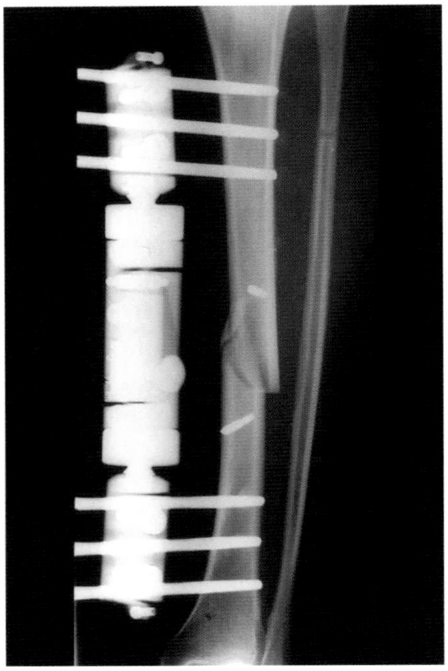

Figure 1.

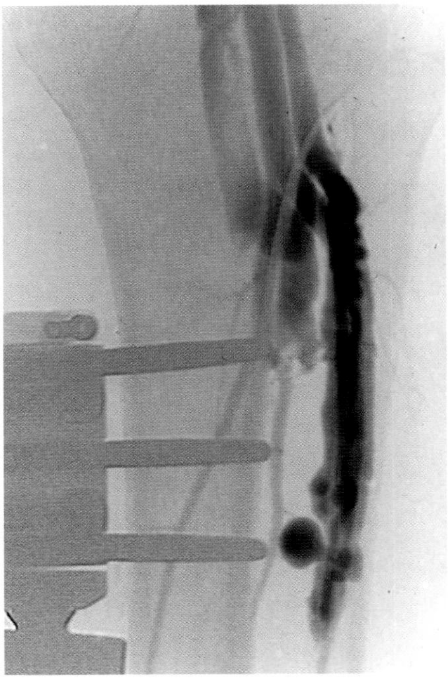

Figure 2.

Chapter 12

Major iliofemoral venous thrombosis, phlegmasia, and caval filters

Anthony Watkinson FRCS FRCR, Consultant Radiologist
Bruce Campbell MS FRCP FRCS, Professor and Consultant Surgeon
Royal Devon and Exeter Hospital and Peninsula Medical School,
Exeter, UK

Introduction

Most patients with deep vein thrombosis (DVT) of the legs are managed confidently by general physicians and others using anticoagulation and conservative measures including compression hosiery. This chapter addresses various forms of severe lower limb DVT about which vascular surgeons and radiologists may be asked for advice, including:

- major iliofemoral DVT with gross leg swelling;
- phlegmasia caerulea (and alba) dolens;
- the need for inferior vena caval filters.

Major iliofemoral DVT

There are two distinct types of iliofemoral DVT. The first occurs when calf DVT propagates proximally: thrombus is often poorly adherent to the vein wall and the potential for massive pulmonary embolisation (PE) is high. The second type involves thrombus originating in the iliac vein with distal propagation and sometimes caval extension (when the risk of PE is increased). Primary iliac vein thrombosis results from extrinsic compression, typically by a gravid uterus, enlarged lymph nodes, the iliac artery; or from intrinsic vein wall abnormalities such as webs or spurs, often associated with chronic compression [1].

Both forms of iliofemoral DVT involve large volumes of thrombus, and complete spontaneous recanalisation with restoration of normal vein function is unlikely. However, the iliac venous segment is functionally simple and restoration of patency may be sufficient to re-establish normal venous return from the leg.

Conventional treatment of acute iliofemoral DVT

A course of adequate anticoagulant therapy reduces the risk of fatal PE and of recurrent venous thrombosis, but is relatively ineffective in preventing post-thrombotic syndrome. Systemic thrombolysis can lead to more rapid and more complete venous recanalisation than anticoagulation alone. An association has been demonstrated between early recanalisation and preservation of venous valvular competence with reduction in the severity of post-thrombotic syndrome. The options for thrombolytic and other means of eliminating thrombus are presented below.

Phlegmasia caerulea (and alba) dolens

Severe and extensive iliofemoral DVT associated with complete thrombosis of the major leg veins causes a grossly swollen and painful leg which is typically pale - phlegmasia alba dolens (PAD) - although it may be erythematous. If thrombosis extends into venules and capillaries with secondary development of acute arterial ischaemia then phlegmasia caerulea dolens (PCD) results. The mechanism of this arterial compromise is mainly hydrostatic, resulting from a massive increase in the capillary hydrostatic pressure with outpouring of fluid and gross interstitial oedema. When there is little or moderate compromise of the arterial circulation, PCD may be reversible; frequently, however, there is progress to venous gangrene over 24-48 hours (Figure 1).

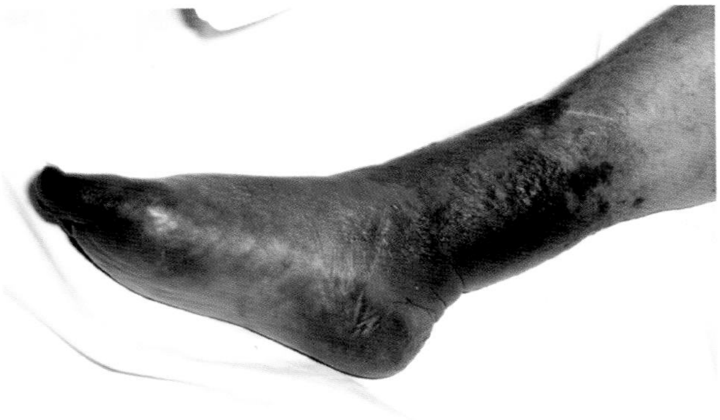

Figure 1. Venous gangrene following phlegmasia caerulea dolens.

PCD is most common in the fifth and sixth decades, has equal sex incidence and involves the left leg almost three times more often than the right, probably as a result of left iliac vein compression syndrome. The leg becomes massively swollen with distal cyanosis, often cutaneous bullae, and in venous gangrene with non-blanching, purplish/black mottling of the skin. Pain is typically intense and bursting in nature. Arterial hypotension secondary to hypervolaemia may be severe. Mortality is around 20% and pulmonary embolism occurs in 12-40% of patients.

An underlying hypercoagulable state can be identified in 90% cases - most commonly malignancy or thrombophilia (particularly activated protein C resistance and/or antiphospholipid syndrome).

Management of phlegmasia caerulea dolens

PCD is a medical emergency. Initial management is directed at improving tissue perfusion by aggressive resuscitation with intravenous fluids to treat hypovolaemic shock, and bed rest with high limb elevation (not just with pillows, but with gallows or a special "wedge"). Immediate anticoagulation with intravenous heparin (target APTT 1.5-2.0) prevents further thrombus propagation. In early cases these measures may produce clinical improvement within 12-24 hours (Figure 2). In severe or advanced PCD, conservative measures are insufficient, and more aggressive treatment may be considered, such as thrombolysis and/or thrombectomy.

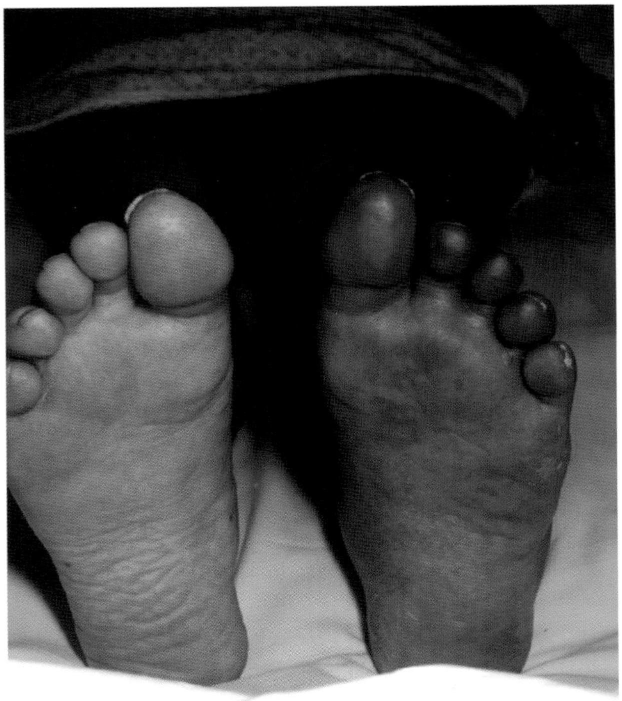

Figure 2. Venous gangrene in a patient with malignant disease who responded to anticoagulation and elevation and the foot recovered without surgical intervention.

Thrombolytic therapy for major iliofemoral DVT and phlegmasia

Systemic thrombolytic therapy

Systemic thrombolytic therapy in acute DVT reduces the incidence of post-thrombotic syndrome compared with heparin alone. Its efficacy is related to the duration of thrombosis and the initial thrombus burden. It has had disappointing results in the treatment of extensive iliofemoral thrombosis and phlegmasia, because of the large volume of thrombus. The risk of bleeding complications, such as stroke, has also limited use of this technique.

Local-regional thrombolytic therapy

Thrombolytic agents are delivered directly into the thrombus, maximising local doses whilst minimising the systemic effects and haemorrhagic complications. Two approaches have been adopted. The first is catheter-directed regional therapy, infusing the thrombolytic drug directly into the thrombus via percutaneous catheters. An advantage of this method is that the entire venous system may be evaluated before starting therapy. The second technique is flow-directed regional therapy, in which high-dose infusion of thrombolytic is given into an ipsilateral dorsal foot vein. Most of the flow is directed into the deep venous system via tourniquets. This method is more time-consuming, requires higher doses of thrombolytics, but allows more effective treatment of the smaller crural veins. Thrombolytic therapy is most effective in the acute thrombus (<3 days) and is largely ineffective in thrombus older than 4 weeks.

The delivery catheter is usually placed either from the contralateral femoral vein (if patent) or from the internal jugular vein (or both). Because of the high risk of pulmonary embolism during the treatment it is advisable to place a temporary filter in the infrarenal IVC via either of these approaches, though this is controversial. The infusion catheter can safely be passed through the filter and embedded into the thrombus. Historically, the most widely used thrombolytic agent has been urokinase, but currently, tissue plasminogen activator (tPA) is most popular.

Early series of catheter-directed thrombolysis reported complete or substantial recanalisation rates of 60-83%. The National Venous Thrombolysis Registry in the USA provides the largest published series to date; 287 patients (303 legs) from multiple centres were followed-up 1 year after catheter-directed thrombolysis [2]. Complete thrombolysis was achieved in 31% and partial (>50%) thrombolysis in 52% of patients. The procedure was more successful in acute DVT and those with no previous history of DVT. The 12-month primary patency rate was 80% - better in iliofemoral than femoropopliteal segments. The overall rate of valvular reflux was 58%, but was only 28% in those who underwent complete thrombolysis. There was an 11% incidence of major bleeding (requiring transfusion) and 16% of minor bleeding. Procedure-related mortality was 0.4%. Other complications included sepsis and traumatic valvular incompetence.

Intra-arterial thrombolysis

Delivery of thrombolytic agent via intra-arterial catheters to the affected limb has been reported in PCD [3]. This approach delivers thrombolysis to the capillary and venular thrombus. Relief from pain and swelling may be rapid (within 6-12 hours) and dramatic. Combining this with intravenous thrombolysis addresses thrombus both in the large veins (iliofemoral) and the microcirculation. Further experience is required of this combined approach to confirm these initial good outcomes.

When should thrombolysis be used in iliofemoral DVT and phlegmasia?

This decision is less straightforward than simple review of the literature suggests. The good results described above for thrombolysis in iliofemoral DVT are largely based on case series (some now rather dated), which are uncontrolled and which represent the work of enthusiasts. While it is clearly possible to obtain excellent outcomes in selected patients, experience of case selection and of the practicalities of lysis for massive DVT is limited in many hospitals. Apart from interventional radiology expertise, intensive

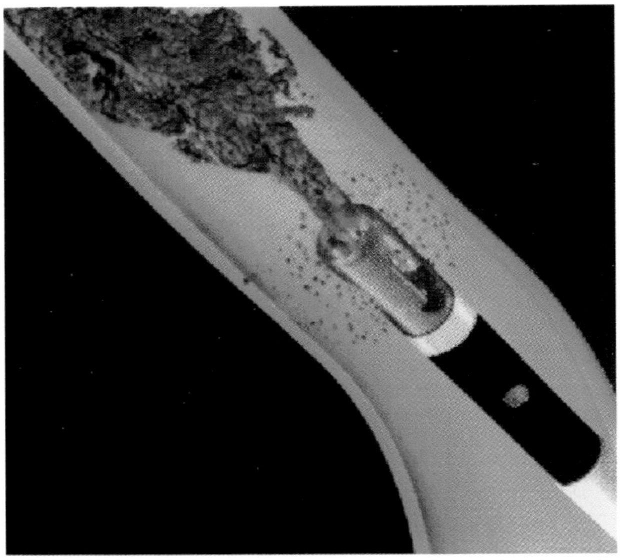

Figure 3. Rotational thrombectomy device (Amplatz).

monitoring of patients is required with clear protocols and arrangements to deal expeditiously with complications. Serious bleeding is a risk and this needs to be balanced against the potential benefits of thrombolysis, compared with simple anticoagulation.

Many patients with phlegmasia are very ill (often with malignant disease), and have a dismal prognosis. They may be poor candidates for thrombolysis and a proportion are most appropriately managed by palliative care only. If venous gangrene has supervened and the situation has stabilised on anticoagulants then continued conservative management is often best. If the patient recovers, the amount of tissue loss may be minimal because the purple/black discoloration of venous gangrene is largely superficial, while the deeper tissues remain viable.

Percutaneous mechanical thrombectomy

Percutaneous mechanical thrombectomy (PMT) refers to the use of percutaneous devices that may work by mechanical dissolution, fragmentation and/or aspiration. The combination of catheter-directed thrombolytic therapy and PMT offers the possibility of rapid ablation of venous thrombus, particularly in situations where there are contra-indications to aggressive or prolonged thrombolytic therapy. In extensive DVT, PMT can restore a venous channel, debulk thrombus and increase the surface area of thrombus exposed to lysis.

PMT carries a risk of fragment embolisation, but meticulous aspiration and recirculation techniques, pharmacological thrombolytics and protective inferior vena cava (IVC) filters can reduce the size of the particles reaching the lungs. PMT devices can themselves, however, cause damage to venous valves resulting in chronic venous insufficiency and the post-thrombotic syndrome. There is evidence that proper techniques such as introducing the device via large conduits and with the direction of flow can reduce such damage.

There are several commercially available devices, but no prospective trials exist comparing their efficacy or complication rates in the venous system (Figure 3).

Surgical venous thrombectomy

Surgical thrombectomy can clear thrombus from major veins, but will not clear thrombosed venules or capillaries, so limiting its effectiveness in PCD. Early series of thrombectomy performed within 10 days of onset in iliofemoral thrombosis (without PCD or venous gangrene) reported 85% patency rates and minimal symptoms of the post-thrombotic syndrome. Later studies, however, found high rethrombosis rates and significant morbidity from late post-thrombotic syndrome on long-term follow-up. There have been suggestions of improved outcomes with use of adjunctive arteriovenous fistulae and attention to relieving proximal venous obstruction in the common iliac veins [4].

Phlegmasia and impending venous gangrene present possible indications for venous thrombectomy. However, anecdotal experience is discouraging and there is little recent literature to promote use of venous thrombectomy. The suggestion that failure of anticoagulant therapy is an added indication seems irrational, because further thrombosis is most likely (Figure 4).

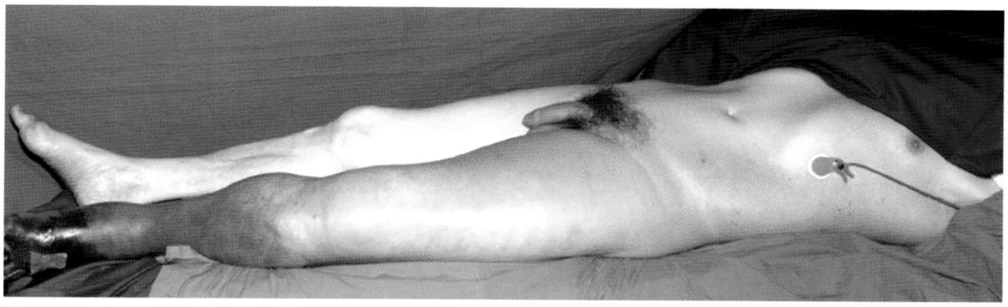

Figure 4. This patient with venous gangrene was treated by surgical thrombectomy but there was no sustained improvement and he died.

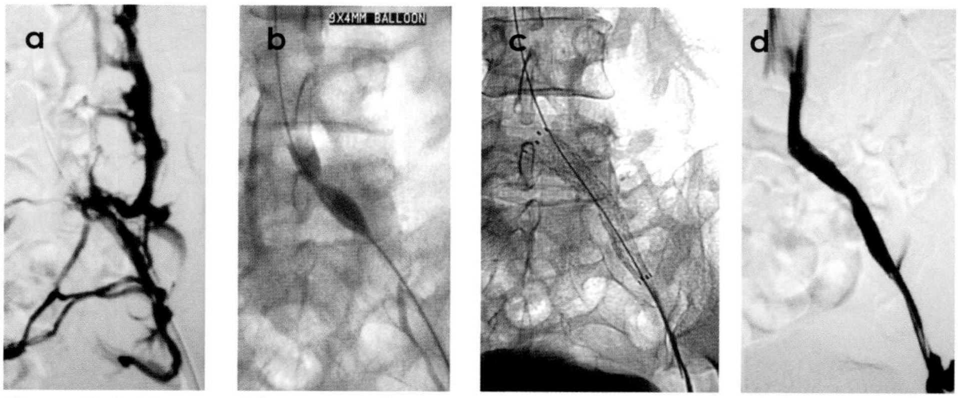

Figure 5. A 45-year-old woman with a previous left DVT presented with a swollen leg with unsightly vulval and upper thigh varices. a) A digital subtraction venogram via a sheath in the left common femoral vein demonstrated a tight stenosis/occlusion of the left common iliac vein with collateral flow consistent with a May-Thurner lesion. b) The left common iliac stenosis/occlusion has been traversed and dilated to 12mm. (A tight waist is visible in the balloon). c) A 1mm self-expanding nitinol stent (Memotherm, Bard UK) has been positioned across the previous narrowing in the left common iliac vein. d) Completion venogram demonstrates rapid flow into the IVC through a patent stent. At 22-month follow-up the patient has marked improvement in her symptoms and the stent remains patent.

Endovascular management of venous lesions exposed by thrombolysis

Malignant iliocaval obstruction is a common cause of refractory DVT, and may benefit from stent placement after thrombo-ablation. May-Thurner syndrome (chronic pulsatile compression of the proximal left common iliac vein by the overlying right common iliac artery or aortic bifurcation, resulting in an intraluminal venous spur, web or membrane) is an increasingly recognised cause of left iliac vein thrombosis, particularly in young patients and is another indication for venous stenting [1] (Figure 5).

Various endovascular stents have been used effectively in the treatment of post-thrombotic iliocaval stenoses. Self-expanding stents seem the best; they can be oversized and left to expand passively. They will recoil and re-expand if temporarily deformed or compressed. Preliminary balloon dilatation and complete stenting of the previously occluded segment should be performed until any pressure gradient is obliterated. Cutting balloon angioplasty may have a role in the treatment of chronic severe venous stenosis and resistant periphlebitis.

Table 1. Indications for IVC filter insertion [7].
Absolute indications
High risk for thrombo-embolism with contra-indication to anticoagulation
Recurrent thrombo-embolic disease despite anticoagulation therapy
Significant complication of anticoagulant therapy
Inability to achieve adequate anticoagulation (despite patient compliance)
Relative indications
Large, free-floating iliocaval thrombus
Thrombo-embolic disease with poor cardiopulmonary reserve
Poor compliance with medications
Severe ataxia; at risk of falls on anticoagulation therapy
During venous thrombolysis
Renal cell cancer with renal vein or IVC involvement

Iliocaval angioplasty and/or stenting should be followed by at least 3 months of anticoagulation to prevent early rethrombosis before the stent is endothelialised. Technical success in longstanding venous iliac occlusions can be achieved in over 90% of procedures with primary patency at 19 months of 80% [5].

Inferior vena caval filters

Anticoagulation remains the most effective primary treatment for lower limb DVT. In a minority of patients, however, anticoagulation will be contra-indicated, will fail or will result in complications. Treatment used to include open surgical interruption of the inferior vena cava below the renal veins by suture plication ("sieving") or external clip placement. These procedures carried significant morbidity and mortality.

The first endoluminal filter was introduced in 1967 (the Mobin-Uddin umbrella filter). Composed of six stainless steel struts coated with a heparin-impregnated fenestrated silastic membrane, the filter was inserted via venotomy with its apex pointing inferiorly. Problems included IVC thrombosis (60%) and migration (0.4%). The Greenfield filter, introduced in 1974, was conical and had superior flow characteristics and hence lower rates of thrombosis. The first percutaneous insertion of a Greenfield filter was in 1984. Since then, development of smaller calibre delivery systems and low profile filters has reduced complications of insertion such as haemorrhage and thrombosis. Most modern filters are made of titanium or nitinol (nickel titanium alloy) - materials that are non-ferromagnetic, eliminating the risk of movement during magnetic resonance scanning. There are currently no good prospective data comparing the efficacy of the various available devices. The Society of Interventional Radiology in the USA has recently published reporting guidelines, in an attempt to standardise future studies and allow valid meta-analysis [6].

Insertion is percutaneous under local anaesthesia without the need for a cut down. The usual portal of entry is the femoral vein, or less commonly, the internal jugular vein. With the smaller nitinol filters the antecubital vein can be used.

Indications for IVC filter insertion

Strict criteria should be applied when assessing patients for caval filter insertion, as there are significant associated risks. These can be divided into absolute and relative indications (Table 1) [7].

Patients with a contra-indication to anticoagulation should be managed with a caval filter alone. In certain cases, a combination of a filter and anticoagulation may be desirable, such as in patients with severe cardiopulmonary compromise. Each case should be considered individually. There is evidence to suggest that the presence of large free-floating iliocaval thrombus is associated with a much higher risk of PE (50%) when compared with occlusive thrombus (15%), despite anticoagulation. The use of IVC filter protection during DVT thrombolysis remains contentious, but is routinely practised in the authors' institution. The only absolute contra-indications to IVC filter insertion are complete IVC thrombosis and lack of access to the IVC. The lack of long-term performance data should make clinicians reluctant to place permanent devices in young patients.

Currently, there is a trend, particularly in North America, to place prophylactic IVC filters in patients who do not yet have thrombo-embolism, but are at high risk by virtue of associated conditions, such as traumatic injury or malignancy [8-9]. These patients also have a relatively high risk of complications from anticoagulation. Studies have identified a subgroup of trauma patients who may be at a 50-fold increased risk of thrombo-embolic events, including those with brain or spinal cord injuries and those with pelvic or lower limb long-bone fractures. Some favourable results have been reported from the use of filters in these patients, but the results remain inconclusive [8-9].

Complications of IVC filter insertion

Recurrent PE has been reported in about 2-5% of patients; however, many recurrent PEs may be subclinical and the true incidence is likely to be higher. One reason can be unusual sources of emboli including the arm veins (particularly associated with central venous catheters) and the right atrium. Most IVC filters will trap large, life-threatening clots, but smaller clots may pass through unhindered. Clot within the filter itself may also become a source of emboli, resulting from *de novo* thrombus, trapped emboli from the lower limb veins or thrombus propagating up the IVC. The incidence of filter-related IVC thromboses varies from 0-28% in reported series. Technical failures, such as incomplete filter expansion, tilting or migration, or failure to recognise thrombus above the position of the filter at time of deployment may also account for recurrent PE.

Complications are reported in between 4% and 11% of procedures and include bleeding, infection, pneumothorax, air embolism, delivery system complications (such as guide wire entrapment) and suboptimal filter deployment. Reported delayed complications include filter migration into the heart, IVC penetration and filter fracture [7].

Recent IVC filter trials

Decousus *et al* reported in 1998 the first prospective randomised controlled trial using IVC filters [10]. Four hundred patients with venography-proven DVT were randomised to receive anticoagulants alone or anticoagulants with one of four types of IVC filter. The results are summarised in Table 2. Filters were effective in preventing PE but there was no improvement in overall mortality rate, possibly because fatal PE is quite rare. There was an increased risk of recurrent DVT at 2 years with filters. No comparison was made between the four different types of IVC filter used. The data may not apply to patients who need filters because they cannot receive anticoagulants.

A number of large, population-based, multicentre studies have looked retrospectively at outcomes of IVC filter placement, showing early protection against life-threatening PE but a non-significant reduction in unadjusted in-hospital mortality, no significant difference in readmission rates for PE, low morbidity and few complications. Leg swelling was more common in patients who received no anticoagulation.

Temporary or retrievable filters

Some patients require only temporary protection against thrombo-embolic events. Indications include the treatment of iliofemoral DVT with catheter thrombolysis, known DVT with a short period of contra-indication to anticoagulant therapy, prophylaxis after major trauma and free-floating thrombus. The long-term effects of permanent IVC filters are

Table 2. Results of PREPIC (Prevention du Risque d'Embolic Pulmonaire par Interruption Cave) Study [10].

Result	Anticoagulation alone (n=200)	Anticoagulation and IVC Filter (n=200)	Odds Ratio (95% CI)	P Value
At 12 days				
Recurrent PE	9(4.8)	2 (1.1)	0.22 (0.05-0.90)	0.03*
Recurrent fatal PE	4 (2.1)	0 (0.0)	-	0.12
Mortality	5 (2.5)	5 (2.5)	0.99 (0.29-3.42)	0.99
Cumulative at 2 years				
Recurrent PE	12 (6.3)	6 (3.4)	0.5 (0.19-1.33)	0.16
Recurrent fatal PE	5 (2.6)	1 (0.6)	0.22	0.22
Recurrent DVT	21 (11.6)	37 (20.8)	1.87 (1.10-3.20)	0.02*
IVC filter thrombosis	-	16 (9.0)	-	-
Mortality	40 (20.1)	43 (21.6)	1.10 (0.72-1.70)	0.65

* $p<0.05$

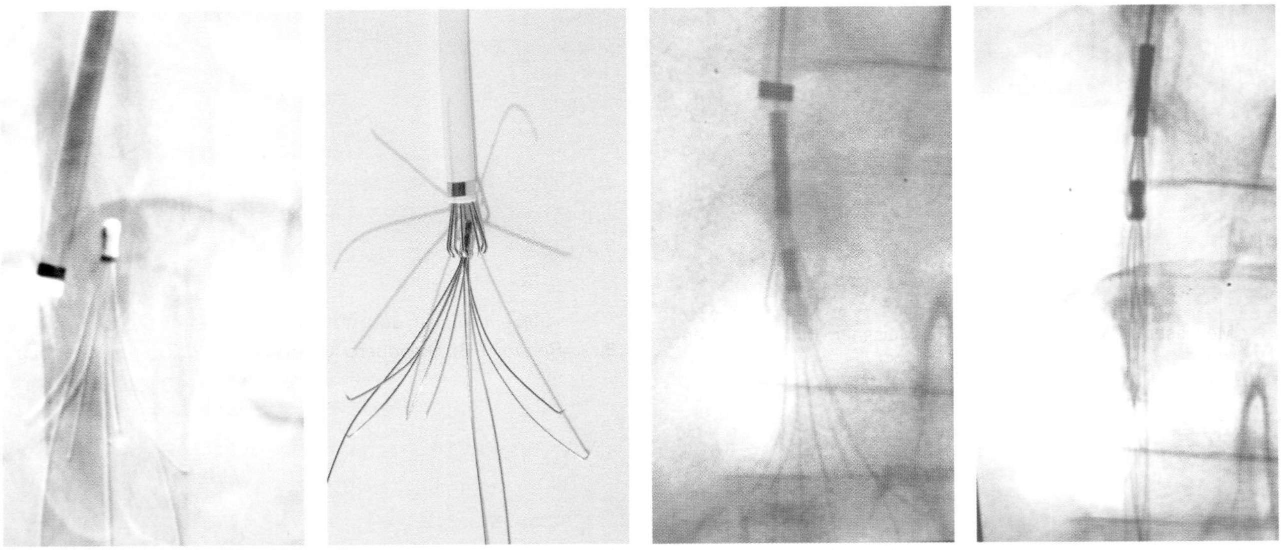

Figure 6. Removeable IVC filter (Pyramed UK Ltd). Series showing filter retrieval using a jugular vein approach 56 days after insertion.

Note: Figures 3, 5 and 6 are reproduced with permission from Elsevier. Watkinson A, Platts A. In: *Vascular & Endovascular Surgery*, 3rd Edition. Beard JB, Gaines P, Eds: (in press), © 2005 Elsevier Ltd.

uncertain. This has led to the development of filters that can be removed once the risk of embolism has passed (Figure 6). Certain temporary filters remain attached to an accessible transcutaneous catheter or wire. They have a similar design to the permanent filters, but have modified caval attachment sites. The disadvantages are that these require a second procedure to remove them and the transcutaneous catheter or wire is a potential pathway for infection. Alternatively, attempts have been made to remove permanent filters before there is endothelialisation of the filter struts to the IVC wall. "Tulip" filters can be retrieved via the right internal jugular vein using a retrieval snare through an 11 French sheath up to 3 weeks after insertion. Other more recently introduced retrievable IVC devices can be left in place for up to 60-90 days before removal.

Problems with removing filters include deciding when this can safely be done and what should be done if a large clot is found on the filter at the time of planned removal. The options for the latter include thrombolysis before filter removal or leaving the filter in place.

Key points

- **Thrombolysis may have a particular place in major iliofemoral DVT because the burden of thrombus is large and post-thrombotic syndrome is relatively common with conventional management.**
- **Phlegmasia caerulea dolens involves thrombosis of major veins and of the microcirculation, with subsequent arterial compromise. Combined venous and arterial thrombolysis may be successful, but advanced cases with venous gangrene may best be treated conservatively.**
- **Iliac vein stenoses exposed after treatment of DVT should be dealt with by balloon angioplasty, often with stenting.**
- **Vena caval filters reduce the early risk of PE, but may increase the longer-term risk of recurrent DVT and leg swelling. Newer temporary filters that can be left in place for several weeks may offer advantages.**

References

1. Hurst DR, Forauer AR, Bloom JR, *et al.* Diagnosis and endovascular treatment of iliocaval compression syndrome. *J Vasc Surg* 2001; 34: 106-13.
2. Mewissen MW, Seabrook GR, Meissner MH. Catheter-directed thrombolysis for lower extremity deep venous thrombosis: report of a national multicenter registry *Radiology* 1999; 211: 39-49.
3. Comerota AJ, Aldridge SC, Cohen G, *et al.* A strategy of aggressive regional therapy for acute iliofemoral venous thrombosis with contemporary venous thrombectomy or catheter-directed thrombolysis. *J Vasc Surg* 1994; 20: 244-54.
4. Eklof B, Kistner RL. Is there a role for thrombectomy in iliofemoral venous thrombosis? *Semin Vasc Surg* 1996; 9: 34-45.
5. Razavi MK, Hansch EC, Kee ST, *et al.* Chronically occluded inferior venae cavae: endovascular treatment. *Radiology* 2000; 214: 133-8.
6. Grassi CJ, Swan TL, Cardella JF. Quality improvement guidelines for percutaneous permanent inferior vena cava filter placement for the prevention of pulmonary embolism. *J Vasc Intervent Radiol* 2003; 14: S271-S275.
7. Kinney, TB. Update on inferior vena cava filters. *J Vasc Intervent Radiol* 2003; 14: 425-40.
8. Rogers FB, Strindberg G, Shackford SR, *et al.* Five-year follow-up of prophylactic vena cava filters in high risk trauma patients. *Arch Surg* 1998; 133: 406-12.
9. McMurty AL, Owings JT, Anderson JT, *et al.* Increased use of prophylactic caval filters in trauma patients failed to decrease overall incidence of pulmonary embolism. *J Am Coll Surg* 1999; 189: 314-20.
10. Decousas H, Leizorovicz A, Parent F, *et al.* A clinical trial of vena caval filters in the prevention of pulmonary embolism in patients with proximal deep-vein thrombosis. *N Engl J Med* 1998; 338: 409-15.

Chapter 13

Pelvic congestion syndrome

Simon G Darke MS FRCS, Consultant Vascular Surgeon
Royal Bournemouth Hospital, Bournemouth, UK

Introduction

It is only proper to concede that this author has never knowingly seen a patient with pelvic congestion syndrome (PCS), so this is written from a status of ignorance in terms of previous personal experience. However, this is not necessarily a disadvantage. Uncertainty and controversy prevail on the management of this condition, so there is merit in starting with an open mind free from any pre-existing conceptions or prejudices.

What information exists on PCS is essentially anecdotal. The literature will be reviewed and an attempt made to interpret this issue as objectively as possible from a vascular surgical perspective. Three illustrative cases kindly contributed by JVRG members with an established interest in this condition are incorporated.

Definition

Although not that common, visible pelvic, vulval and upper thigh varices arising from incompetent ovarian or internal iliac veins, are a familiar entity in the practice of vascular surgery. They may be primary or recurrent. They may be painful; occasionally, it would seem disproportionately so, and they can be difficult to manage. More usually, these varices occur quite independently, but on occasions they would seem to accompany what is termed the pelvic congestion syndrome. Furthermore, the latter syndrome in a major proportion of patients presents with no visible varices. It is important at the outset to recognise both this association and distinction.

PCS is characterised by patients complaining of what might loosely be described as "gynaecological symptoms." There is a commonly occurring and readily recognisable group of patients in gynaecological practice presenting with chronic pelvic pain and dyspareunia for which no clear pathological cause can be found. The exclusion of identifiable pathology is usually on the basis of a normal laparoscopy [1-3]. More recently, a normal pelvic ultrasound examination may complement or replace this [2]. Within the UK, roughly half the patients undergoing laparoscopy for gynaecological reasons do so primarily for pain of this nature and in about two thirds of these no clear gynaecological cause is identified [3]. Disorders of menstruation and urological symptoms may also occur, and psychological disorder frequently accompanies this situation but it is generally not clear as to whether this is as a consequence of, or a causative factor [1-3]. A number of therapeutic strategies have been tried, but the effectiveness of these remains uncertain [2].

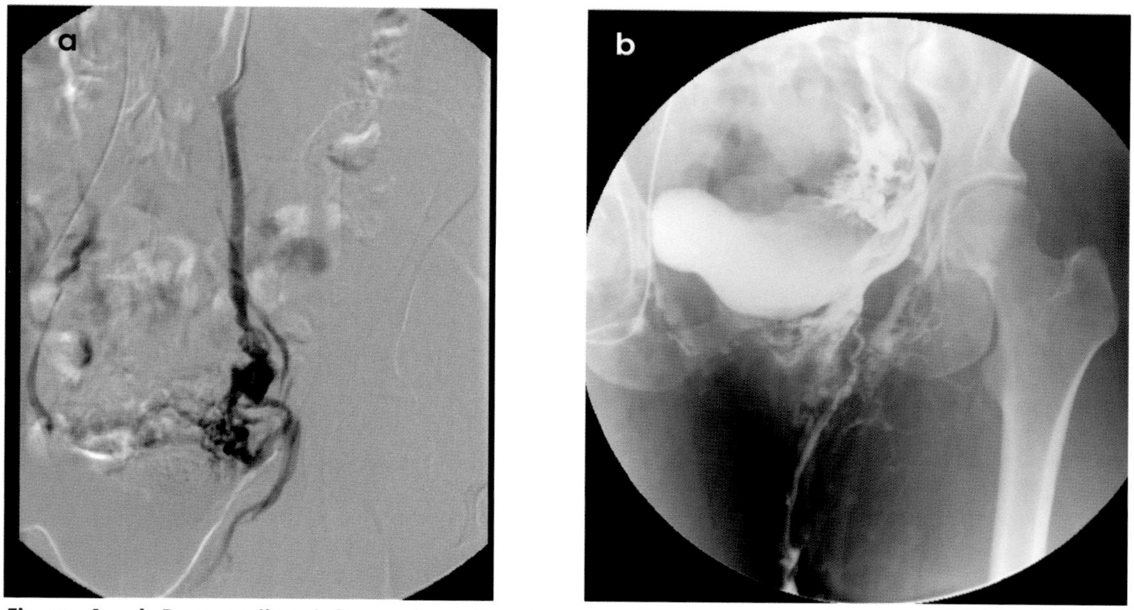

Figure 1. a) Descending left ovarian digital subtraction venogram in a woman with painful perineal varicose veins. b) Conventional venogram image showing reflux into the pudendal veins. Courtesy of Mr. M Gough and Dr. R Fowler.

Against this background, some of these patients have demonstrable incompetent and varicose ovarian and pelvic veins. Among the treatment options, therefore, it has been postulated that symptoms may be relieved by ablation of these incompetent veins [1]. This chapter will focus on this aspect.

Historical background

A possible link between pelvic pain and ovarian varicosities was considered before the middle of the 19th Century. This was particularly in the left ovarian vein, cited as comparable to a testicular varicocoele [4]. Focus in more recent times within the UK came from a seminal paper by Beard and associates in 1984 from St. Mary's Hospital, London. They were among the first to make a detailed and structured study of this possible association, although conceding that many others had previously made what were anecdotal but similar observations. This paper was a major factor in bringing the concept into contemporary thinking and practice [3]. Transuterine pelvic phlebography was carried out on women undergoing investigation for a variety of gynaecological complaints: 45 women with otherwise unexplained pelvic pain and a provisional diagnosis of PCS; 10 women had established pelvic pathology and a further eight who were undergoing laparascopic sterilisation were regarded as controls. The pelvic and ovarian veins were imaged and assessed according to ovarian vein size, time for clearance of dye from out of the pelvis, and appearance of the ovarian veins themselves in terms of varicosity. These features were combined to produce a score. The group of women diagnosed as having PCS had statistically significantly higher scores than the controls, although in one third of the former the pelvic veins were found to be normal. When present, this venous congestion, as it was termed, was unrelated to parity or the menstrual cycle.

Subsequent to that, and also from St. Mary's, John Hobbs with his established interest in venous disease focused further attention on this difficult subject [1]. In his overview in 1990, he records that the occurrence of tubo-ovarian varicosities had been recognised as long ago as the 19th Century. More latterly they were frequently seen at laparotomy or laparascopic examinations. In terms of imaging, initially at least, venography often via selective renal vein catheterisation was used to demonstrate reflux into the ovarian and pelvic veins (Figure 1).

There were sporadic early attempts to test the theory of symptom relief by ablating the apparently offending varices; one of the first major series reported was by Lechter [5]. Over a 5-year interval 1986-1991, 28 women were identified from the gynaecological practice of colleagues. The characteristics of these women were that they all had pelvic pain and 20 complained of dyspareunia. Nine also had vulval varices. No gynaecological pathology could be found to account for their symptoms. Laparoscopy was used to diagnose the presence of ovarian varices. Twenty-three underwent ligation of both ovarian veins and in 20 this was performed transabdominally and combined with hysterectomy. In three patients ligation was performed by a retroperitoneal exposure. All women reported short-term relief of their symptoms.

Current perspectives

In current gynaecological practice there remains the problem of undiagnosed and persistent pelvic pain and dyspareunia. In a significant proportion of these women this might be associated with ovarian vein reflux that is potentially treatable. Furthermore, against this historical background there has been the emergence of a number of investigative and therapeutic techniques that have potential in the management of these women. There are advances in ultrasound imaging of the organs of the pelvis to exclude obvious pathological features and colour Doppler ultrasound to interrogate the ovarian and pelvic venous circulation [6]. Similarly, CT has become progressively more sophisticated to address both these aspects [7]. In addition, laparascopic interventions have allowed not only the diagnosis of ovarian and pelvic varices, but their ligation without open surgery [8]. Endovenous transcatheter procedures are now used for selective venography and also embolic ablation of ovarian and pelvic veins [9-12].

With these technical advances has come information about the specificity and sensitivity of pelvic venous reflux in women with PCS. From the original work of Beard it would seem that about two thirds of women with pelvic pain have demonstrable venous incompetence. In another more recent study by Park *et al* [6], ultrasound was undertaken. In fact the prime objectives were to validate the use of ultrasound to identify ovarian vein reflux by comparing it with venography. In this study, 139 women with clinically suspected PCS underwent ultrasound to assess their ovarian veins; reflux was found in 74 (53%). Thirty-two of these went on to ovarian venography as part of the validation exercise and in all reflux was confirmed on venography. It could be argued, however, that reflux may have been missed on the original ultrasound and might have been demonstrable on venography, so this 53% could be an underestimate. Frustratingly, the larger subsequent and more contemporary series fail to record the proportion of women that were investigated with clinical PCS and that had normal ovarian and pelvic veins [7-9]. The best estimate is that ovarian/pelvic vein reflux is found in about half.

The question remains how many apparently normal and asymptomatic women of similar age and parity have ovarian vein reflux? In the ultrasound/venography comparative series alluded to above, reflux was found on ultrasound in four of 16 normal control patients [6]. A recent CT study specifically set out to challenge the significance of ovarian vein reflux [10]. A consecutive series of scans that had been performed for other reasons, were reviewed retrospectively. Incompetent and dilated ovarian veins were found in 16 of 34 women aged between 18 and 46 years, so a best estimate might be that about a third to a half of normal asymptomatic women of comparable age have pelvic venous reflux.

Results of intervention

The first issues with respect to intervention are method, risks and short- and long-term technical success. Not surprisingly, early reports were exclusively of open operative procedures, either by an extraperitoneal or transperitoneal approach, often accompanied by hysterectomy [1,4,5]. More recent reports employed laparoscopic ligation [11] or percutaneous transcatheter techniques with embolising coils, or a mixture of enbrucilate and lipiodized oil (Figure 2). The immediate success in closing the offending varices with this technique is reported consistently as over 90%. Inadvertent pulmonary embolisation of coils and glue are

reported, but without any serious clinical consequences [7-9,12].

Less has been written about the possible recurrence of ovarian varicosities after closure by any method. Instinctively, a vascular surgeon might feel that recurrence is likely considering well-established experience of varicose veins in the leg, particularly given the complex and rich nature of the pelvic venous circulation. Irrespective of any other consideration, the ovary has to establish some alternative route of venous drainage. In this respect, Venbrux *et al* [8] reported follow-up of women who had intensive coil and sclerosant transcatheter therapy to the ovarian and internal iliac veins and found recurrence in three out of 56 patients followed-up for at least 12 months. There do not seem to be any longer follow-up reports.

Finally, comes the question of symptomatic relief. There are no randomised controlled trials of intervention for PCS. Venbrux and Lambert [12] have reviewed much of what has been reported, principally following ovarian coil embolisation. This they feel at the present time is the method of choice for achieving technical objectives. Most reports reviewed included single or small numbers of patients, but the overall impression was that symptoms are durably relieved/improved in 50-80%. They rightly point out that these are uncontrolled studies and there is a significant need for a controlled trial.

There have been three recent studies of catheter embolisation, predominantly of the left ovarian vein. Maleux *et al* in 2000 reported 58% symptomatic improvement at mean follow-up of 20 months in a series of 41 women. There was no difference in outcome between the 32 women undergoing left ovarian vein embolisation compared to the nine who had bilateral embolisation [7]. Venbrux and colleagues in 2002 reported their own experience in more detail. They found statistically significant relief of symptoms as assessed by a 65% reduction in Visual Analogue Scores of pain perception at a mean follow-up of 22 months [8]. More recently, d'Archambeau and De Schepper from Antwerp have reported a personal series of 66 women; 48 of those originally treated were followed-up. In 42, only the left ovarian vein had

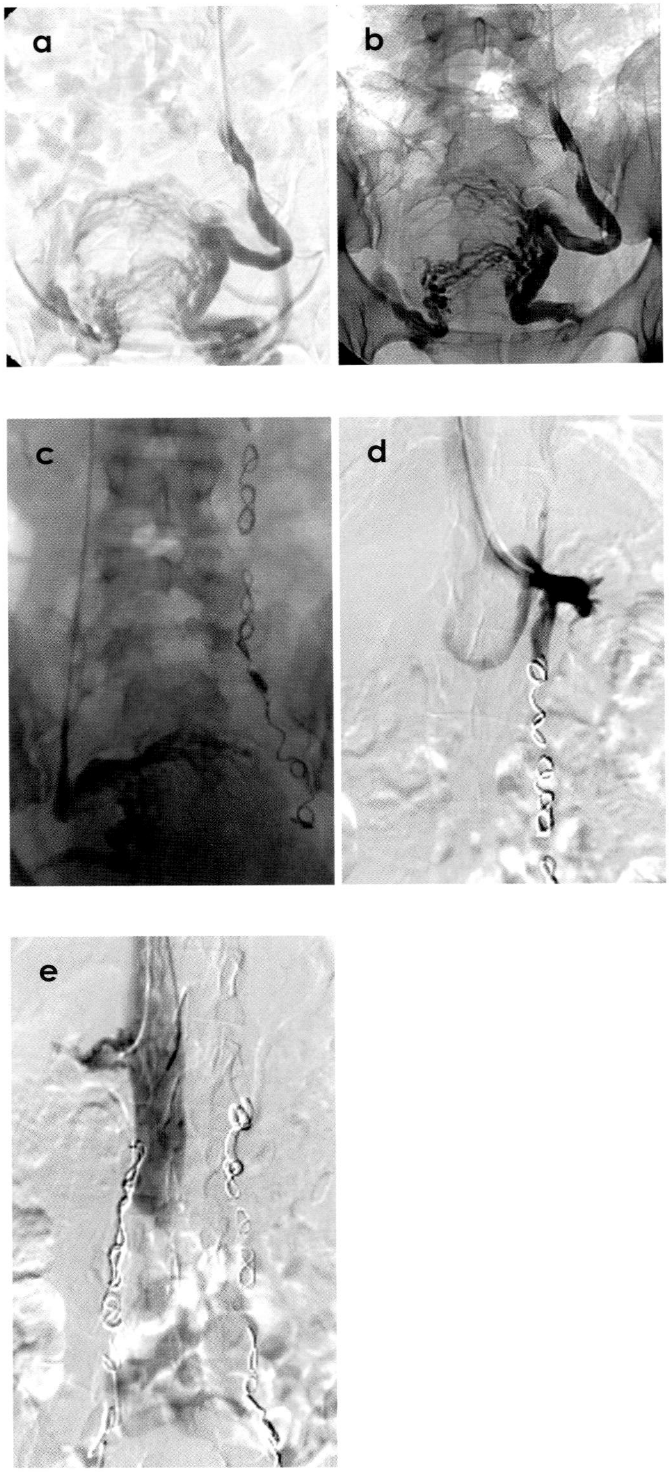

Figure 2. A 38-year-old woman with painful vulval varices on standing. a) & b) Descending left ovarian venograms. c-e) Embolisation with a total of nine coils 10 and 20mm diameter via the antecubital vein. Symptoms were relieved. Courtesy of Dr. J Hancock and Dr. S Travis.

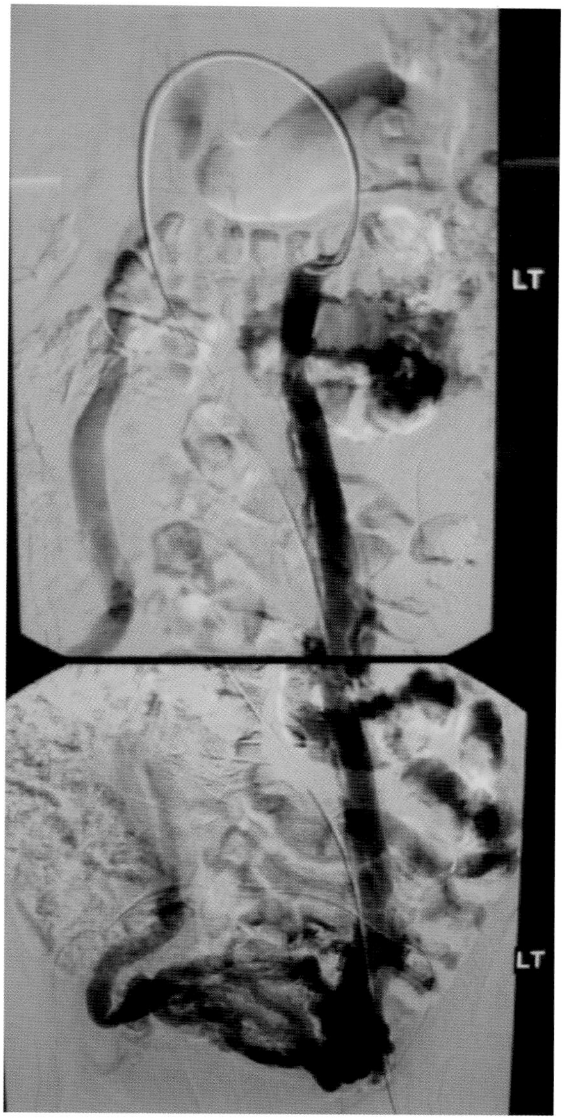

Figure 3. Multiparous woman with symptoms of PCS, and painful left pudendal veins. Selective venogram shows drainage of the left kidney is via the renal pelvis veins and up the right ovarian vein. There was a 5mmHg pressure drop across the left renal vein, thought to be due to compression by the superior mesenteric artery ("nutcracker phenomenon"). Symptoms were relieved completely by laparoscopic left ovarian vein ligation. Courtesy of Mr. B Braithwaite.

been coil embolised. At mean follow-up of 43 months, symptomatic improvement was recorded in 75% of women. These authors also allude to the possible anatomical phenomenon of compression of the left ovarian vein between the superior mesenteric artery and the aorta, the so-called nutcracker phenomenon [9]. Anecdotally, this has also been noted by contemporary colleagues who have found a measurable pressure difference across the left renal vein (Figure 3). (Watkinson A 2004, Braithwaite BD 2004, personal communications).

Since none of the series has a control group, it remains uncertain what could be expected in women managed with more conservative measures. Although not necessarily comparable, in a prospective randomised controlled trial that compared medroxyprogesterone acetate therapy with supportive counselling, both groups had a reduction in pain of about 50%. Similar rates of pain relief were found in the other control groups of a number of other randomised trials studying a variety of interventions [2].

Discussion

Venous disease is notoriously difficult to investigate for several reasons. Often what is apparently clinically significant morphology may be found in individuals completely free from symptoms. This lack of specificity casts doubt on any correlation with clinical state. Venous reflux is primarily based on imaging and is difficult to quantify. Comparable groups of venous disease entities are difficult to recruit, thus limiting the potential to establish a suitable cohort of patients for randomised trials. Venous disease is inherently chronic with a potential to recur after intervention, which means that follow-up of clinical outcomes must be long term to be valid. This condition of PCS is typical of these dilemmas.

On the one hand, PCS is a well-recognised clinical syndrome characterised by subjective symptoms. Some of the women have refluxing pelvic veins, usually the left ovarian. This incompetence, however, is also evident in some normal women. The ovarian veins can now be ablated relatively non-invasively and safely, usually with coil or other catheter-based embolisation. This is followed in the medium term by symptomatic relief in some, but certainly not all women, an outcome that may be somewhat better than conservative measures alone. Against this background it is not surprising that this practice does not seem to have gained wide application. A recent Cochrane Review on the management of PCS failed even to mention ovarian/pelvic venous incompetence as a possible cause [2].

On the other hand, there are the publications and convictions of several respected contemporary clinicians, although they are the first to admit that evidence remains anecdotal. Protagonists, including a number within the UK, cite the massive size of some of these ovarian veins, comparable to the inferior vena cava. There is little doubt among vascular surgeons about the existence of visible and painful vulval and perineal veins that arise from reflux within the pelvis. If these occur why should there not be painful veins within the pelvis too? Indeed, it is likely that a vascular surgeon will be involved in management of patients with painful and visible perineal veins. The relationship between these and PCS is uncertain, although it is clear that either problem can occur independently. Isolated pelvic pain and dyspareunia are likely to fall within the province of the gynaecologist and interventional radiologist and there is only a limited estimate as to what proportion of these will have ovarian and iliac vein reflux.

It will be apparent that Level I and II evidence regarding PCS is lacking. What is needed is a thorough investigation of a representative consecutive series of women from gynaecological practice with these symptoms, in whom other causes have been excluded. These patients then need to be investigated systematically, probably with ultrasound initially to establish the prevalence of ovarian reflux and any link with visible perineal veins. Ideally, women with apparently significant incompetence should be randomised into a control group with conservative management or a group with ovarian vein ablation. Until this is undertaken doubts and uncertainties will continue.

Acknowledgement

The author would like to thank Mr. M Gough and Dr. R Fowler, The General Infirmary at Leeds, Dr. J Hancock and Dr. S Travis, Consultant Vascular Radiologists, Royal Cornwall Hospitals Trust, and Mr. B Braithwaite, Queen's Medical Centre, Nottingham, for kindly providing the Figures.

Key points

- **Pelvic pain, dyspareunia and other gynaecological and psychological symptoms for which no obvious cause can be found is a well-recognised problem, often termed the pelvic congestion syndrome.**
- **In possibly half of these women, incompetent pelvic and ovarian veins can be demonstrated by venography, ultrasound or CT, particularly on the left side. These findings have been also reported in apparently normal asymptomatic women of similar age.**
- **In about a third of these women, painful visible perineal and vulval varices may be evident as well.**
- **Intervention to ablate these incompetent ovarian/iliac veins either by open surgery, laparoscopy or transcatheter endovenous embolisation is accompanied by medium-term relief of symptoms in about 75% of patients. This may be somewhat better than the outcome of more conservative supportive treatment.**
- **Protagonists of this concept cite the large size of these ovarian veins. Additionally, the occurrence of painful visible veins arising from incompetent pelvic veins is well recognised, but how these relate to the full syndrome is uncertain.**
- **A structured and systematic randomised controlled trial is needed.**

References

1. Hobbs JT. The pelvic congestion syndrome. *Br J Hosp Med* 1990; 43: 200-6.
2. Stones RW, Mountfield J. Interventions for treating chronic pelvic pain in women (Cochrane Review). In: *The Cochrane Library*, Issue 3, 2004. John Wiley and Sons Ltd, Chichester, UK.
3. Beard RW, Highman JH, Pearce S, Reginald PW. Diagnosis of pelvic varicosities in women with chronic pelvic pain. *Lancet* 1984; ii: 946-9.
4. Railo JE. The pain syndrome in ovarian varicocoele. *Acta Chir Scand* 1968; 134: 157-9.
5. Lechter A. Pelvic and vulvar varices: pelvic congestion syndrome. In: *Varicose veins and telangiectasias; diagnosis and treatment.* Bergan JJ, Goldman MP, Eds. Quality Medical Publishing Inc, St. Louis, Missouri, 1993: 353-69.
6. Park SJ, Lim JW, Ko YT, *et al.* Diagnosis of pelvic congestion syndrome using transabdominal and transvaginal sonography. *Am J Roentgenol* 2004; 182: 683-8.
7. Maleux G, Stockx L, Wilms G, Marchal G. Ovarian vein embolization for the treatment of pelvic congestion syndrome: long-term technical and clinical results. *J Vasc Intervent Radiol* 2000; 11: 859-64.
8. Venbrux AC, Chang AH, Kim HS, *et al.* Pelvic congestion syndrome (pelvic venous incompetence): impact of ovarian and internal iliac vein embolotherapy on the menstrual cycle and chronic pelvic pain. *J Vasc Intervent Radiol* 2002; 13: 171-8.
9. D'Archambeau O, Maes M, De Schepper AM. The pelvic congestion syndrome: role of the "nutcracker phenomenon" and results of endovascular treatment. *JBR-BTR* 2004; 87: 1-8.
10. Rozenblit AM, Ricci ZJ, Tuvia J, Amis ES. Incompetent and dilated ovarian veins: a common CT finding in asymptomatic parous women. *Am J Roentgenol* 2001; 176: 119-22.
11. Grabham JA, Barrie WW. Laparoscopic approach to pelvic congestion syndrome. *Br J Surg* 1997; 84: A1264.
12. Venbrux CA, Lambert DL. Embolization of the ovarian veins as a treatment for patients with chronic pelvic pain caused by pelvic venous incompetence. *Curr Opin Obstet Gynaecol* 1999; 11: 395-9.

Case vignette

Foam sclerotherapy for Klippel-Trenaunay syndrome

Philip Coleridge-Smith DM FRCS, Consultant Vascular Surgeon, The Middlesex Hospital, London, UK

This 28-year-old man with Klippel-Trenaunay syndrome affecting his right leg had surgery for large varices affecting the lateral aspect of the thigh and calf on three previous occasions. He presented with large symptomatic varices affecting the distal calf and foot (Figure 1).

Duplex ultrasonography showed that he still had a large incompetent lateral limb vein that was filling his calf and foot varices. He also had several large (4-5mm) incompetent perforating veins in his thigh and a similar number in the calf that contributed to reflux in the lateral limb vein. The angioma did not extend into the muscles of the leg. The cutaneous part of his angioma faded considerably as he reached adult life and was not a cosmetic problem.

He was managed by ultrasound-guided foam sclerotherapy comprising a course of four sessions. The incompetent lateral limb vein and associated varices in the thigh were treated first, followed by those in the calf and finally the foot (Figure 2). At follow-up 1 year later only one perforating vein showed evidence of recurrence. This was small in diameter (3mm) and easily dealt with by further foam injection.

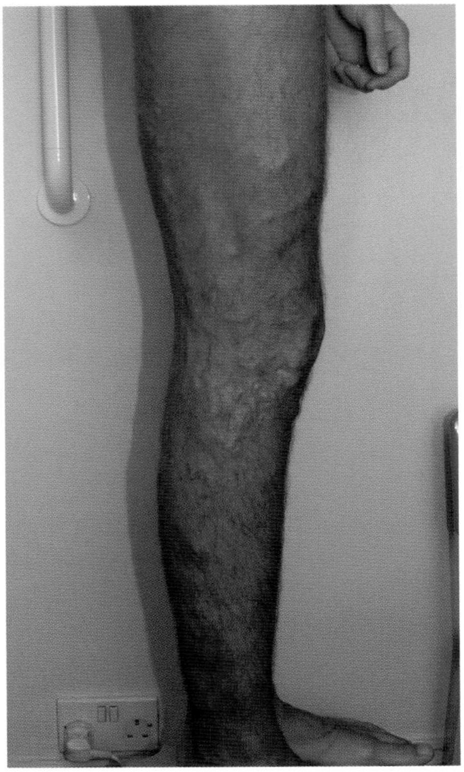

Figure 1.

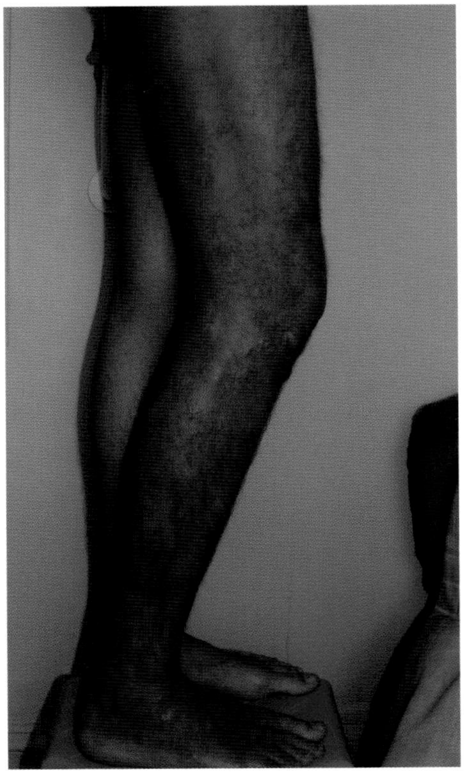

Figure 2.

Chapter 14

Klippel-Trenaunay syndrome

Rhys L Thomas BSc MB BS, Senior House Officer in Surgery
Royal Surrey County Hospital, Guildford, UK

Alun H Davies MA DM FRCS, Reader in Surgery and Consultant Surgeon
Imperial College School of Medicine, Charing Cross Hospital, London, UK

Introduction

Klippel-Trenaunay syndrome (KTS) is a rare congenital condition comprising a triad of capillary malformations (manifesting as port-wine stains), large venous malformations or varicosities, and bone and soft tissue hypertrophy affecting one or more limbs [1,2,3]. Both sexes are affected equally and there appears to be no ethnic or geographical variation, athough it is reported that more than one family member can be affected [2].

Historical perspective

Naevus variqueus hypertrophique (varicose osteohypertrophic naevus) was described in 1900 by two French physicians who identified a constellation of abnormalities including port-wine stain, varicose veins/venous anomalies and bone/soft tissue hypertrophy as the commonest features. A number of rare features have since been described [2]. In 1974, Bourde suggested that a persistent embryonic vascular system in the foetus was a contributing factor, Servelle (1985) suggested venous hypertension secondary to deep vein agenesis, atresia or hypoplasia [1] based on findings in a series of 768 operative cases, whereas Baskerville [3] (1985) and Young (1988) suggested mesodermal developmental abnormalities. This final theory explains the three features of KTS, whereas a persistent embryological vascular system may have a role in increased limb circumference, length and vascular histological changes, which may later develop into clinical varicosities and capillary malformations [1]. It is accepted that the presence of arteriovenous fistulae excludes the diagnosis of KTS [3], these being a feature of Parkes-Weber syndrome. Some, however, include the disease in a conglomeration of features, including arteriovenous fistulae; the disease is then known as Klippel-Trenaunay-Weber syndrome. More recently, Tian implicated increased transcription of a mutated angiogenic factor (VG5Q) in the development of KTS [4].

Clinical presentation

Of 252 cases reviewed by Jacob between 1956 and 1995, 63% of patients had all three of the cardinal features and 37% had two [2]. Almost all patients had obvious capillary malformation, i.e. port-wine stains (98%), 72% had severe varicosities and 67% had limb hypertrophy. The commonest sites of the abnormalities were the legs (88%), whereas approximately one quarter of the patients had thoracic

Table 1. Signs and symptoms in patients with Klippel-Trenaunay syndrome. (Modified with permission from Jacob *et al,* 1998 [2]).

Signs and symptoms	Patients %
Capillary malformation (port-wine stains)	98
Soft-tissue/bone hypertrophy	94
Varicosity	72
Lateral	56
Medial	19
Suprapubic	1
Pain	37
Bleeding	17
Superficial thrombophlebitis	15
Cellulitis	13
Rectal bleeding	12
Lymphatic malformation	11
Lymphoedema	10
Hyperpigmentation	8
Ankle ulcers	6
Verrucae	6
Hyperhidrosis	5
Deep vein thrombosis	4
Induration	4
Pulmonary embolism	4
Limb numbness	2
Other	27

involvement. The features of KTS are illustrated in Table 1 [2].

Capillary malformations

The capillary malformations are usually red-purple in colour, flat and irregularly distributed (Figure 1). They may or may not blanch on direct pressure and do not regress spontaneously. When located on the torso, they rarely cross the midline and the majority are located on the same side as the affected leg (85%). In children, high output cardiac failure and anaemia may occur. In severe cases, thrombocyte sequestration occurs, leading to defective fibrinolysis, clotting and haemolysis. When bleeding occurs the condition can be fatal and is known as Kasabach-Merritt syndrome. Approximately 30-40% of children with KTS present in this way [5]. It should be noted that when high-output cardiac failure is present in the adult, the diagnosis of Parkes-Weber is more likely, as this may be secondary to arteriovenous shunting.

Varicosities

The varicosities in KTS are rarely obvious at birth, but develop as the child begins to walk. Adult patients generally complain of fatigue, leg heaviness and swelling. There may be bleeding, thrombophlebitis (19-45%), cellulitis and lymphoedema. In 68% of patients the lateral vein of the thigh (Vein of Servelle) is present [3]; the sciatic vein may also persist. The veins are large and tortuous with absent valves

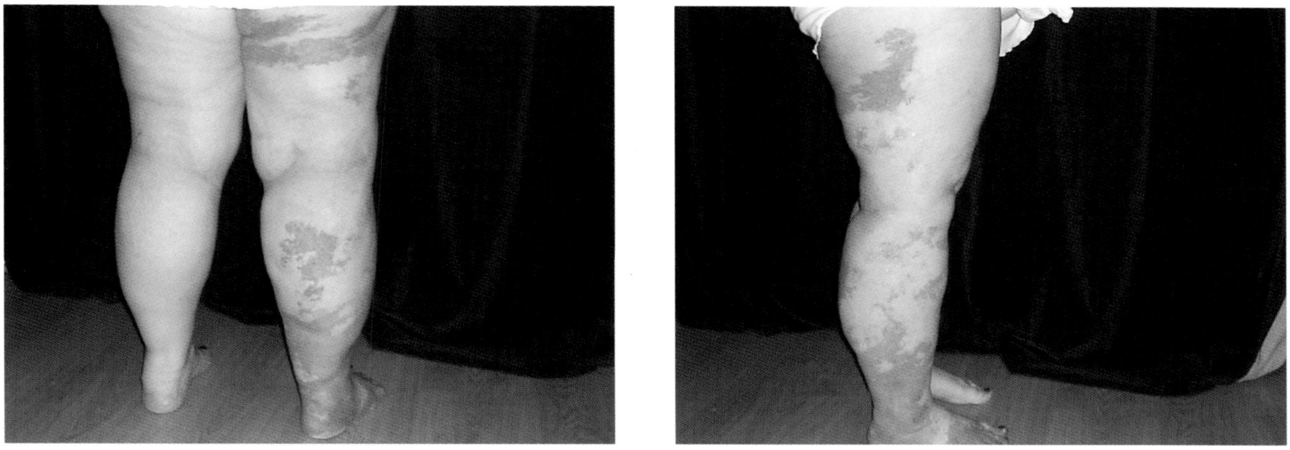

Figure 1. Extensive port-wine stains on the right calf and thigh of a woman with Klippel-Trenaunay syndrome.

(Figure 2). The large lateral vein drains into deep veins at variable distances from their origin, and may drain via the gluteal veins into the internal iliac vein [3]. In 70-90% of patients there is unilateral leg involvement, athough both legs and arms may be affected. Deep venous anomalies chiefly involve the popliteal and superficial femoral veins, which may be absent, hypoplastic or aneurysmal [2]. The femoral and iliac veins may also be affected, as well as the inferior vena cava (Table 2). Where deep venous hypertension exists, secondary varicosities may result in rectal bleeding and haematuria due to rectal or bladder wall malformations. Oesophageal variceal bleeding is rare, but reported.

Limb hypertrophy

Limb hypertrophy is variable and unpredictable in its rate of overgrowth, athough it is complete at the time of epiphyseal closure [2]. The affected limb may be shorter, or have increased circumference, or it may be grossly enlarged (Figure 3). Limb length discrepancy may reach 5cm, with similar values in girth. The increased leg length is due to long bone lengthening and can lead to unphysiological gait with poor posture and scoliosis of the spine unless corrected [1]. Where upper limb length disparity exists, the problem is seldom severe enough to require intervention.

Table 2. Venographic findings of 30 patients with Klippel-Trenaunay syndrome. (Modified with permission from Jacob *et al,* 1998 [2]).

Vein	Normal	Absent	Hypoplastic	Aneurysmal	Not seen
Common iliac	22	3	-	-	5
External iliac	24	3	-	-	3
Common femoral	27	3	-	-	-
Deep femoral	16	-	-	-	14
Superficial femoral	29	4	2	1	4
Popliteal	16	-	2	11	1
Tibial	19	1	1	2	7

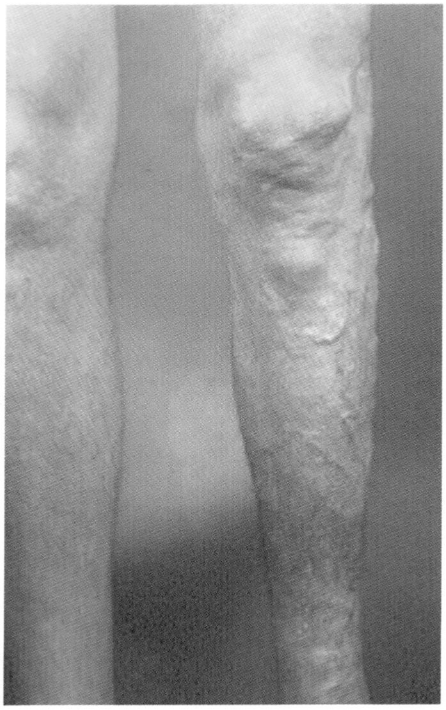

Figure 2. Varicosities on the lateral aspect of the leg in this patient with KTS. Reproduced with permission from The Ronald O. Perelman Department of Dermatology, NYU School of Medicine. Hale EK. Klippel-Trenaunay syndrome. Dermatology On-line 2002; 8(2): 13.

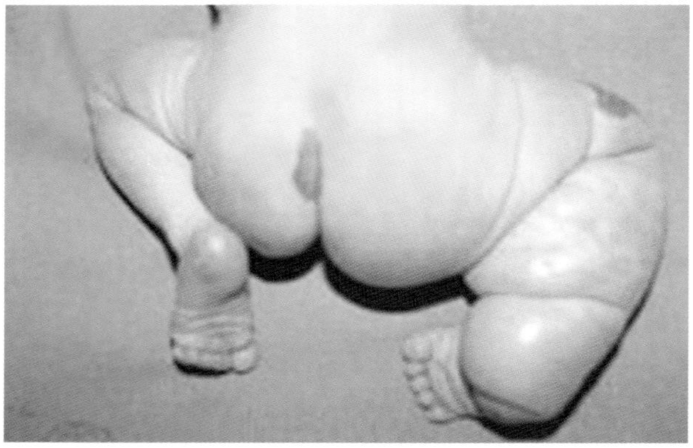

Figure 3. Gross right limb hypertrophy in a baby with Klippel-Trenaunay syndrome. There are also naevi visible overlying the sacrum and on the right thigh. Reproduced with permission from Israel Alfonso MD.

Additional features

Other presenting features in children include pain and thrombophlebitis. Congestive cardiac failure, gangrene of the affected extremity and cellulitis are rare [5]. A variety of skeletal, cardiovascular and soft tissue abnormalities have been reported in KTS [2] and recurrent pulmonary embolism, gross urological and pelvic abnormality and mediastinal cavernous haemiangioma have been described. It is also noteworthy that thrombo-embolic episodes are extremely common in KTS patients: up to 22.4% in one series [3].

Management

Capillary malformations

Lightly coloured capillary malformations are treated conservatively with cosmetic camouflage. Dark naevi may be treated with pulsed dye lasers that penetrate the dermis at 6-week intervals. The result, however, is often disappointing, requiring several courses of treatment. Surgical excision may be necessary if skin breakdown and ulceration occur, though the affected area often heals poorly [1].

Varicosities

Varicosities and venous malformations should be treated conservatively where possible, symptomatic relief being the prime objective. Graduated compression stockings should be prescribed for venous hypertension, insufficiency and lymphoedema. Recurrent cellulitis may be managed with prophylactic antibiotics.

Sclerosing agents

Percutaneous use of sclerosing agents such as sodium tetradecyl sulphate or absolute alcohol may be used to diminish the size of cavernous venous malformations through endothelial irritation. This requires general anaesthesia and results in skin breakdown in up to 50% of procedures [2]. In a recent series of 11 patients, 64% of whom were referred following varicose vein surgery, an ultrasound-guided protocol of foam sclerotherapy using 3% sodium tetradecyl sulphate produced good cosmetic results, with minimal recurrence of varicosities over 5 years [6]. These patients were treated under sedation and local anaesthetic.

Surgical intervention

Duplex imaging, venography (Figure 4) or MRI should be performed to evaluate the varicosities and to ensure deep venous system patency. Surgery is reserved for selected patients and should be avoided for cosmesis. Superficial vein ligation and stripping may relieve local symptoms, though recurrence of symptoms and varicosities is common. Stripping of large veins should be avoided if the deep veins are atretic or absent [2], since the varicosities and associated symptoms are liable to recur or worsen. CT may also reveal pelvic vascular anomalies.

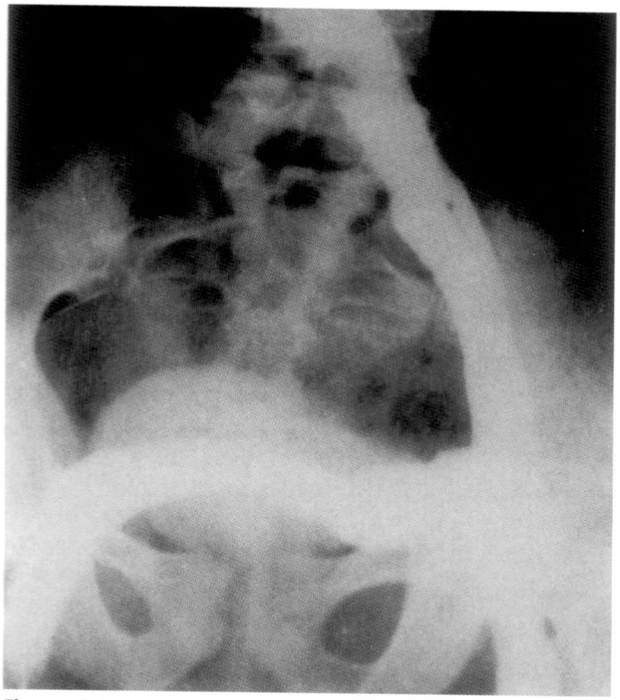

Figure 4. Venogram showing occluded right iliac vein. There is instead a dilated suprapubic vein crossing the symphysis pubis to the left common femoral vein. Reproduced with permission from the Texas Heart Institute Journal, © 1999, Texas Heart Institute [7].

Limb hypertrophy

As for venous malformations, limb hypertrophy should also be dealt with individually. Limb lengths should be monitored with serial scanograms or CT. Conservative treatment includes shoe lifts for posture and gait if the discrepancy is less than 2cm; if greater, limb-shortening procedures should be considered. These include epiphyseal fusion to halt growth in the longer limb, femoral or tibial shortening and epiphyseal stapling, though this is considered to be less reliable. In the rare instance, digit amputation may improve a functional deficit [1].

Management - additional features

Lymphoedema should be managed with pneumatic compression stockings and education regarding skin hygiene. Manual lymphoedema treatment (massage and drainage) should be performed in conjunction with elevation. If severe, surgical debulking of excess skin and subcutaneous tissue may be considered. In view of the propensity to thrombo-embolic disease, surgical patients should always be anticoagulated and patients with KTS should be advised to avoid oral contraceptives and hormone replacement. In the absence of thrombo-embolic disease however, long-term anticoagulation is not thought to be necessary [2]. Where cellulitis is a feature, patients should be treated with antibiotics, either recurrently or prophylactically.

Key points

- **Klippel-Trenaunay syndrome includes a triad of features: capillary malformations, venous malformations and bone and soft tissue hypertrophy.**
- **Symptoms include fatigue, bleeding, cellulitis, lymphoedema and thrombophlebitis.**
- **Treatment is primarily conservative and for symptoms, but may involve laser treatment, sclerotherapy, vein ligation and stripping and orthopaedic procedures for severe limb length discrepancy.**
- **There is increased risk of thrombo-embolic disease. Prophylactic anticoagulation should be employed at times of increased risk, such as surgery. Oral contraceptives and hormone replacement therapy should be avoided.**

References

1. Capraro PA, Fisher J, Hammond DC, Grossman JA. Klippel-Trenaunay syndrome. *Plastic Reconstr Surg* 2001; 109: 2052-60.
2. Jacob AG, Driscoll DJ, Shaughnessy WJ, *et al.* Klippel-Trenaunay syndrome: spectrum and management. *Mayo Clin Proc* 1998; 73: 28-36.
3. Baskerville PA, Ackroyd JS, Lea Thomas M, *et al.* The Klippel-Trenaunay syndrome: clinical, radiological and haemodynamic features and management. *Br J Surg* 1985; 72: 232-6.
4. Tian XL, Kadaba R, You SA, *et al.* Identification of an angiogenic factor that when mutated causes susceptibility to Klippel-Trenaunay syndrome. *Nature* 2004; 427: 640-5.
5. Samuel M, Spitz L. Klippel-Trenaunay syndrome: clinical features, complications and management in children. *Br J Surg* 1995; 82: 757-61.
6. Sorensen S, McDonagh B, Cohen A, *et al.* Management of venous malformations in Klippel-Trenaunay syndrome with ultrasound-guided foam sclerotherapy. *Phlebology* 2005; in press.
7. Kutsal A, Lampros TD, Cobanoglu A. Right iliac vein agenesis, varicosities and widespread hemangiomas. *Texas Heart Inst J* 1999; 26: 149-51.

Chapter 15

Subcutaneous calcification in leg ulcers

Simon D Parvin MD FRCS, Consultant Vascular Surgeon
Royal Bournemouth Hospital, Bournemouth, UK

Introduction

Leg ulcers are extremely common, and consume large amounts of resource. Broadly speaking, their aetiology falls into one of seven groups (Figure 1). They may then be exacerbated by co-existent disease such as diabetes, heart failure leading to peripheral oedema, malnutrition and varicose veins. The majority of ulcers are healed easily once malignancy and vasculitis have been ruled out, and adequate arterial circulation ensured. Next, good granulation tissue must be encouraged by excluding oedema (by bandaging or leg elevation). Occasionally when the ulcer base is chronic, it may be so thickened as to prevent growth of good granulation tissue. Here, excision of the ulcer base back to fresh subcutaneous tissue which bleeds freely will promote healing. When the ulcer is very large, a skin graft may significantly reduce the time needed to achieve healing, once good granulation tissue is present. The problem has usually been keeping the ulcer healed once healing has been achieved.

A small number of ulcers fail to heal despite this proven regimen. Possible causes include non-compliance with treatment, incorrect diagnosis at the outset, and rarely, the presence of subcutaneous calcification.

When present, subcutaneous calcification prevents epithelium from growing over exposed calcified plaque, and thereby prevents final healing.

Historical review

There are few publications on the aetiology and management of leg ulcers with subcutaneous calcification [1,2]. Since 1960 only about five articles have directly addressed this problem. The frequency is difficult to estimate, and probably relates to the use of lower limb X-ray [3]; it might approach 10% of women with chronic venous insufficiency [4]. The rare causes of subcutaneous calcification are shown in Table 1 [5-10]. Previous treatment by injection sclerotherapy has been suggested as a possible cause [3]. The pathophysiology is unclear particularly when calcium and phosphate levels are usually normal. Tissue necrosis due to inflammation may increase alkalinity which might then lead to calcium precipitation. Alkaline phosphatase released by damaged lysosomes may also facilitate the calcification [6].

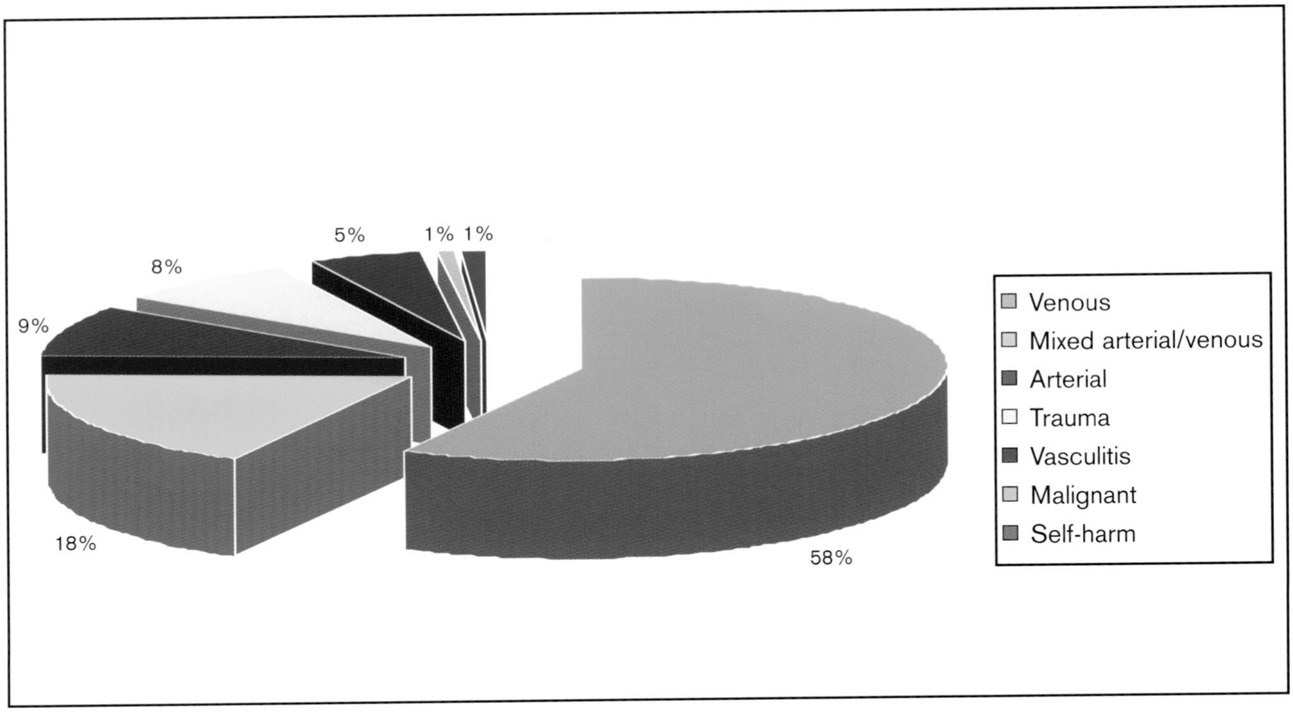

Figure 1. Causes of leg ulcers.

Table 1. Rare causes of subcutaneous calcification in ulcers.
Primary hyperparathyroidism
Secondary hyperparathyroidism
Trauma
Malignant tumours
Pseudoxanthoma elasticum
Ehler-Danlos syndrome
Mixed connective tissue disease [5]
Scleroderma
Systemic lupus erythematosus [6,7]
Radiation overdose [8]
In association with venous hypertension in the leg [9,10]

Clinical presentation

History

Subcutaneous calcification may be present for many years and cause no problems at all provided the skin remains intact. Skin breakdown, usually the result of minor trauma, leads to a chronic non-healing ulcer. In the majority of cases, there are the classical signs of venous hypertension in the lower leg. Most patients will have been treated for long intervals in the community. Ulcers often come close to healing, but then break down again.

Examination

Presentation is typically with a chronic ulcer with thickened fibrotic base and subcutaneous calcification in and around the base and edge of the ulcer. This may not be visible, but is palpable (Figure 2). There is significant surrounding skin damage with lipodermatosclerosis. There are islands of epithelium within the ulcer surrounded by slough. The arterial circulation is usually normal.

On palpation, the surrounding skin feels hard and unyielding. Pressure in one area may distort the skin elsewhere if it is particularly rigid. In severe cases, it feels as though there is bone within the skin. Closer examination of the ulcer base or edge reveals yellowish flakes of calcium. On palpation with a finger, the calcium feels gritty and flakes may sometimes be dislodged.

Investigation and management

The key to the management of this condition is to think of the diagnosis. A plain X-ray will confirm the extent of the problem. Calcification is clearly visible and may extend far away from ulcerated areas around the circumference of the calf (Figure 3). Measurement of serum calcium, phosphate and alkaline phosphatase should be checked, but are likely to be normal.

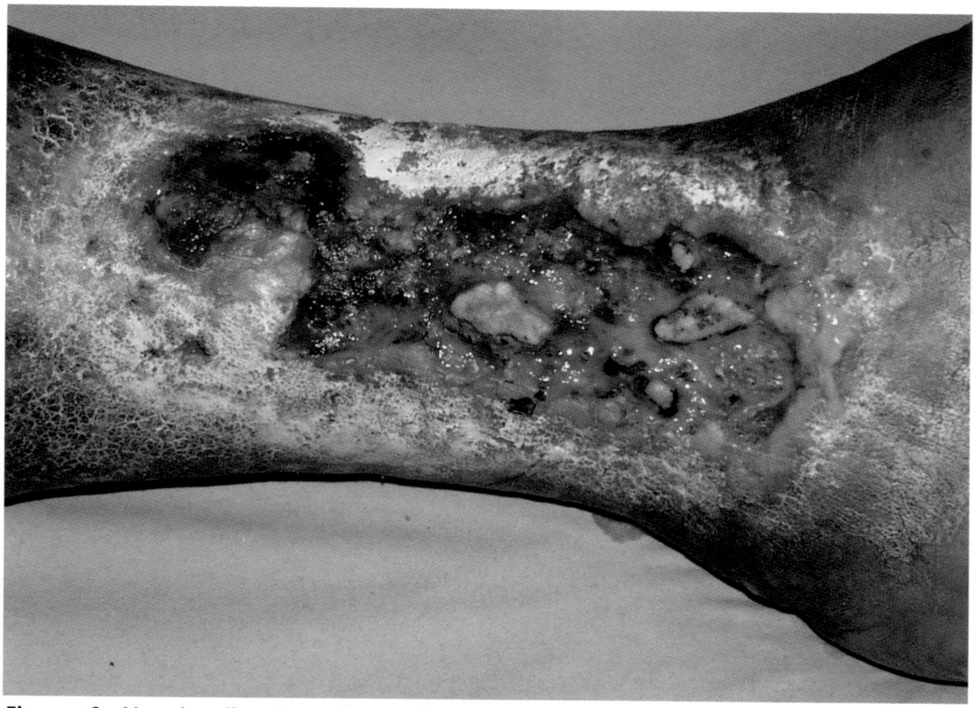

Figure 2. Non-healing leg ulcer with a fibrous base and islands of epithelium. Calcium deposits are palpable within and around the ulcer.

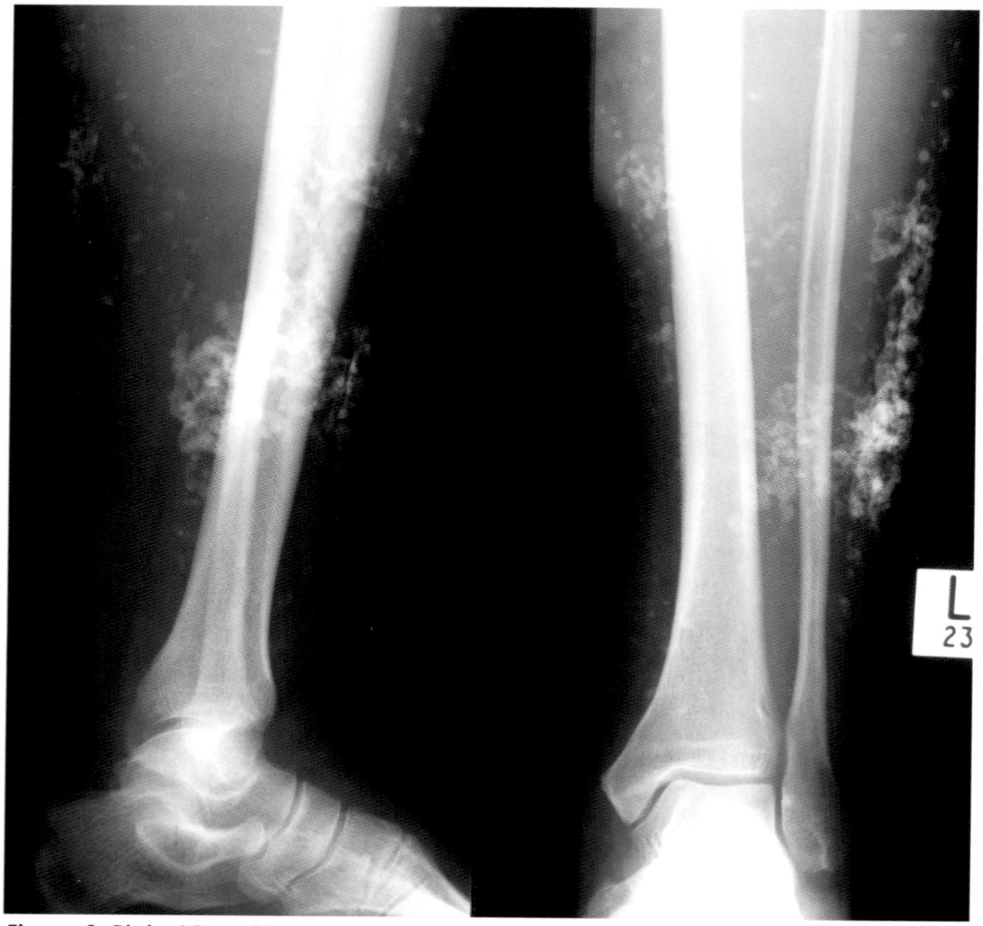

Figure 3. Plain AP and lateral X-ray of the leg showing extensive calcification.

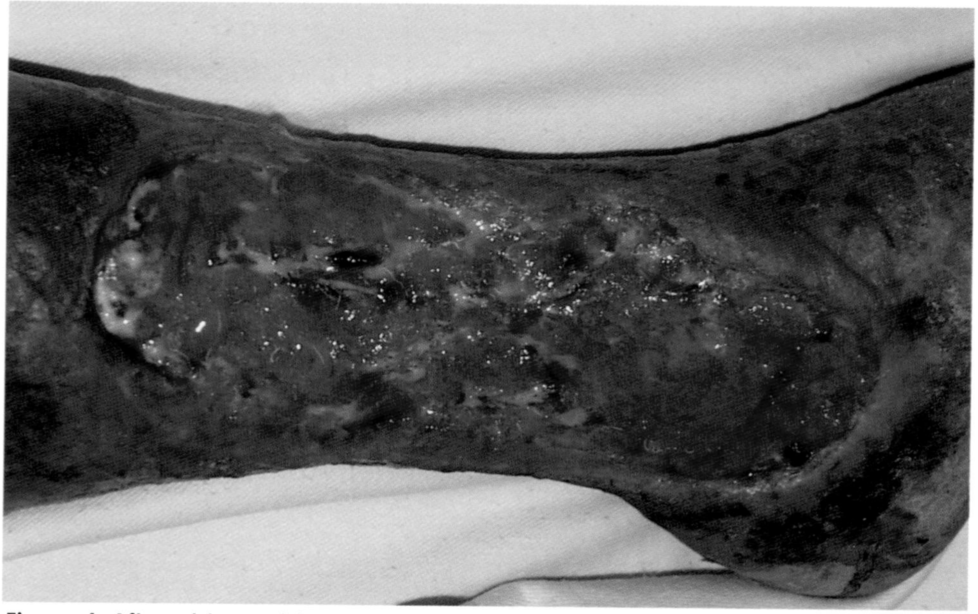

Figure 4. After wide excision back to healthy tissue, with signs of good granulation.

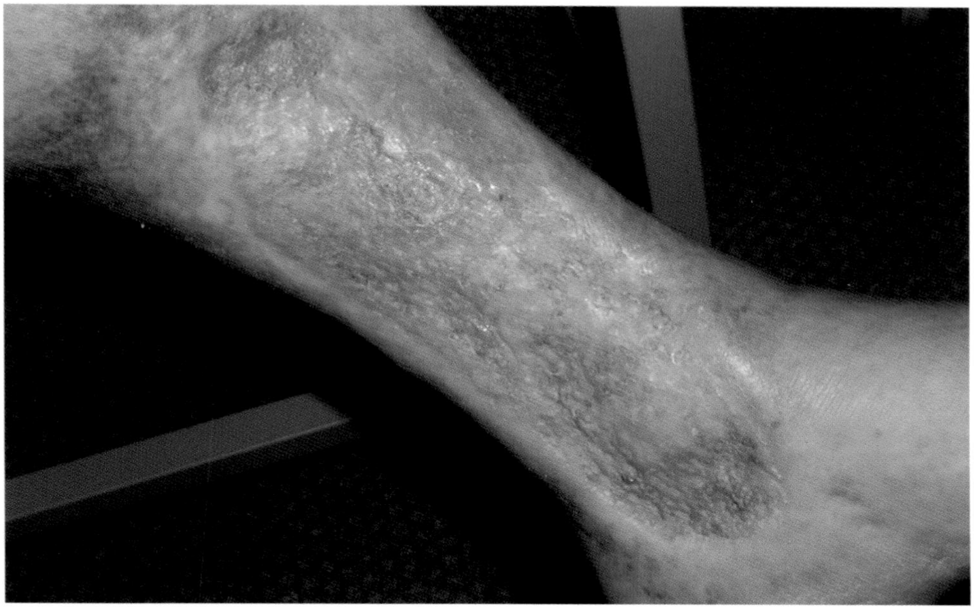

Figure 5. Successful skin grafting.

Surgery

Surgical debridement is the essential first step in management [1,2]. It is not necessary to remove all the calcification, but it is important to ensure that there is no calcium left in the base or at any point in the edge of the ulcer. Sometimes, it is better to remove all the skin from immediately above malleolar level up to mid calf (Figure 4). This is particularly the case when there is widespread ulceration with very extensive skin damage. Once the ulcer is fully granulated, a skin graft can be used to advance healing [10] (Figure 5).

Key points

- **If an ulcer won't heal, consider a plain X-ray to exclude subcutaneous calcification.**
- **Calcified tissue should be excised widely to normal non-calcified subcutaneous tissue.**

References

1. Peled I, Bar-Lev A, Wexler MR. Subcutaneous calcifications of the lower limbs. *Ann Plastic Surgery* 1982; 8: 310-3.
2. Pathy AL, Rae VR, Falanga V. Subcutaneous calcification in venous ulcers: report of a case. *J Dermatol Surg Oncol* 1990; 16: 450-2.
3. Sundquist AB, Kurien VA, Duke M. Subcutaneous calcification of the legs in chronic venous insufficiency. *Conn Med* 1966; 30: 41-2.
4. Lippman J, Goldin RR. Subcutaneous ossification of the legs in chronic venous insufficiency. *Radiology* 1960; 74: 279-88.
5. Itoh O, Nishimaki T, Itoh M, Ohira H, Irisawa A, Kaise S, Kusakawa R. Mixed connective tissue disease with severe pulmonary hypertension and extensive subcutaneous calcification. *Internal Medicine* 1998; 37: 421-5.
6. Nomura M, Okada N, Okada M, Yoshikawa K. Large subcutaneous calcification in systemic lupus erythematosus. *Arch Dermatol* 1990; 126: 1057-9.
7. Park YM, Lee SJ, Kang H, Cho SH. Large subcutaneous calcification in systemic lupus erythematosus: treatment with oral aluminium hydroxide administration followed by surgical excision. *J Korean Med Sci* 1999; 14: 589-92.
8. Lewis VJ, Holt PJ. Subcutaneous calcification following high-dose radiotherapy. *Br J Derm* 2004; 150: 1049-50.
9. Bennison J, Morales A. Subcutaneous calcifications in leg ulcers. *Arch Dermatol* 1964; 90: 314-8.
10. Pathy AL, Falanga V. Subcutaneous calcification in venous ulcers: report of a case. *J Dermatol Surg Oncol* 1990; 16: 450-2.

Case vignette

Marjolin's ulcer

Frank CT Smith BSc MD FRCS FRCS (Ed) FRCS (Glas), Consultant Senior Lecturer, Bristol Royal Infirmary, UK

A squamous cell carcinoma developed in a venous ulcer that had been present for many years in this elderly woman. In the presence of an adequate arterial blood supply, the tumour was excised widely and skin grafted.

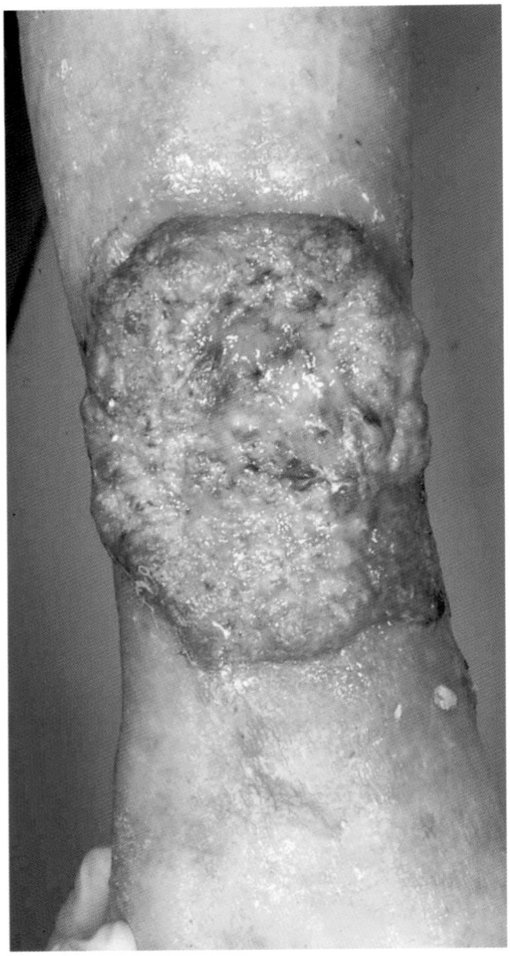

Chapter 16

Carotid and vertebral artery dissection

Demosthenes Dellagrammaticas MB ChB MRCS, Research Fellow
Michael J Gough ChM FRCS, Consultant Vascular Surgeon
The General Infirmary at Leeds, Leeds, UK

Introduction

Carotid and vertebral artery dissections are a relatively rare cause of transient cerebral ischaemia or stroke. Advances in imaging techniques, however, have increased the number of ante-mortem diagnoses of dissections and raised awareness that a significant number of cervical artery dissections produce minimal symptoms or remain asymptomatic. Symptoms occur following either aneurysmal dilatation or stenosis/ occlusion of the affected artery.

Epidemiology

Whilst dissections account for a small number of all strokes, they may be responsible for up to 25% of strokes in young/middle-aged patients, with a peak incidence in the 5th decade [1-3]. They may occur at any age, including childhood, with an estimated annual incidence of 2.5-3 per 100,000 for spontaneous carotid dissection and 1-1.5 per 100,000 for vertebral artery dissection [4,5]. Men and women are affected equally. Trauma is also an important cause of cervical artery dissection and is responsible for 20-50% of cases.

Anatomy

Although dissection can occur in any artery, the extracranial cervical arteries, in contrast to the intracranial vessels, appear particularly prone. This presumably relates to their relative mobility and their proximity to bony structures. The internal carotid artery (ICA) is most commonly involved; dissection of the common carotid artery (CCA) is rare and usually occurs in association with an aortic dissection. The origin of the dissection most commonly occurs in the pharyngeal portion of the ICA rather than at the usual sites of atherosclerotic plaques. In the vertebral arteries the proximal and distal segments are relatively mobile and dissection is more likely there.

Pathophysiology

Following the initial intimal tear, blood is forced between the layers of the arterial wall producing an intramural haematoma within the tunica media. The haematoma may extend subsequently towards either the adventitia or the intima. The former may result in aneurysmal dilatation, whilst the latter may compromise the arterial lumen leading to stenosis or occlusion. A double lumen develops if flow re-enters the lumen at a point distal to the initial tear. It is unclear

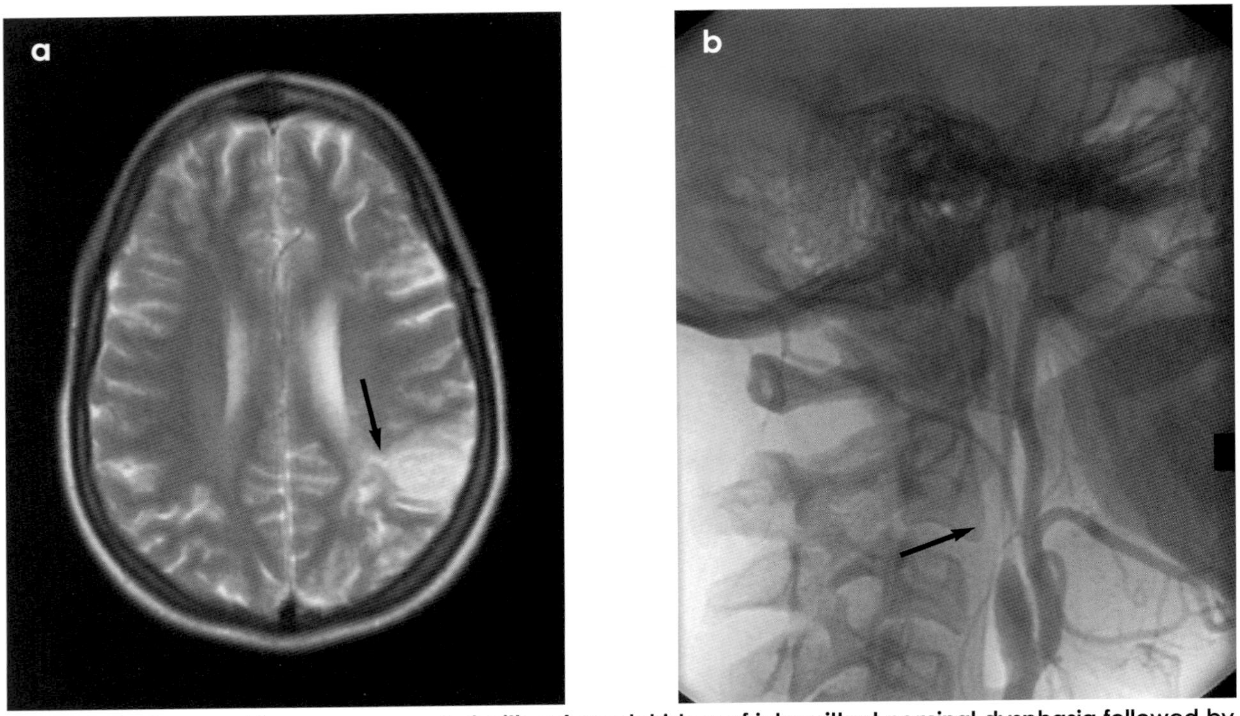

Figure 1. A 19-year-old woman presented with a 4-week history of intermittent nominal dysphasia followed by 2 weeks of increasing weakness of her right arm. a) The MRI was reported as showing a space-occupying lesion (arrow) but craniotomy and biopsy indicated a cerebral infarction. b) A duplex ultrasound demonstrated a small ICA with low-flow velocities suggestive of dissection which was confirmed by angiography (arrow). Antiplatelet therapy was prescribed and the patient made a full recovery. She subsequently developed an acute monoarthritis and livedo reticularis raising the possibility of an underlying connective tissue abnormality.

whether the primary event leading to dissection is the intimal tear or a primary intramural haematoma from the vasa vasorum, with subsequent rupture into the arterial lumen. It is likely that both occur [5,6].

Predisposing factors

Genetic

Some patients with cervical artery dissection may have an underlying arterial wall abnormality, including inherited vascular conditions such as Marfan's syndrome, Ehlers-Danlos Type IV syndrome, alpha-1 antitrypsin deficiency, osteogenesis imperfecta and autosomal dominant polycystic kidney disease [7,8]. Although these clearly defined anomalies are only recognised in a minority of patients, others may have a clinically suspicious but uncharacterised connective tissue disorder (Figure 1). This may explain familial clustering in up to 5% of cases [9]. Further, some familial cases have been associated with multiple cutaneous lentigines, bicuspid aortic valves and angiolipomatosis. This implicates a defect in the development of neural crest tissue in a predisposition to dissection, given the common development of the arterial media, melanocytes and aortic valve cusps.

Other associated conditions may include homocysteinaemia (no specific genotype identified), fibromuscular dysplasia, and cystic medial necrosis (Figure 2). However, these vessel wall abnormalities are non-specific and are found in various arterial diseases. Similarly, although changes in the ultrastructure of collagen have been suggested, no particular genetic defect is identified in most patients with dissection.

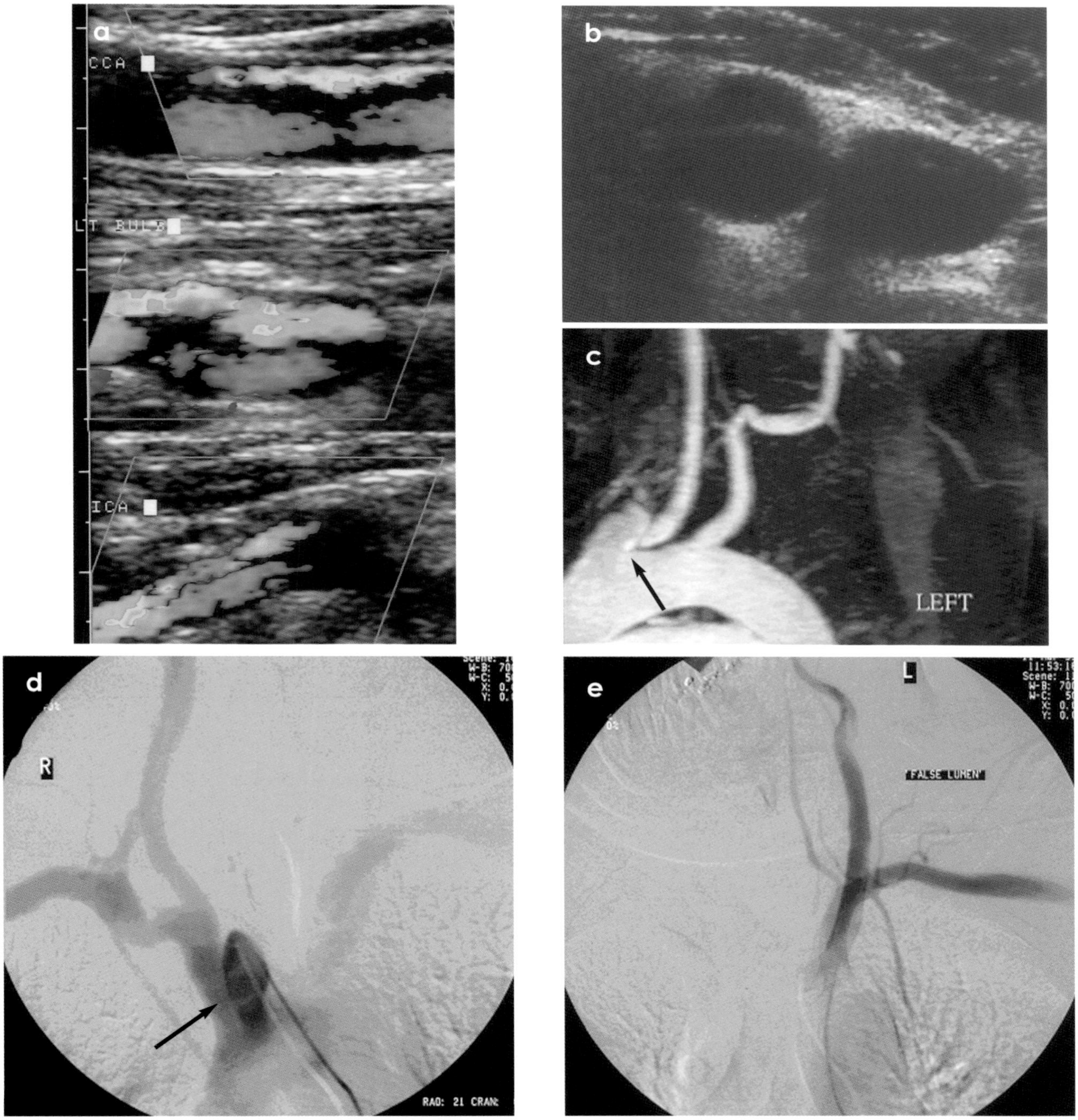

Figure 2. A 65-year-old hypertensive man developed a sudden headache and right arm monoparesis lasting less than 24 hours. A cerebral CT was normal but ultrasound was reported as showing a >70% left ICA stenosis. He was referred for carotid endarterectomy. a) & b) Repeat ultrasound revealed a double lumen within the CCA extending into the ICA. An intimal flap was visible on the transverse images. c) d) & e) MRA and arch aortography were considered to show a saccular aneurysm of the aortic arch close to the origin of the innominate artery (IA) (arrows) and confirmed the false lumen in the CCA. At operation (performed for risk of aneurysm rupture or stroke) dissections of both the IA and CCA were confirmed. The aortic arch was normal. Both arteries were divided at their origins and oversewn and an 18 x 9mm bifurcated dacron graft was anastomosed to the ascending aorta and the distal ends of the IA and CCA. Subsequent progress over 5 years has been unremarkable. Histology of the aortic arch/innominate artery revealed cystic medial degeneration.

Environmental

Conventional risk factors for vascular disease (hypertension, hypercholesterolaemia, smoking) do not seem to have a major role in the pathogenesis of cervical artery dissection; atherosclerosis is uncommon in these patients [5]. Recent general or focal head and neck trauma (road traffic accidents, sporting injuries) is a feature of some cases whilst others may present with possible minor trauma as a potential precipitating event. The latter include bouts of coughing, sneezing, vomiting, the Heimlich manoeuvre, chiropractic manipulation and other sudden neck movements that may cause sufficient stretching of the artery to result in a dissection. Nevertheless it is difficult to exclude an underlying structural defect of the arterial wall in all of these patients.

More recently, it has been suggested that an infectious trigger may be important in some patients. This hypothesis is based on case control studies, indicating an increased incidence of upper respiratory tract infections, various other infections such as gastro-enteritis and a seasonal variation with a peak incidence in autumn. The mechanisms by which infection may be relevant are unclear.

Clinical features

The mode of presentation depends upon the artery affected, although many dissections remain asymptomatic or present with minimal symptoms initially. Local symptoms typically precede cerebral symptoms by hours or days, allowing a window of opportunity for definitive diagnosis and intervention. Confirmation of the diagnosis has become easier with advances in non-invasive vascular imaging.

Internal carotid artery

Local symptoms

The commonest local symptom is sharp pain, localised to the neck or radiating to the jaw, pharynx or face. Others include a throbbing headache, ipsilateral Horner's syndrome without anhidrosis (sweat fibres accompany the external carotid artery), due to stretching or compression of peri-arterial sympathetic fibres, pulsatile tinnitus, and cranial nerve palsies, particularly affecting the lower cranial nerves such as the hypoglossal nerve. The presence of such a lesion with concomitant pain should alert the clinician to the possibility of dissection.

Cerebral symptoms

Cerebral ischaemic symptoms may range from a transient ischaemic attack, including amaurosis fugax, to a major cerebral infarction and stroke. The classic triad of neck pain, Horner's syndrome and cerebral or retinal ischaemia only occurs in one third of patients [5]. Contrary to expectation, strokes are more likely to be embolic in nature than due to hypoperfusion. This is supported by the pattern of ischaemic lesions, which are typically in the distribution of the major basal cerebral vessels rather than in watershed areas.

Common carotid artery

When symptomatic, CCA dissection may also present with ipsilateral cervical pain. Horner's syndrome and cranial nerve lesions do not occur, although other neurological symptoms are similar to those associated with ICA dissection but are less common. This may reflect the additional contribution to cerebral perfusion via cross-neck collaterals from the contralateral external carotid artery.

Vertebral artery

Local symptoms

Pain in the ipsilateral neck and lateral occiput is commonly described and typically precedes any cerebral symptoms. Motor deficits or pain in the ipsilateral upper arm due to compression of the cervical spinal nerve roots have also been described.

Cerebral symptoms

Transient ischaemic attacks are uncommon following vertebral artery dissection with most symptoms resulting from a lateral medullary infarction

(Wallenberg's syndrome: diplopia, swallowing difficulties, clumsiness, gait ataxia, sensory deficits - Figure 3). The thalamus, cerebellum or cerebral hemispheres in the distribution of the posterior circulation may also be affected. A rare complication of vertebral artery dissection is isolated ischaemia of the cervical spinal cord.

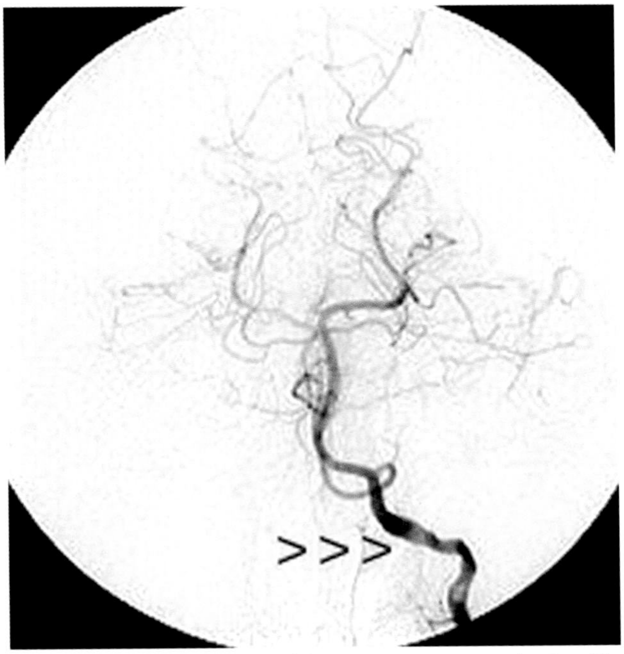

Figure 3. A 43-year-old woman presented with vertigo, vomiting, numbness of the left side of the face, transient swallowing difficulty, diplopia and clumsiness. This had been preceded by pain in the left neck of 3 weeks' duration. Clinical examination and a cerebral MRI scan were consistent with a posterolateral medullary infarction (Wallenberg's syndrome) and angiography confirmed a spontaneous vertebral artery dissection which, when re-imaged after 3 months of warfarin therapy appeared normal.

Diagnosis

Clinical suspicion that prompts suitable imaging is the key to accurate diagnosis. Failure to recognise the appropriate symptoms may lead to an incorrect diagnosis and inappropriate management (Figure 1).

Duplex ultrasound imaging

Colour-flow duplex ultrasound has the advantage of visualising the arterial wall and lumen, as well as providing haemodynamic information. This may be combined with transcranial Doppler to assess the distal effects of a stenosis or occlusion on cerebral perfusion and to detect embolic events.

A characteristic stenosis or tapered occlusion in association with an intramural haematoma or a double lumen separated by an intimal flap are found in fewer than a third of patients, although abnormal flow patterns are seen in at least 90% [10]. These include high-resistance flow (low-flow velocity, increased pulsatility index) in the ipsilateral CCA, stump flow in the carotid bulb or staccato flow (high-resistance obstructive flow: reduced systolic flow, absent or reduced diastolic flow) in the ICA. The absence of atherosclerotic disease may also support the diagnosis of dissection. Although similar flow abnormalities may be seen in the vertebral arteries, detection of morphological abnormalities is less likely. When an ultrasound examination is suspicious of dissection it should be followed by definitive imaging.

Ultrasound imaging is also useful in the follow-up of dissections to monitor recanalisation of stenoses and occlusions that occurs in the majority of patients.

Magnetic resonance imaging (MRI)

On T1- and T2-weighted cross-sectional MRI, an intramural haematoma may be seen as a crescentic area of hyperintensity surrounding a narrowed lumen, whilst 3-D time-of-flight magnetic resonance angiography (MRA) may demonstrate a tapered occlusion or stenosis (string sign) of the artery. Despite reported sensitivities and specificities in the order of 84-95% and 99%, differentiation of intraluminal thrombus from slow flow may be difficult on MR and the sensitivity for detection of aneurysmal dissection may be low. Some of these limitations may be overcome by contrast-enhanced MRA.

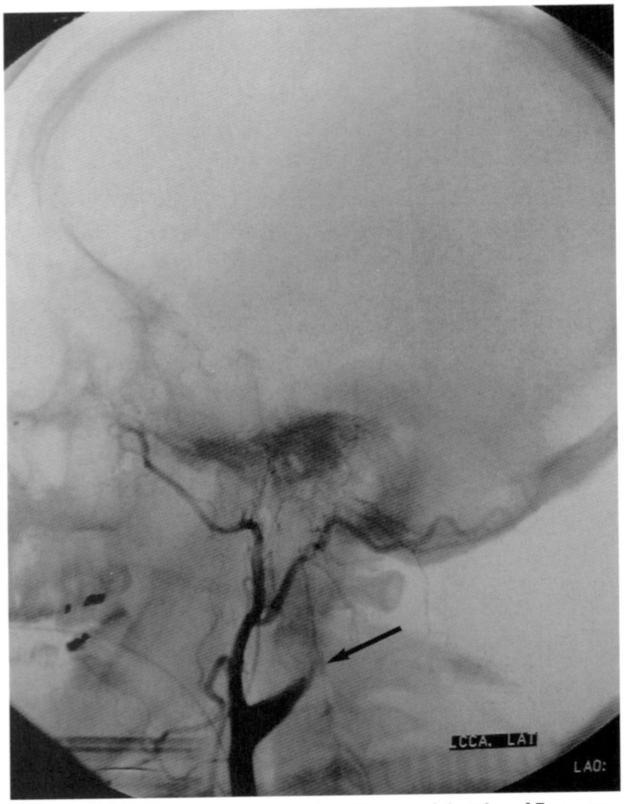

Figure 4. Following a road traffic accident a 45-year-old male developed a right upper limb monoparesis which progressed to a hemiplegia. Angiography demonstrated a tapered occlusion of the left ICA (flame sign) (arrow). Following 3 months of anticoagulation there was an improvement in the neurological signs, although the ICA remained occluded.

Angiography

Intra-arterial catheter angiography is still regarded as the reference standard for the diagnosis of cervical artery dissection. It also demonstrates underlying anomalies such as fibromuscular dysplasia or vessel tortuosity. In the ICA, the most frequent finding is an irregular, tapered string sign which extends from 2-3cm distal to its origin to the base of the petrous bone, with abrupt reconstitution of the vessel lumen. A double lumen, the pathognomonic finding in dissection, or a tapered occlusion (flame sign) is seen in 10% and 20%, respectively (Figure 4). Aneurysmal dilatation (typically a saccular aneurysm leading to the misdiagnosis of a pseudo-aneurysm) is most commonly seen in the subcranial ICA. Vertebral artery dissections are most common at the level of the first and second cervical vertebrae. A double lumen or an intimal flap is rarely seen.

Computed tomography (CT)

One series reported a high sensitivity and specificity for helical CT in detecting stenosis or occlusion due to ICA dissection. Characteristically, there is eccentric luminal narrowing of the artery and an increase in its external diameter. However, the role of CT in the diagnosis of dissection requires further evaluation.

Prognosis

Approximately 70% of patients that present with local signs attributable to ICA dissection will develop symptoms of cerebral ischaemia. The subsequent outcome depends on the severity of the initial ischaemic insult, although more than two thirds make a good functional recovery and mortality is less than 5%. The use of less invasive imaging has increased the numbers of minimally symptomatic or even asymptomatic dissections that are identified and thus the prognosis appears to be improving.

Less invasive imaging has also allowed easy monitoring of the natural history of cervical artery dissections and it is apparent that recanalisation of severe stenoses and occlusions occurs in up to 90% and 75%, respectively. Further, a third of aneurysms decrease in size. Nevertheless, although aneurysm rupture has not been reported in extracranial cervical dissections, persisting aneurysms may cause recurrent ischaemic events for several years following their development.

Recurrent dissection of an affected artery is rare, although dissection may occur in a previously unaffected artery in the same patient. The estimated risk is 1% per year and is more likely in patients with an inherited arteriopathy such as Ehlers-Danlos syndrome (see Chapter 7, Ehlers-Danlos syndrome).

Finally, a persistent headache or cervical pain is not uncommon, although in most patients this resolves within 1 week.

Treatment

The optimum management for cervical artery dissections is unclear. Anticoagulation, antiplatelet drugs, endovascular treatment and surgery have all been advocated in different situations, although there are no controlled studies to compare outcome following these various strategies.

Conservative

Most dissections heal spontaneously and conservative management with 3-6 months of systemic anticoagulation (heparin followed by warfarin) is most frequently adopted. Some authors have suggested that this might delay healing or promote extension of the dissection and have recommended antiplatelet therapy as an alternative. In a recent Cochrane Review there was no evidence that either regimen was superior and in the absence of any control studies there did not appear to be any sound basis for either treatment [11]. A large study of 116 patients similarly showed no difference in outcome events between these treatment options [12].

The rationale for anticoagulation is based on evidence from transcranial Doppler and cross-sectional imaging studies, suggesting that most cerebral events after dissection are thrombo-embolic. However, a recent study using diffusion-weighted MRI has indicated that both haemodynamic and thrombo-embolic factors may be important in stroke following ICA dissection.

Serial non-invasive imaging should be performed to assess dissection healing as part of conservative therapy.

Endovascular treatment

Advances in endovascular techniques have led to enthusiasm for treating cervical artery dissections. This may be appropriate when symptoms persist despite anticoagulation, where there is a risk of stroke due to hypoperfusion, or when local symptoms are unremitting. Options include intra-arterial or intravenous thrombolysis for which promising results have been reported following ICA or middle cerebral artery occlusion [13] or endovascular stenting, which at least in small series, appears to have excellent results [14,15].

In general, endovascular treatment should be reserved for complicated cases where the risk of stroke is considered high.

Surgical treatment

The indications for surgical treatment are the same as those for endovascular therapy. In the largest operative series, patients were offered surgery when a high-grade stenosis or aneurysm persisted after a median of 9 months of anticoagulation. Most were treated by ligation of the affected artery followed by *in situ* bypass; a small number underwent thrombo-endarterectomy and patch closure. In patients where an ICA dissection extended beyond the base of the skull, ligation or clipping of the artery was performed [16]. Others have suggested that the latter might be combined with intracranial-extracranial bypass, although endovascular treatment may be more appropriate. In general, surgical treatment is technically demanding and associated with significant morbidity. Careful anatomical assessment is vital before intervention is contemplated.

Key points

- Cervical artery dissections are a significant cause of cerebral ischaemic events in young patients.
- Subtle and variable local symptoms commonly precede the cerebral event.
- Clinical suspicion warrants initial assessment with ultrasound or magnetic resonance but the definitive diagnosis is usually confirmed by arteriography or magnetic resonance angiography.
- Conservative treatment is appropriate for most patients.
- Follow-up assessment by magnetic resonance angiography determines the length of treatment.
- Endovascular therapy or surgery might be required for patients with recurrent symptoms, enlarging aneurysms or complicated dissections.

References

1. Bogousslavsky J, Despland PA, Regli F. Spontaneous carotid dissection with acute stroke. *Arch Neurol* 1987; 44: 137-40.
2. Cerrato P, Grasso M, Imperiale D, *et al.* Stroke in young patients: etiopathogenesis and risk factors in different age classes. *Cerebrovasc Dis* 2004; 18: 154-9.
3. Dziewas R, Konrad C, Drdger B, *et al.* Cervical artery dissection - clinical features, risk factors, therapy and outcome in 126 patients. *J Neurol* 2003; 250: 1179-84.
4. Schievink WI, Mokri B, Whisnant JP. Internal carotid artery dissection in a community Rochester, Minnesota, 1987-1992. *Stroke* 1993; 24: 1678-80.
5. Schievink WI. Spontaneous dissection of the carotid and vertebral arteries. *N Engl J Med* 2001; 344: 898-906.
6. Guillon B, Livy C, Bousser MG. Internal carotid artery dissection: an update. *J Neurol Sci* 1998; 153: 146-58.
7. Schievink WI, Michels VV, Piepgras DG. Neurovascular manifestations of heritable connective tissue disorders A review. *Stroke* 1994; 25: 889-903.
8. Vila N, Millan M, Ferrer X, Riutort N, Escudero D. Levels of alpha1-antitrypsin in plasma and risk of spontaneous cervical artery dissections: a case-control study. *Stroke* 2003: E168-9.
9. Schievink WI, Mokri B, Piepgras DG, Kuiper JD. Recurrent spontaneous arterial dissections: risk in familial versus nonfamilial disease. *Stroke* 1996; 27: 622-4.
10. Logason K, Hardemark HG, Barlin T, *et al.* Duplex scan findings in patients with spontaneous cervical artery dissections. *Eur J Vasc Endovasc Surg* 2002; 23: 295-8.
11. Lyrer P, Engelter S. Antithrombotic drugs for carotid artery dissection. *Cochrane Database Syst Rev* 2003(3): CD000255.
12. Beletsky V, Nadareishvili Z, Lynch J, Shuaib A, Woolfenden A, Norris JW. Cervical arterial dissection: time for a therapeutic trial? *Stroke* 2003; 34: 2856-60.
13. Leistner S, Hartmann A, Marx P, Koennecke HC. Successful thrombolytic treatment of intracranial carotid occlusion due to dissection. *Eur Neurol* 2001; 45: 284-5.
14. Bergeron P, Khanoyan P, Meunier JP, Graziani JN, Gay J. Long-term results of endovascular exclusion of extracranial internal carotid artery aneurysms and dissecting aneurysm. *J Intervent Cardiol* 2004; 17: 245-52.
15. Assadian A, Senekowitsch C, Rotter R, Zolss C, Strassegger J, Hagmuller GW. Long-term results of covered stent repair of internal carotid artery dissections. *J Vasc Surg* 2004; 40: 484-7.
16. Muller BT, Luther B, Hort W, *et al.* Surgical treatment of 50 carotid dissections: indications and results. *J Vasc Surg* 2000; 31: 980-8.

Chapter 17

Carotid body tumour

M Shafique Sajid FRCS, Clinical Vascular Fellow
Daryll M Baker PhD FRCS, Consultant Vascular Surgeon
Royal Free Hospital, London, UK

Introduction

The carotid body is a 3-5mm sized organ located in the adventitial layer of the common carotid artery at the bifurcation. As a chemoreceptor organ it detects blood pCO_2, pO_2 and pH, and initiates reflex changes in cardiovascular and respiratory activity. When a tumour develops it remains encapsulated within the adventitia.

Carotid body tumours (CBT) are the commonest neoplasms that derive from embryological neural crest tissue, called paragangliomas. They are closely related to phaeochromocytomas. CBT present as encapsulated, firm round masses within the adventitia of the bifurcation of the common carotid artery. They are usually asymptomatic, but large masses may encroach upon the parapharyngeal space and produce pressure symptoms. They are rare tumours, but comprise the majority (60-70%) of head and neck paragangliomas. Most CBT are benign, but malignant transformation can occur.

Incidence and geographical perspective

CBT has an incidence of 1 in 30,000. This is higher in patients with chronic obstructive pulmonary disease and people living at high altitude, such as Peru or New Mexico. The peak age of incidence is between 45-55 years and the sex distribution is equal. Some 7-15% of paragangliomas are familial and 90% of these are CBT, with autosomal dominant inheritance. Familial CBT present at a younger age and can be associated with other types of paragangliomas. About 25% of inherited cases are bilateral compared with only 3% of sporadic forms.

Historical aspects

Von Haller first described the carotid body in 1743. In 1762, Heller introduced the term glomus tumour and this was re-established by Guild in 1953. Reigner attempted excision of a CBT in 1880, but the patient died. Maydl also attempted CBT excision in 1886 but this patient developed a stroke. The first successful CBT excision was performed by Albert in 1889. Kohn first introduced the term paraganglioma in 1903. In 1950, Mulligan proposed the term chemodectoma to

Stage I	Stage II	Stage III
Confined between carotid bifurcation.	Starts encircling carotids.	Tumour encircles carotids completely and extends beyond them.

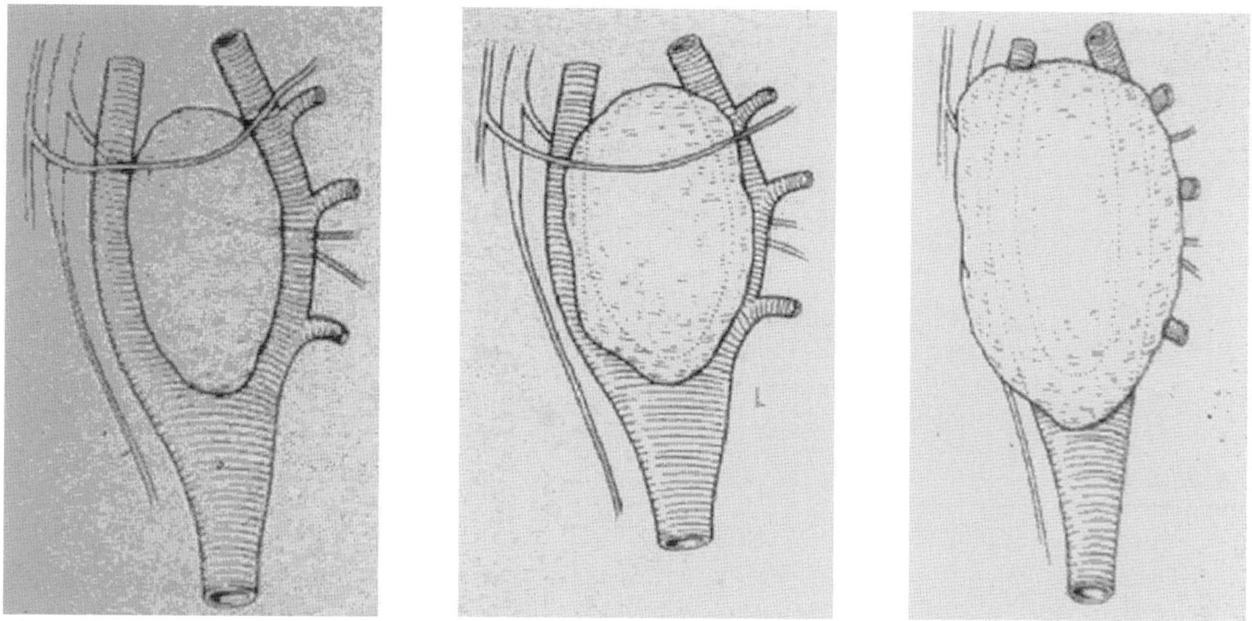

Figure 1. The Shamblin classification of carotid body tumours based on tumour position and extension.

reflect the origin from chemoreceptor tissue. Based on the work of Glenner and Grimley the term paraganglioma is now the most widely used to classify CBT [1].

Classification

CBT can be classified as follows:

- Sporadic: these comprise 80-90% of CBT, are more common in women and 10% are bilateral. Some 6-12% are malignant.
- Hyperplastic: these include about 3-5% of all CBT and have equal sex distribution. They are more common in people living at altitude and with lung disease; they are rarely malignant but are generally (90%) bilateral.
- Familial: this group constitutes 7-9% of all CBT, one third are bilateral and a quarter are malignant. They occur at a younger age and with equal sex incidence. Screening of high-risk individuals is recommended from the age of 16-18 years.

Surgeons prefer the anatomical classification that describes the position of the tumour with respect to the carotid bifurcation. The Shamblin classification also predicts how difficult the operation will be to remove the CBT and the rate of complications (Figure 1).

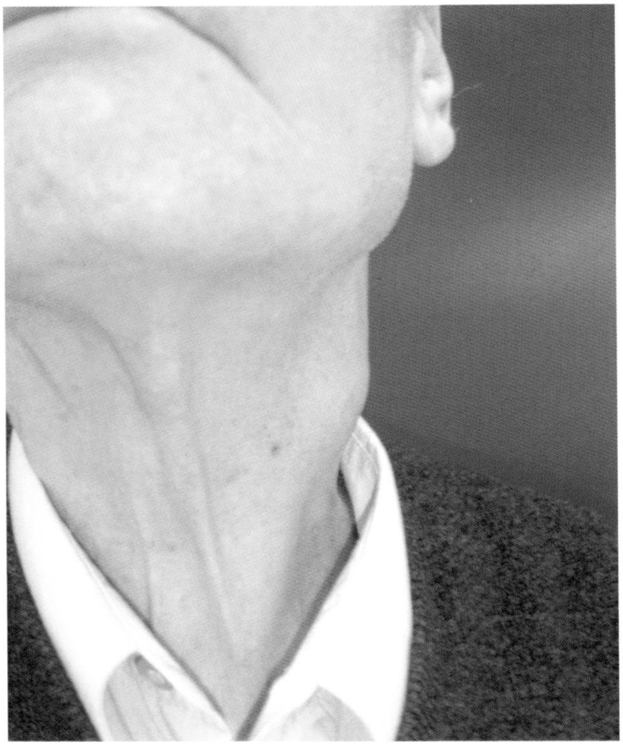

Figure 2. Carotid body tumour presenting as an asymptomatic lump in the neck.

Histopathology

CBT is a well defined, lobulated solid mass with a fibrous pseudocapsule. The size varies between 1-8cm. The external surface is tan-gray and the cut surface shows many blood vessels. Both light and electron microscopy reveal a biphasic pattern identical to that seen in other paragangliomas consisting of two cell types: chief cells and sustentacular cells. These cells form clusters called zenballen by Kohn. Nuclear pleomorphism and cellular hyperchromatism are common. Often there are areas of spindle cells called sarcomatoid foci. The stroma surrounding the two cell lines consists of a mixture of nerve fibres, endothelial cells and vascular pericytes.

Clinical presentation

CBT usually presents as a painless, slow-growing lump in the side of the neck (Figure 2). Most are asymptomatic, but a few cause pressure symptoms such as dysphagia, tongue paresis, dysphonia, stridor, dyspnoea or hoarseness. Cranial nerves IX-XII are most commonly involved. Rarely, a patient may present with focal neurological symptoms such as transient ischaemic attack. When a CBT contains functioning tissue or has an associated functioning paraganglioma such as a phaeochromocytoma, hypertension, blushing and palpitations may occur. The carotid body tumour syndrome consists of attacks of bradycardia, hypotension and loss of consciousness caused by compression of the carotid bifurcation by tumour.

Examination reveals a smooth, mildly tender, firm lump, usually in the anterior triangle of the neck. The characteristic feature of a CBT is that it is mobile in lateral directions but immobile vertically. There is often a palpable thrill or an audible bruit over the lump. Symptoms from a functioning tumour may also be elicited.

Investigation

Duplex ultrasound is the simplest and most accurate investigation to identify (and follow-up) CBT. On ultrasound it appears as an oval, heterogeneously hyperechoic solid mass in the neck that splays the carotid bifurcation. The vascularity of the tumour can also be defined [2]. Encasement of the carotid vessels can be visualised by transoesophageal ultrasound imaging.

CT can demonstrate tumours above 8mm in diameter as a soft tissue mass in the carotid space giving homogeneous and intense enhancement following intravenous contrast injection. Splaying of the carotid vessels is very suggestive of CBT. The main value of CT is to exclude the presence of other associated head and neck tumours.

On MRI, CBT typically exhibit low signal intensity with standard spin-echo, short TR/TE and long TR/short TE sequence, and high signal intensity with long TR/TE sequence. So, MRI can identify lesions smaller than 5mm [3]. Homogenous intense enhancement is also seen after intravenous contrast

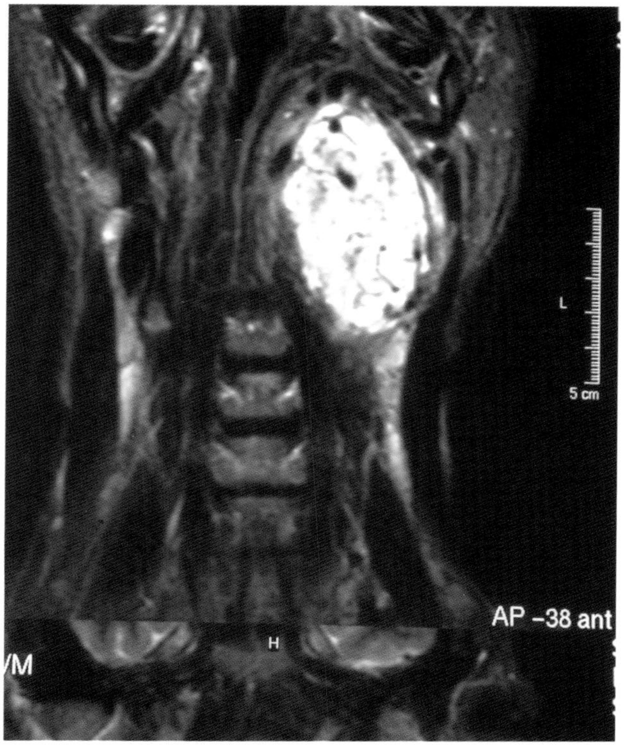

Figure 3. MR image showing a vascular carotid body tumour.

that demonstrates excessive vascularity of the tumour and gives rise to a "salt and pepper" appearance (Figure 3).

Angiography shows a hypervascular mass lying at the carotid bifurcation with splaying of the carotids (Figure 4). It can also depict enlarged feeding arteries, an intense tumour blush and early draining veins. Many surgeons prefer pre-operative angiography before planning a resection [2].

Other possible investigations include Indium-111 labelled octreotide imaging, which reliably detects tumours greater than 1.5cm in diameter, but is insensitive for tumours less than 1cm in diameter. It has been used as a screening investigation in familial disease and to help differentiate CBT from other nerve sheath tumours. It can identify other similar paragangliomas elsewhere in the body and gives an indication as to their functional activity. Positron emission tomography is also reported to be very accurate in the diagnosis of paragangliomas, including CBT. However, it is rarely used since it gives little data about surrounding structures and seldom adds to the information gained from other investigations.

Treatment

There is no conservative treatment for CBT; radiotherapy and drugs have no effect. Small tumours in elderly patients may be left alone and simply observed; it is unlikely they will grow to cause complications within the patient's lifetime. The risk of local complications as the tumour enlarges means that surgery is the treatment of choice for most CBT. For the best outcomes, a vascular specialist should undertake the procedure when the tumour is small [4,5]. In the past many tumours were referred after surgical biopsy had been done to make the diagnosis. This can be disastrous, as severe bleeding ensues. Modern diagnostic imaging should make this obsolete. Accurate pre-operative disease staging enables pre-operative planning of the procedure, and medical and anaesthetic optimisation is an advantage. Some surgeons believe that pre-operative embolisation of feeding vessels can reduce the vascularity of a CBT and hence operative blood loss, but this remains unproven in controlled trials [3].

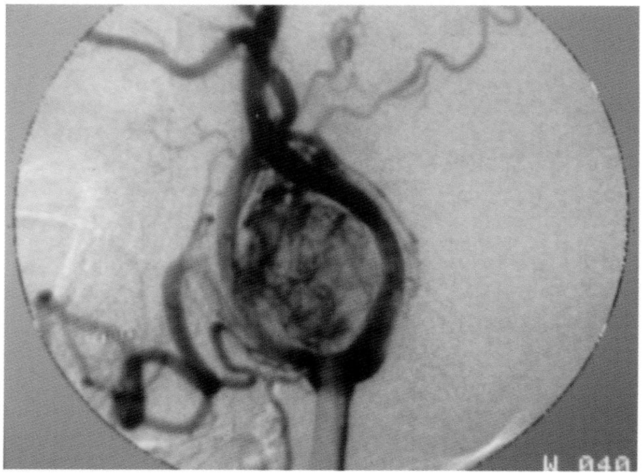
Figure 4. Digital subtraction angiogram showing a hypervascular carotid body tumour splaying the carotid bifurcation.

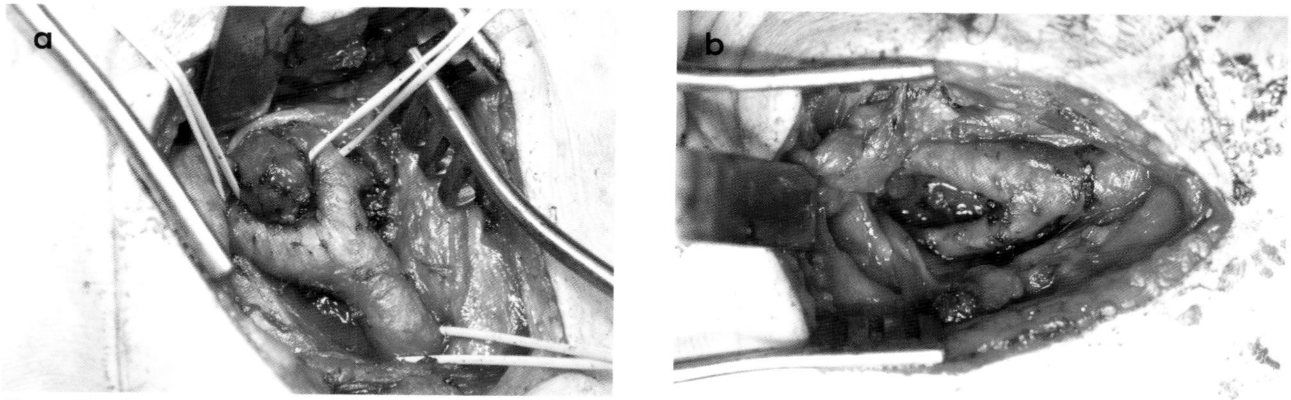

Figure 5. Operative illustration of removal of a small carotid body tumour. a) During dissection, the carotid vessels are all taped. b) After removal of the tumour. Courtesy of Mr. SD Parvin.

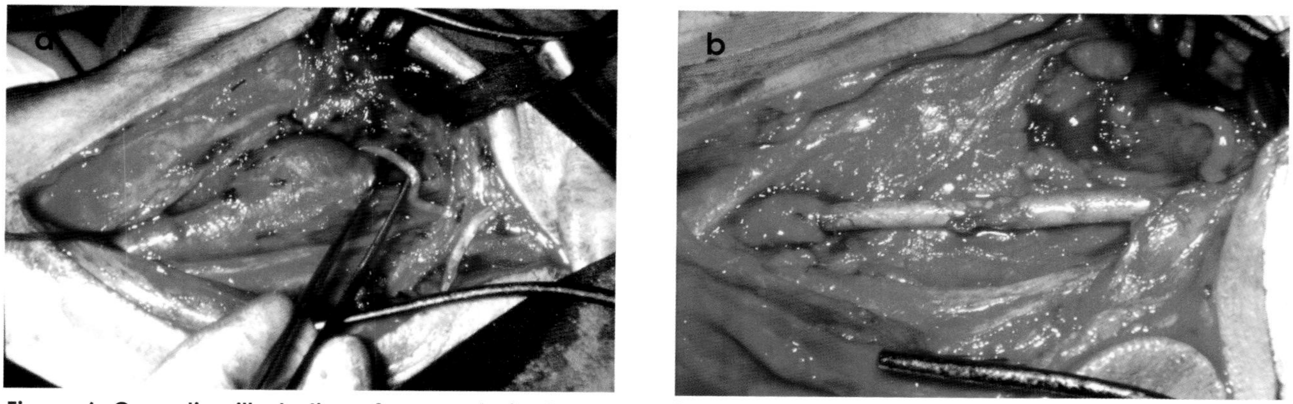

Figure 6. Operative illustration of removal of a large carotid body tumour that required sacrifice of the carotid bifurcation. a) During dissection. b) Continuity is restored with an interposition long saphenous vein graft. Courtesy of Professor A Mansfield.

Surgery involves a wide exposure of the carotid vessels and the surrounding cranial nerves. All the individual structures are dissected and taped to achieve arterial control. The CBT is dissected out along the "bloodless" subadventitial plane (the white line) as the CBT lies within adventitia, using careful diathermy excision and ligatures (Figure 5). Occasionally, the tumour is so extensive, or the carotid artery is damaged during dissection, such that the carotid vessels have to be sacrificed and a reversed saphenous vein graft is used to restore arterial continuity (Figure 6). A carotid shunt will be necessary during this procedure to avoid a stroke [6].

Complication rates are higher for large tumours that require extensive surgery [7]. These include the following:

- *Cranial nerve palsy.* This has an incidence of 18-44% and, unlike after carotid endarterectomy, is permanent in 50%. Hypoglossal nerve palsy produces a clumsy tongue, vagus nerve palsy causes hoarseness, and glossopharyngeal nerve palsy results in dysphagia or choking. Sympathetic nerve damage can result in Horner's syndrome.
- *Airway compromise.* This can occur particularly when manoeuvres such as mandibular subluxation or nasotracheal intubation are required for extensive tumours and is the result of haematoma, laryngeal oedema or vocal cord paresis [8].
- *Stroke.* The overall postoperative stroke and death rate in large series is about 6%.

Most patients have an uncomplicated recovery after surgery for CBT performed by an expert team. Recurrence rates are low (6%), and generally occur only after excision of large or familial tumours. Following successful resection the prognosis is the same as for an age- and sex-matched individual. The need for duplex follow-up is questionable in sporadic cases, but is required for familial CBT.

Acknowledgement

The authors would like to thank Mr. SD Parvin, Royal Bournemouth Hospital, and Professor A Mansfield, St. Mary's Hospital, London, for kindly providing Figures 5 and 6 respectively.

Key points

- Carotid body tumours are rare, but they are still the commonest of the head and neck paragangliomas.
- There are distinct sporadic and familial forms.
- Duplex ultrasound imaging is effective in making the diagnosis, but angiography and CT or MRI are helpful to plan surgery.
- Excision is indicated for most tumours, but the surgery is not risk-free and the best results are achieved by a specialist team.

References

1. van der Mey AG, Jansen JC, Baalen JM. Management of carotid body tumors. *Otolaryngol Clin North Am* 2001; 34: 907-24.
2. Muhm M, Polterauer P, Gstottner W, *et al.* Diagnostic and therapeutic approaches to carotid body tumors. Review of 24 patients. *Arch Surg* 1997; 132: 279-84.
3. Westerband A, Hunter GC, Cintora I, *et al.* Current trends in the detection and management of carotid body tumors. *J Vasc Surg* 1998; 28: 84-93.
4. Barros D'Sa AAB, Harkin DW, McIlrath E, McBride RJ. One vascular surgeon's experience in managing carotid body tumours. *Br J Surg* 2003; 90: A507.
5. Patetsios P, Gable DR, Garrett WV, *et al.* Management of carotid body paragangliomas and review of a 30-year experience. *Ann Vasc Surg* 2002; 16: 331-8.
6. Maxwell JG, Jones SW, Wilson E, *et al.* Carotid body tumor excisions: adverse outcomes of adding carotid endarterectomy. *J Am Coll Surg* 2004; 198: 36-41.
7. Dardik A, Eisele DW, Williams GM, Perler BA. A contemporary assessment of carotid body tumor surgery. *J Vasc Endovasc Surg* 2002; 36: 277-83.
8. Iafrati MD, O'Donnell TF Jr. Adjuvant techniques for the management of large carotid body tumors. A case report and review. *Cardiovasc Surg* 1999; 7: 139-45.

Chapter 18

Carotid aneurysms

Geoffrey Gilling-Smith MS FRCS, Consultant Vascular Surgeon
Royal Liverpool University Hospital, Liverpool, UK

Rao Vallabhaneni MD FRCS, Endovascular Fellow
Malmö University Hospital, Malmö, Sweden

Introduction

Although rare, aneurysms of the extracranial carotid arteries are important. They are almost never benign and if left untreated will almost inevitably cause pain, swelling, cranial nerve palsy and/or haemorrhage. Large aneurysms are in general more difficult to treat than small ones and early diagnosis and treatment are therefore essential.

Aneurysmal dilatation of the carotid artery was first reported in the late 17th Century. Since then, almost 1000 cases have been reported in the surgical literature. Most reports have been of single cases or small series with only seven reports of more than 25 patients each [1-7]. It is clear from these that the aetiology, clinical presentation and management of carotid aneurysm have changed considerably over the last 50 years. Nonetheless, there are some common themes and important lessons to aid the surgeon who is faced with such a problem.

This chapter will focus on the incidence, aetiology, diagnosis and management of both true and false aneurysms of the extracranial carotid arteries. Aneurysms of the intracranial arteries are more common, but are usually managed by neurosurgeons and neuroradiologists and will not be considered further.

Incidence

The true incidence of carotid aneurysm remains unknown [1]. Aneurysms of the carotid artery do not feature with any prominence as incidental findings in autopsy studies and they have been estimated to account for no more than 0.4% of all peripheral aneurysms [3]. Aneurysms are being found more frequently with increased use of CT and MRI to investigate pathology in the head and neck, but there is no evidence that the incidence of true aneurysms is increasing. The incidence of false aneurysms, however, is almost certainly increasing with the increase in violent penetrating trauma to the neck.

Aetiology

True aneurysms are most commonly atherosclerotic and involve the carotid bifurcation or proximal internal carotid artery. Although more common in men than in women (male: female ratio 2:1), male preponderance is much less than with other peripheral aneurysms. The male to female ratio for aortic aneurysm, for example is 10:1, while that for popliteal aneurysm is 30:1. True aneurysms of the carotid artery are also less frequently associated with aneurysmal dilatation at other sites than are most peripheral aneurysms.

Multiple aneurysms have been reported in only 15-20% of patients with a carotid aneurysm, while multiple aneurysms are found in between 60-90% of patients with femoral or popliteal aneurysms.

True aneurysmal dilation may also occur secondary to infection (see Chapter 33, Mycotic aneurysms). *Salmonella*, *Klebsiella*, *E. Coli*, *Proteus* and *Yersinia* have all been reported to cause mycotic aneurysm of the carotid artery. Syphilitic aneurysm of the carotid artery has been reported, but is now very rare. Occasionally, *Staphylococcus aureus* infection of the tonsil can spread to involve the carotid artery. This can result in profuse oropharyngeal bleeding during surgery to drain a "tonsillar abscess".

Other causes of true aneurysmal dilatation of the carotid artery include fibromuscular dysplasia, Marfan's syndrome, cystic medial necrosis and idiopathic medial arteriopathy. Carotid aneurysms have also been documented in early life. In the absence of other aetiological factors, such aneurysms are referred to as congenital aneurysms.

False aneurysms of the extracranial carotid arteries are most commonly caused by penetrating trauma to the neck, attempts at percutaneous cannulation of the internal jugular vein, cervical radiotherapy and/or surgery to the neck. Carotid arterial surgery is more likely to be complicated by a false aneurysm if the artery is closed with a synthetic patch [7] (see Chapter 32, Infection following aortic and carotid surgery).

Fracture of the mandible may occasionally result in a false aneurysm (if the artery is penetrated by a fragment of bone), but blunt trauma is more likely to cause dissection than false aneurysm. If left untreated however, dissection results in late aneurysmal dilatation in up to 30% of cases. If both artery and vein have been injured, a false aneurysm may be associated with an arteriovenous fistula.

Clinical presentation

The clinical presentation of a carotid aneurysm depends on its aetiology, location and size. Small aneurysms may remain clinically silent. As the aneurysm enlarges, however, the development of a mass usually results in signs and symptoms.

Aneurysms involving the common carotid artery may present as a pulsatile mass in the anterior triangle of the neck. Aneurysms involving only the internal carotid artery may also present as a mass if the carotid bifurcation is relatively low. If the bifurcation is situated higher in the neck, the aneurysm may be masked by the overlying cervical fascia. Such aneurysms are more likely to present as swellings in the throat where the pharyngeal constrictors offer little resistance. Carotid aneurysm should always be considered in the differential diagnosis of a mass in the neck, posterolateral pharynx or tonsillar fossa. A history of previous surgery or trauma to the neck should prompt inclusion of false aneurysm in the differential diagnosis.

Pain within the swelling is a common symptom. It may be associated with headache and dizziness. Embolisation of aneurysm thrombus may result in hemispheric or ocular symptoms such as amaurosis fugax, retinal infarction, transient ischaemic attack (TIA) or stroke. Such symptoms are more common in patients with true aneurysms than in those with false aneurysms.

Aneurysms may also present with symptoms due to stretching or compression of adjacent structures, particularly cranial nerves. Thus, auricular pain, facial pain, hoarseness of voice, Horner's syndrome and fifth or sixth cranial nerve palsy have all been reported. Compression of the pharynx can result in dysphagia.

Rupture of true aneurysm is very rare but infected or false aneurysms can present with bleeding into the throat or epistaxis. Infected aneurysms can present with tenderness, inflammation and/or systemic sepsis.

Elongation and tortuosity of the common carotid artery in the root of the neck is often mistaken for carotid aneurysm. Other differential diagnoses include lymphadenopathy, branchial cyst and carotid body tumour.

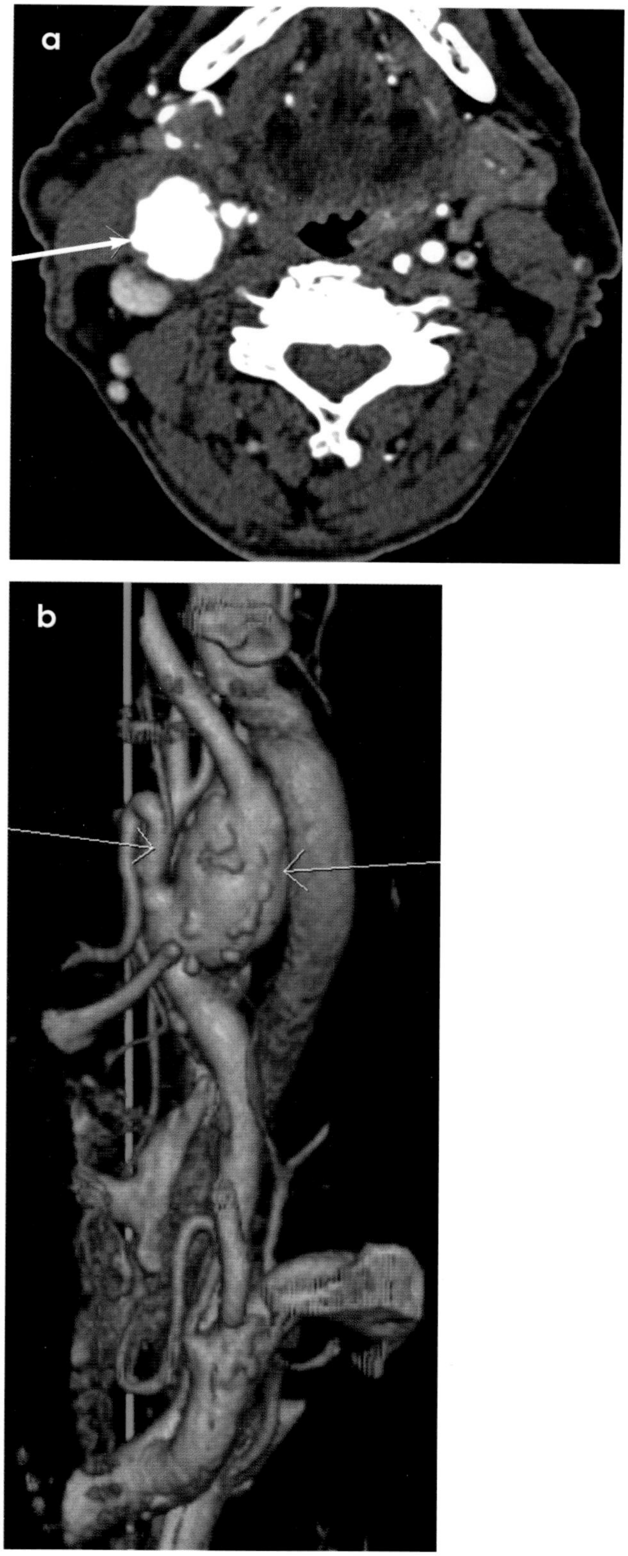

Figure 1. a) CT scan revealing a large false aneurysm of the right internal carotid artery (arrow). b) Reconstructed CT image of the false aneurysm (arrows).

Investigation

The purpose of investigation is to confirm the diagnosis and to delineate the vascular anatomy in order to plan surgical or endovascular treatment.

The diagnosis can usually be confirmed on Duplex imaging, but CT or MRI may be useful to define the extent of the lesion and relation to adjacent structures (Figure 1). In the past, digital subtraction angiography was performed prior to any intervention, but magnetic resonance angiography with 3D reconstruction is now the preferred modality for defining the vascular anatomy. MR is non-invasive and permits appreciation of more than just the arterial lumen.

Management

Intervention is required in most cases to relieve symptoms and/or prevent complications such as cranial nerve palsy, rupture and bleeding. The choice of intervention will depend on the aetiology, location and size of the aneurysm, as well as the availability of surgical and endovascular skills.

Surgical treatment

Hunterian ligation

Simple ligation of the carotid artery proximal and distal to the aneurysm is now rarely performed because of the unacceptably high incidence of postoperative stroke and death [8]. A variety of methods has been proposed to ascertain whether or not the collateral circulation within the brain is adequate to permit safe ligation of the internal carotid artery but none has proved reliable. Even if ligation is tolerated in the short term, cerebral infarction can occur up to several days later [8]. In most cases, therefore, open resection and reconstruction or endovascular therapy are the treatments of choice.

Resection of the aneurysm

It may sometimes be possible to resect a small aneurysm of the internal carotid artery and restore arterial continuity by simple end-to-end anastomosis

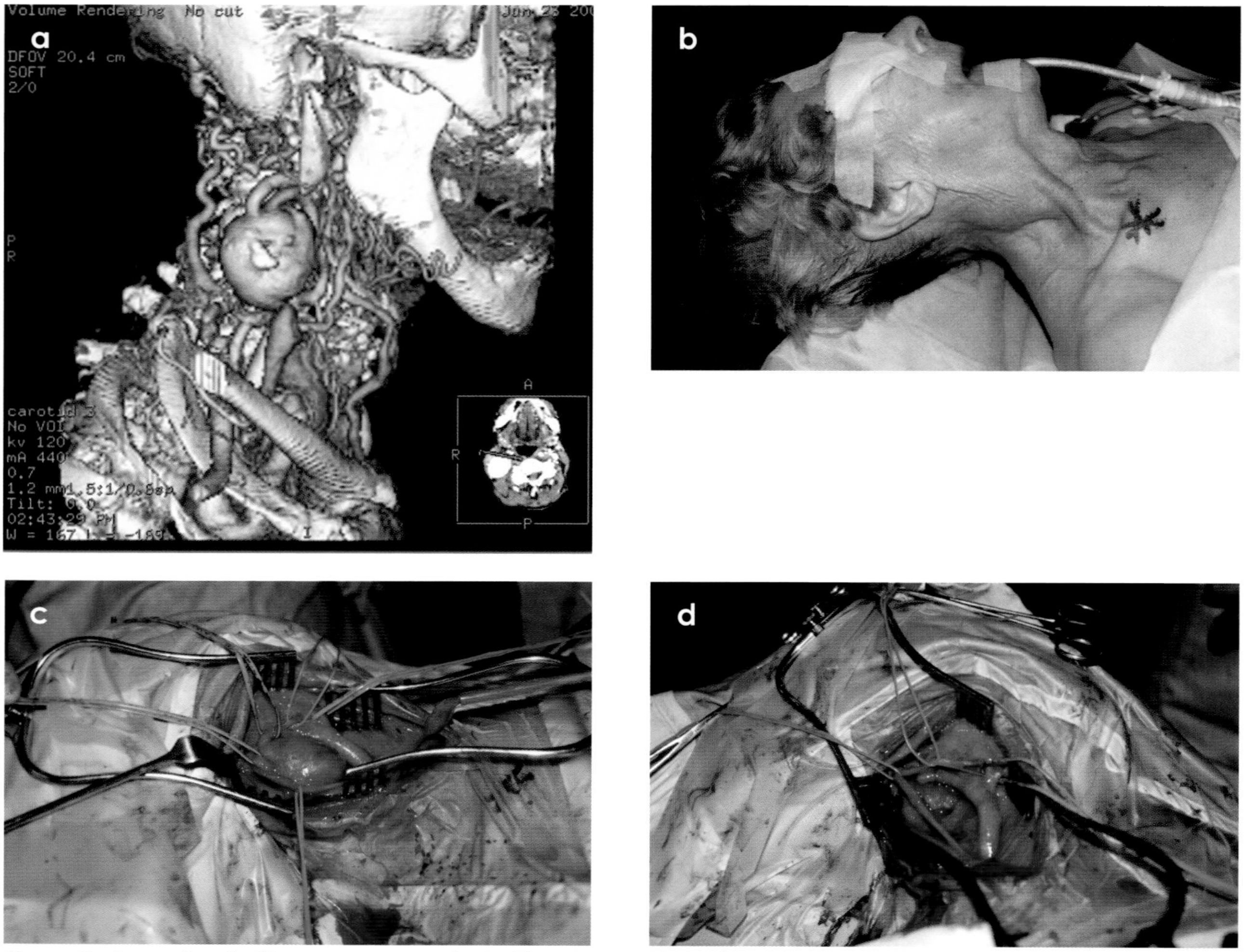

Figure 2. A previously fit woman presented with new onset deafness in her right ear. Examination revealed a pulsatile mass in the neck. Duplex imaging demonstrated a large carotid aneurysm but the anatomy could not be defined. a) A CT reconstruction showed an internal carotid aneurysm with both the inflow and outflow entering the aneurysm from above. b) External appearance of the aneurysm at operation. c) The aneurysm was dissected free from the vagus and hypoglossal nerves (red slings). The inflow and outflow are elongated internal carotid artery (blue slings to left of image). d) After resection of the aneurysm with end-to-end anastomosis of the remaining internal carotid artery. The patient made an uneventful recovery and her deafness resolved. Courtesy of Miss F Meyer.

(Figure 2). Larger aneurysms however, require formal reconstruction, particularly if they involve the bifurcation.

Exposure

Surgical exposure of the aneurysm can be difficult. Manipulation of the aneurysm can result in embolisation of thrombus to the brain, while the risk of injury to the facial, hypoglossal, glossopharyngeal and vagus nerves is high. If the aneurysm extends close to the base of the skull, it may be very difficult to expose and control the internal carotid artery distally. Surgical exposure of the distal internal carotid can be facilitated by division of the posterior belly of digastric muscle, separation of sternocleidomastoid from its attachment and by subluxation of the mandible. The mass of the aneurysm may, however, preclude satisfactory exposure. If pre-operative imaging reveals the aneurysm to lie high in the neck, consideration should be given to endovascular treatment.

Reconstruction

Reversed long saphenous vein harvested from the groin is the conduit of choice, although satisfactory results have been reported with prosthetic grafts [7]. The interposition graft must be tailored to bridge the gap between proximal and distal arterial segments. This can be difficult if a shunt is employed. It is in any case important to place the graft under gentle tension so as to avoid redundancy and kinking once flow is restored.

If the aneurysm involves the origin of the external carotid artery, the reconstruction should if possible be tailored to restore flow into both internal and external carotid arteries. This may require construction of a bifurcated vein graft. Occasionally, however, the external carotid artery can be anastomosed directly onto the internal carotid vein graft.

Cerebral protection

Shunts may be employed routinely or selectively, as in surgery for occlusive disease. If a shunt is employed, the vein graft must first be threaded over the shunt. The proximal anastomosis is fashioned with the shunt *in situ*. Ideally, the distal anastomosis should also be started before the shunt is removed but this can be technically challenging.

It has been argued that the threshold for shunting should be lower than when performing carotid endarterectomy since the procedure is likely to last longer. This does not seem entirely rational; either a shunt is required or it is not. Furthermore, the use of a shunt increases the risk of injury to the distal intima at a site which is unlikely to be accessible should a flap be raised upon restoration of flow. A shunt is also likely to provoke spasm of the vein graft and/or injury to the venous endothelium.

Endovascular treatment

Endovascular techniques can be employed to treat both false and true aneurysms of the extracranial carotid arteries.

False aneurysms

Detachable balloons have been employed to occlude the carotid artery proximal and distal to the aneurysm [8]. This is the endovascular equivalent of Hunterian ligation and equally hazardous. Coils have been employed to induce thrombosis of the aneurysm, but flow though the false lumen before thrombosis can result in embolisation of coils to the brain. The risk of embolisation can be reduced by first placing a bare metal stent across the mouth of the aneurysm and then employing microcatheters to embolise the aneurysm through the stent [9]. This is technically complex and many interventionists find it simpler and quicker to place a covered stent across the arterial defect [10]. This will usually result in rapid and spontaneous thrombosis of the false aneurysm.

A covered stent is particularly useful if the patient is bleeding from a false aneurysm [11] (Figure 3). Although a surgeon's first instinct in such a situation is to operate, haemorrhage into the neck can render intubation very difficult so that rapid exposure and control of the arterial injury may not be possible. If surgery is nonetheless the preferred option, it may be advantageous to place a deflated balloon occluder in the common carotid artery percutaneously via the femoral artery before taking the patient to theatre. Torrential haemorrhage during surgical exposure can then be controlled by temporary inflation of the balloon.

A covered stent can still be employed if the aneurysm is infected [11]. At the very least, such a manoeuvre will provide a temporary solution. Persistent infection despite long-term antibiotic therapy can always be dealt with surgically at a later date when the patient is stable.

True aneurysms

A true aneurysm can be isolated from the circulation by intraluminal deployment of a covered stent graft to bridge the gap between normal artery proximal and distal to the aneurysm. Such an intervention should prevent continued expansion of the aneurysm and/or rupture and haemorrhage. In most cases, however, it will not result in early or significant shrinkage of the aneurysm and it will not therefore relieve symptoms or complications (pain, cranial nerve palsy, venous congestion) that result simply from the mass of the aneurysm.

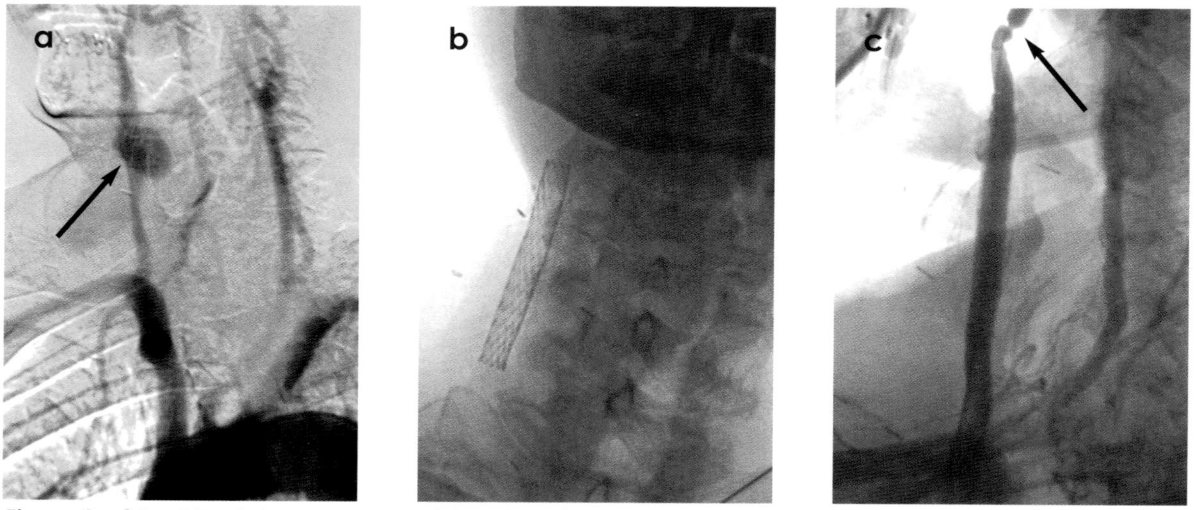

Figure 3. a) Leaking false aneurysm of the distal right common carotid artery secondary to surgery and radiotherapy for cervical malignancy (arrow). b) Treated by placement of a covered stent in the common and internal carotid arteries. c) Angiogram after the procedure. The origin of the external carotid artery is occluded by the stent. Note the spasm of the distal internal carotid artery following stent deployment (arrow).

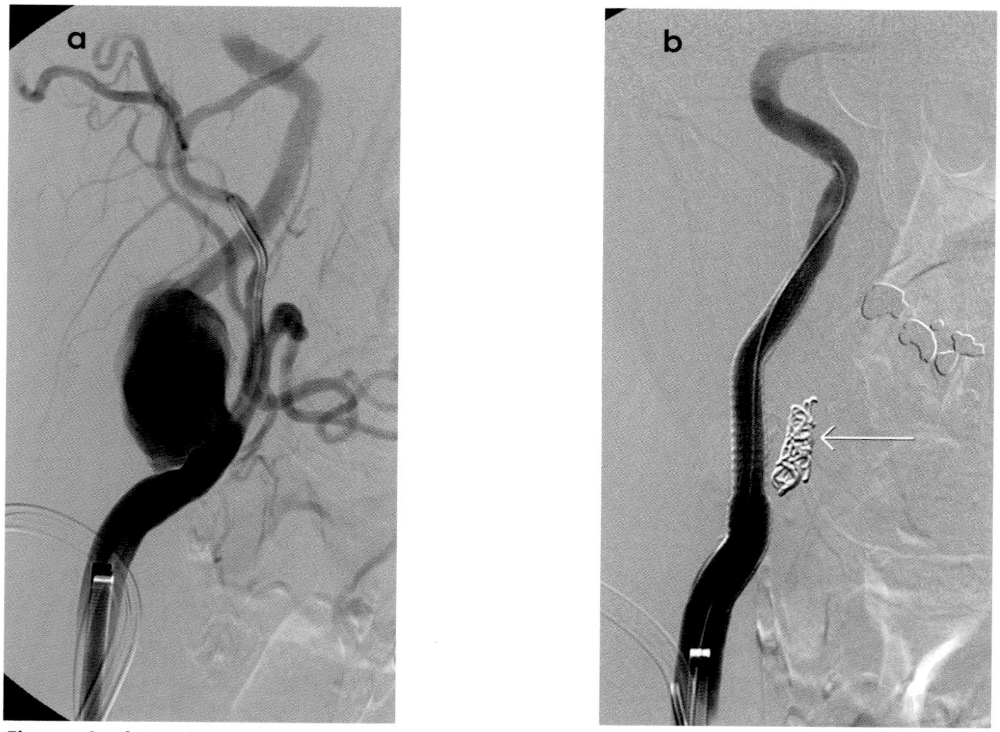

Figure 4. a) Angiogram showing aneurysm of the internal carotid artery. b) Treated by placement of a covered stent in the common and internal carotid arteries. Note occlusion of the external carotid artery by coil embolisation (arrow). This was performed after stent deployment to minimise the risk of embolisation of coils into the internal carotid artery.

In many cases the aneurysm involves the origin of the external carotid artery and this will need to be occluded by coil embolisation (Figure 4) in order to prevent backflow into the aneurysm (endoleak) and persistent pressurisation of the aneurysm. Although technically feasible this adds to the complexity of the procedure and is associated with a risk of embolisation. It may also be argued that occlusion of the external carotid artery is unwise in a patient who may subsequently develop in-stent stenosis and occlusion of the internal carotid artery.

On the other hand, an endovascular approach offers significant advantages in a patient with aneurysmal dilatation of the distal internal carotid artery. In such patients it may be very difficult at open operation to obtain vascular control, particularly if the aneurysm is large. An endovascular approach also minimises the risk of surgical injury to adjacent cranial nerves or veins.

Cerebral protection

There is a widespread belief that cerebral protection reduces the risk of thrombo-embolic complications during balloon angioplasty of atheromatous carotid stenoses. There is in fact no Level I evidence to support this belief (while there is some evidence that cerebral protection may actually increase the risk of embolisation). Despite this, many interventionists believe that cerebral protection should also be employed when treating aneurysms of the extracranial carotid arteries.

It is difficult to discern any logic in this approach. Although carotid aneurysms may be lined with thrombus, the lumen through the aneurysm is usually significantly larger than the native artery, so that passage of a guide wire and delivery system through the aneurysm is unlikely to disrupt aneurysm thrombus. It should be noted in this context that distal embolisation is a very rare complication during endovascular repair of aortic aneurysm, a procedure which is usually associated with significantly more intraluminal manipulation.

In most cases, cerebral protection is more likely to harm than benefit a patient undergoing endovascular therapy for carotid aneurysm. The authors do recognise, however, that cerebral protection may protect the interventionist from anxiety and/or litigation.

Acknowledgement

Figures 1 and 4 reproduced by kind permission of Mats Lindh, Jan Holst and Krassi Ivancev, Malmö University Hospital, Sweden and Figure 2 by Miss F Meyer, Norfolk and Norwich University Hospital, Norwich.

Key points

- Aneurysms of the extracranial carotid artery should in general be treated either to relieve symptoms or to prevent late complications.
- The choice between open surgical and endovascular therapy depends on the indications for intervention, the anatomy of the carotid arteries, the perceived difficulty of an open surgical approach and the availability of appropriate interventional skills.
- Since there are no long-term data on outcomes after endovascular intervention, the choice may also be governed by the age of the patient.

References

1. McCollum CH, Wheeler WG, Noon GP, *et al.* Aneurysms of the extracranial carotid artery. Twenty-one years' experience. *Am J Surg* 1979; 137: 196-200.
2. Pratschke E, Schafer K, Reimer J, *et al.* Extracranial aneurysms of the carotid artery. *Thorac Cardiovasc Surg* 1980; 28: 354-8.
3. Welling RE, Taha A, Goel T, *et al.* Extracranial carotid artery aneurysms. *Surgery* 1983; 93: 319-23.
4. Moreau P, Albat B, Thevenet A. Surgical treatment of extracranial internal carotid artery aneurysm. *Ann Vasc Surg* 1994; 8: 409-16.
5. Zhang Q, Duan ZQ, Xin SJ, *et al.* Management of extracranial carotid artery aneurysms: 17 years' experience. *Eur J Vasc Endovasc Surg* 1999; 18: 162-5.
6. Nair R, Robbs JV, Naidoo NG. Spontaneous carotid artery aneurysms. *Br J Surg* 2000; 87: 186-90.
7. El-Sabrout R, Cooley DA. Extracranial carotid artery aneurysms: Texas Heart Institute experience. *J Vasc Surg* 2000; 31: 702-12.
8. Chaloupka JC, Putman CM, Citardi MJ, *et al.* Endovascular therapy for the carotid blowout syndrome in head and neck surgical patients; diagnostic and managerial considerations. *Am J Neuroradiol* 1996; 17: 843-52.
9. Phatouros CC, Sasaki TY, Higashida RT, *et al.* Stent-supported coil embolization: the treatment of fusiform and wide-neck aneurysms and pseudoaneurysms. *Neurosurgery* 2000; 47: 107-13.
10. Marin ML, Veith FJ, Paanetta, *et al.* Transluminally placed endovascular stented graft repair for arterial trauma. *J Vasc Surg* 1994; 20: 466-73.
11. Macdonald S, Gan J, McKay AJ, *et al.* Endovascular treatment of acute carotid blow-out syndrome. *J Vasc Interv Radiol* 2000; 11: 1184-8.

Case vignette

Carotid thrombus causing crescendo transient ischaemic attacks

Michael Jenkins BSc MS FRCS, Consultant Vascular Surgeon, St. Mary's Hospital, London, UK

A 44-year-old man admitted with right hemisphere crescendo transient ischaemic attacks. Magnetic resonance angiography was reported as normal, but duplex imaging suggested there was fresh thrombus at the carotid bifurcation. At operation, minimally adherent thrombus was removed to reveal normal intima (Figures 1 and 2). Further investigation failed to find the source, but the patient was anticoagulated empirically.

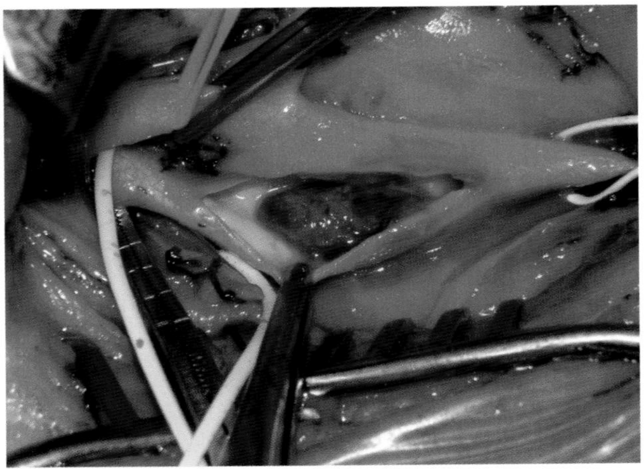

Figure 1.

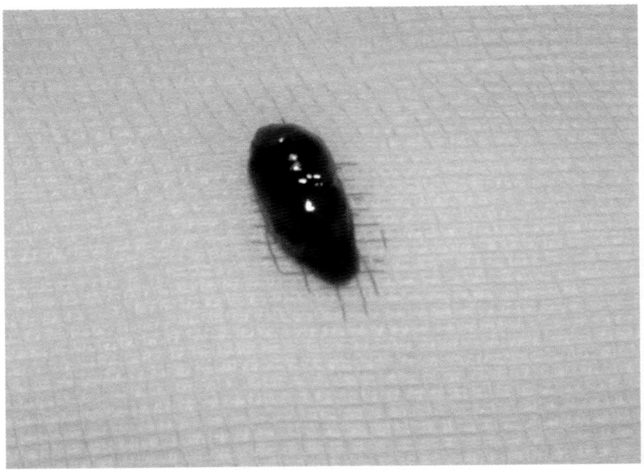

Figure 2.

Chapter 19

Thoracic outlet syndrome

John F Thompson MS FRCS (Ed) FRCS, Consultant Surgeon
Royal Devon and Exeter Hospitals, Exeter, UK

Introduction

The thoracic outlet syndromes (TOS) are probably underdiagnosed [1] and in some centres overtreated [2]. Indiscriminate surgery in this complex area has resulted in a wave of litigation, especially in the USA. The purpose of this chapter is to guide the surgeon in making the diagnosis and treating appropriately. To do this requires a multidisciplinary team so that cases can be discussed and cross-referred if appropriate. Key stakeholders are as follows:

- Vascular surgeons.
- Vascular laboratory.
- Radiologists.
- Neurophysiologists.
- Physiotherapists.
- Orthopaedic surgeons.
- Rheumatologists/occupational health physicians.
- Pain clinic.

The syndromes consist of arterial (A-TOS), neurological (N-TOS) and venous (V-TOS) subsets that often co-exist. Secondary diagnoses may be present independently, such as carpal tunnel syndrome, or have evolved as a consequence of the TOS, such as frozen shoulder or glenohumeral subluxation. The key to successful treatment is to identify and treat alternative diagnoses and to find the dominant component of the TOS. If an anatomical lesion is found that can explain the symptoms, removal of the compression will cure the patient.

Anatomy

The primary anatomical mechanism for the development of TOS is the bony costoclavicular shears that tend to pinch the neurovascular bundle at the thoracic outlet. The subclavian vein lies anterior and is most vulnerable, followed by the artery and lying behind this, the C8/T1 nerve root that will form the ulnar nerve. Thus, venous obstruction (and in severe cases thrombosis), arterial ischaemia and ulnar paraesthesia often co-exist in these cases (Figure 1). Fractures of the clavicle or sternoclavicular dislocation may contribute.

If a cervical rib (0.25% of the population) or band is present, the vein is seldom involved, but the artery and lower trunk of the brachial plexus are stretched over it (Figure 2). This results in wedging of the artery between the rib and the scalenus anterior muscle, with post-stenotic dilatation and aneurysm formation, with the capacity for limb-threatening thrombo-embolism. Bands are often worse than bones!

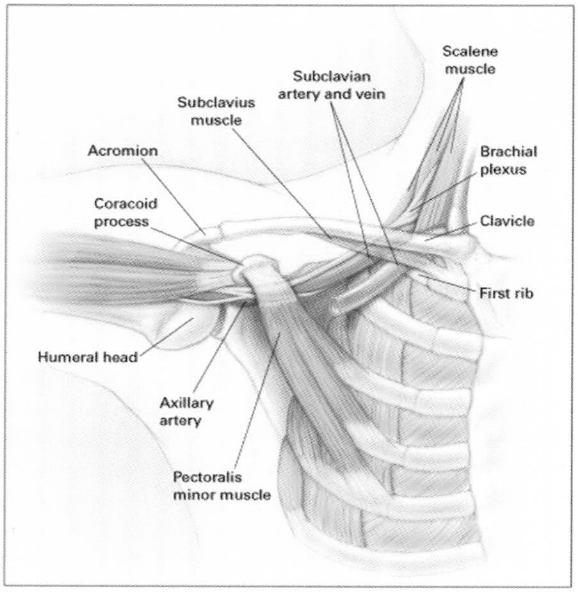

Figure 1. The anatomy of the thoracic outlet.

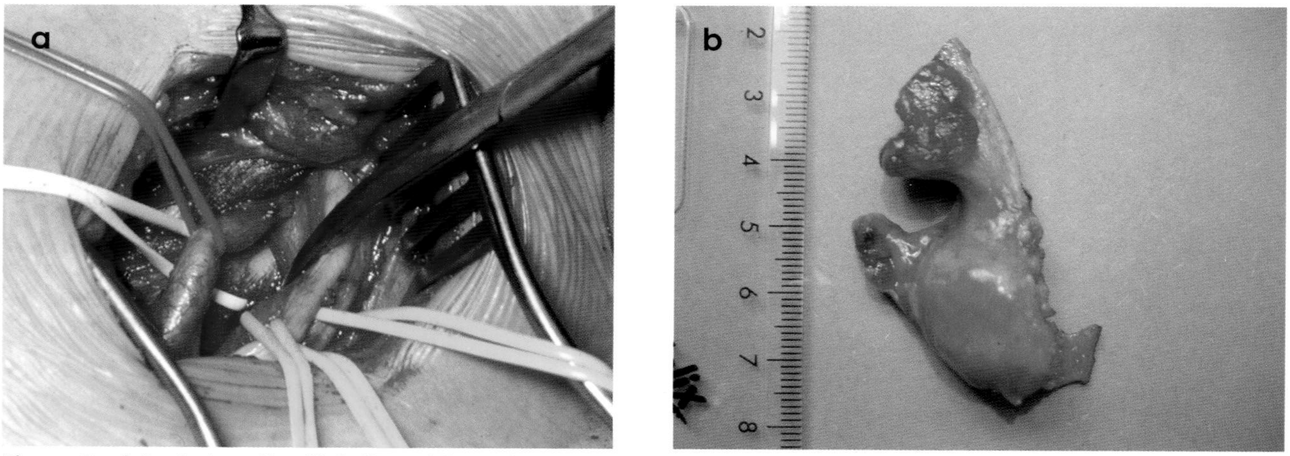

Figure 2. a) Post-stenotic dilatation of the subclavian artery due to compression by the large true synovial joint between a cervical rib and the scalene tubercle. b) The resected rib. The neck and scalene tubercle are nibbled back further after this initial resection.

Neurological involvement is more common than ischaemia in individuals with symptomatic cervical ribs.

Embryologically, the developing upper limb bud takes with it nerves and vessels that pierce the myotomes at the root of the neck. It is not surprising that there are a wide range of neurological syndromes associated with aberrant bands and muscle slips, which may not show clearly on cross-sectional imaging (Figure 3).

Finally, acquired anatomical anomalies may lead to TOS, such as the drooping posture associated with VDU usage, hypertrophy of the subclavius muscle in athletes or repetitive movements such as throwing a ball or playing a musical instrument.

Clinical presentation

Women outnumber men with TOS by 3:1 and the median age at presentation is 36 years. V-TOS is considered in Chapter 20. A-TOS presents with early fatigue of the upper limb when working with the arm elevated which is relieved by dependency. Aneurysms are usually associated with a cervical rib and may be complicated by distal embolism. N-TOS presents as painful paraesthesia in the distribution of the C8/T1 dermatome (little finger, medial half of ring finger and forearm). The symptoms are felt on the palmar aspect, whereas radicular compression results in dorsal pain. The paraesthesia then spreads proximally to the deltoid and trapezius areas with a unilateral occipito-frontal headache that accompanies use of the ipsilateral arm and is relieved by rest. This is due to tension on the dura from the rectus capitis posterior minor muscle when in spasm.

Facial or jaw pain is common; temporomandibular joint dysfunction or dental problems are often

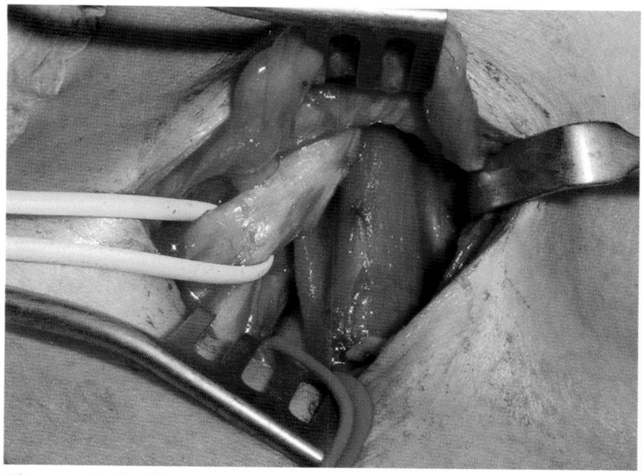

Figure 3. Patient with severe upper plexus pain and paraesthesia on swimming and repetitive movement. Note nerve roots piercing scalenus anterior. Complete resolution after scalenectomy.

misdiagnosed. Grip strength and fine motor function decline as the small muscles waste. In severe cases, the presentation is similar to burnt out carpal tunnel syndrome, with total intrinsic muscle loss. Sensory blunting is present from an early stage; patients tolerate very hot water that their partners find painful.

True upper plexus TOS is very rare and really only applies to abnormal muscles or bands affecting the C5/6 root. C6 pain is more often referred to the wrist from the glenohumeral joint.

There should be a clear relationship between use of the limb and the development of symptoms. Rest usually helps, but in some patients a vicious circle of pain/spasm and more pain supervenes, especially in the controversial or disputed form of TOS that follows whiplash injuries.

Secondary diagnoses are common. They include double crush disorders such as N-TOS with carpal tunnel syndrome, cervical spine pain or cumulative motion disorders. Over time, disuse of the arm can lead to frozen shoulder or glenohumeral subluxation. Pain neurosis is a difficult area. Some genuine patients may be driven mad by their symptoms and the quest for a diagnosis, others may have been neurotic to start with; sensitivity and an open mind are essential for the interested clinician.

Clinical examination

Patients should be examined sitting, with a straight back. The cervical spine is carefully assessed for spasm, abnormal motion segments and root compression. The supraclavicular fossa is viewed from behind. The normal concavity may be absent if a cervical rib or band is present and the subclavian pulse is prominent. Palpation may reveal a cervical rib, but X-rays are essential as many are subtle. Palpation of the brachial plexus may result in paraesthesia and tapping here and over the clavicle may produce tingling in the little finger. The arm is then examined for arthropathy and peripheral nerve compression, especially at the elbow and wrist. The intrinsic muscles of the hand are then examined. The arterial supply to both arms is then checked with blood pressures measurements.

Positional pulse changes are important and may be accompanied by a subclavian bruit that disappears as the artery occludes, but it is vital to appreciate that:

- many normal individuals occlude their pulses during provocative manoeuvres;
- only those with TOS will develop the precise symptoms of which they complain during provocation;
- most patients develop these symptoms very quickly (within 30 seconds);
- ischaemia may co-exist with ulnar paraesthesia, so that European specialists recognise A-TOS whereas Americans consider this a primarily neurological diagnosis;
- in those with a cervical rib, elevation of the limb may lift the artery out of its cleft between the rib and scalene band, so that the pulse is preserved;
- the Roos test (USA), "surrender" position (Germany) or "candlestick" position (France) is very helpful, but should be taken in the clinical context and combined with investigations to amass a body of evidence to support the diagnosis. There is no clear cut test for TOS.

Investigation

Plain radiographs of the cervical spine are vital; MRI often misses subtle bony anomalies. The transverse process of T1 points upwards so that any rib attached to it is a first rib, even if it looks like a cervical rib; that of C7 points downwards, so any rib attached to it is a cervical rib (Figure 4).

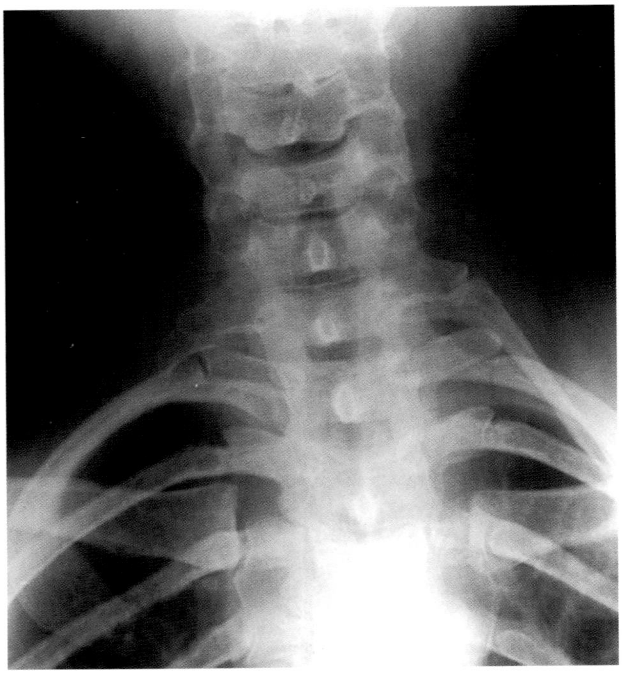

Figure 4. Left complete cervical rib articulating with the first rib. On the right (symptomatic) side the transverse process of C7 has a "crow's beak" appearance. There was a band extending from the tip to the scalene tubercle.

MRI can replace conventional angiography and can also identify cervical radicular compression and exclude rare diagnoses such as a syrinx.

Duplex ultrasonography is performed at rest and in the positions that provoke the TOS, such as holding a hairdryer. Some observations from our practice are:

- Duplex is dynamic. The artery may occlude then open again as the arm is raised.
- The technologist should develop an interest in the history and try to correlate the ultrasound findings with the development of symptoms.
- Venous obstruction is difficult as it is not always possible to identify the subclavian vein if large collaterals are present. The venous reponse to deep inspiration is useful.
- Arterial occlusion is a good surrogate marker for venous narrowing.
- The C8/T8 root lies adjacent to the artery, so arterial compression is also an indication that the root is being compressed.
- Normal subjects can often occlude their arteries, but they remain asymptomatic.

Arteriography is seldom required unless the A-TOS has been complicated by aneurysm or embolus. Venography may be helpful in V-TOS (see Chapter 20, Paget Schroetter syndrome).

Many authors have stated that TOS is a clinical diagnosis, but neurophysiological examination is important. N-TOS causes changes ranging from subtle anomalies in f-wave conduction, through decreases in the sensory action potential in the medial antebrachial cutaneous nerve (C8/T1) to motor unit loss in the hand [3]. These may be diagnostic of TOS when taken in the clinical context. EMG also excludes other diagnoses, acts as a baseline and is vital for medicolegal reasons.

Treatment

A-TOS

In patients with brachial ischaemia, the diagnosis and mechanism is explained and the patient is reassured that the condition is usually not serious. Physiotherapy, losing weight, stopping smoking and improving posture will often help [4]. A period of 6-12 months of active conservative management is essential in the first instance. Failure to respond may be due to occupational stresses, the more severe bony anomalies or injury.

Pre-operatively, the operation of transaxillary first rib resection is explained in detail [5], including the potential complications, and these are documented in

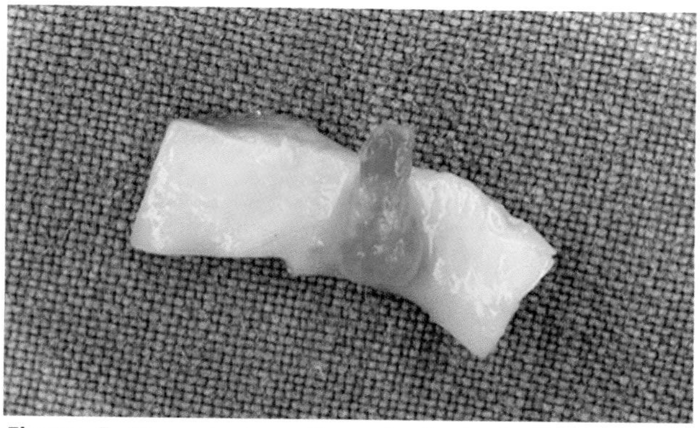

Figure 5. Resected section of subclavian artery with intimal thrombus due to trauma from a cervical rib. Direct anastomosis was possible.

a letter to the family doctor, with a copy to the patient. The final decision to operate is made by the patient at home and after due thought. Key issues for consent include the following:

- Success (relief of primary symptoms) is 80-85%, falling to 75% at 5 years.
- There is a small but significant risk of death, failure to relieve symptoms or making the arm worse. Limb loss has never been reported.
- Bleeding, nerve damage (including phrenic) and thoracotomy are occasionally seen.
- Intercostobrachial neuropraxia is common and may persist.

In patients with aneurysms or thrombo-embolism, surgery is usually mandatory, unless the aneurysm has thrombosed and collateral supply is adequate (rare). The bony anomaly (usually a cervical rib) is resected and arterial supply restored with a graft. Surprisingly, the redundant length of artery left after the resection of a cervical rib is often enough to permit a direct anastomosis (Figure 5). Failing this a short PTFE graft may be required; saphenous vein grafts are used to bypass longer occlusions.

In patients with severe ischaemia or Raynaud's phenomenon, it is simple to locate the second rib neck and to diathermy the sympathetic chain at that point. Alternatively, an endoscopic transthoracic sympathectomy provides an elegant solution.

N-TOS

Patients with N-TOS without muscle wasting and well preserved hand function should be treated conservatively as above. The choice of physical therapist, whether an osteopath, chiropractor or physiotherapist is vital; they must be experienced in dealing with the condition. Neck traction, for example, is very painful and can make the condition worse. The aim is to lengthen the scalene muscles, improve pectoral girdle geometry and to break the cycle of spasm and pain. Injection of local anaesthetic or botulinum toxin into the scalenes may help [6].

Those with pain and muscle wasting associated with a defined anatomical anomaly (usually a cervical rib) rarely respond to physiotherapy. When treatment fails, surgery should be offered to relieve the pain, but motor loss is permanent. Patients with total intrinsic muscle loss in a painless hand do not require operation.

The choice of operation should be directed towards treating the dominant component. If the patient has arterial TOS with a neurological component (An-TOS), a transaxillary rib resection is appropriate, even if a cervical rib is present. If the variant is mainly neurological (N-TOS or Na-TOS) the best approach is supraclavicular because the whole plexus can be explored. The aim is to resect the bony anomaly or band and if this explains the symptoms of which the patient complains, no additional dissection is performed (Figure 6); a policy of removing the scalene muscles, cervical and first ribs leaves the plexus without surrounding structures and makes it vulnerable to scarring and adhesions.

Haemostasis should be meticulous to prevent haematoma formation. The wound is flooded and infiltrated with long-acting local anaesthetic and closed over a vacuum drain. The pleura is often breached and this in fact may be preferable as any blood will drain into the pleural cavity rather than accumulate around the plexus. No separate chest drain is required.

Postoperative physiotherapy is limited to gentle mobility exercises to prevent adhesions and scarring.

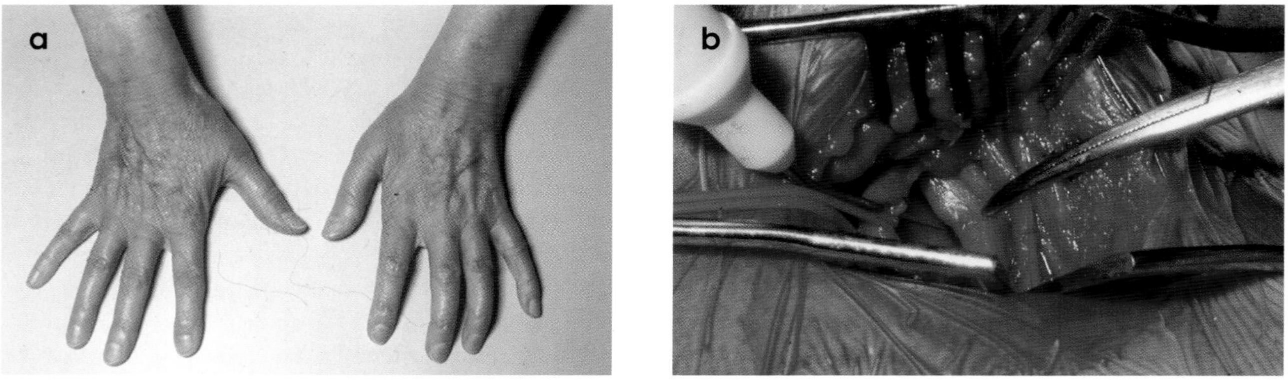

Figure 6. a) Wasted intrinsic muscles in a 58-year-old pianist unable to play with the left hand. b) Supraclavicular scalenectomy and excision of cervical band. Note indented lower trunk; chronically compressed nerve roots do not fire with the nerve stimulator.

Disputed N-TOS

This form of the syndrome refers to the development of symptoms characteristic of TOS after trauma, usually a motor accident with a whiplash injury. Physical signs may not be present and tests are negative. Great care should be taken, as the results of surgery are unpredictable, particularly if litigation is involved and if there is a long history. A careful psychological assessment is important, as is meticulous documentation and risk management [7]. The general approach should be to avoid operating unless the patient is quite clear that the procedure should be considered exploratory and that every non-operative approach has failed. Tertiary referral is a good idea.

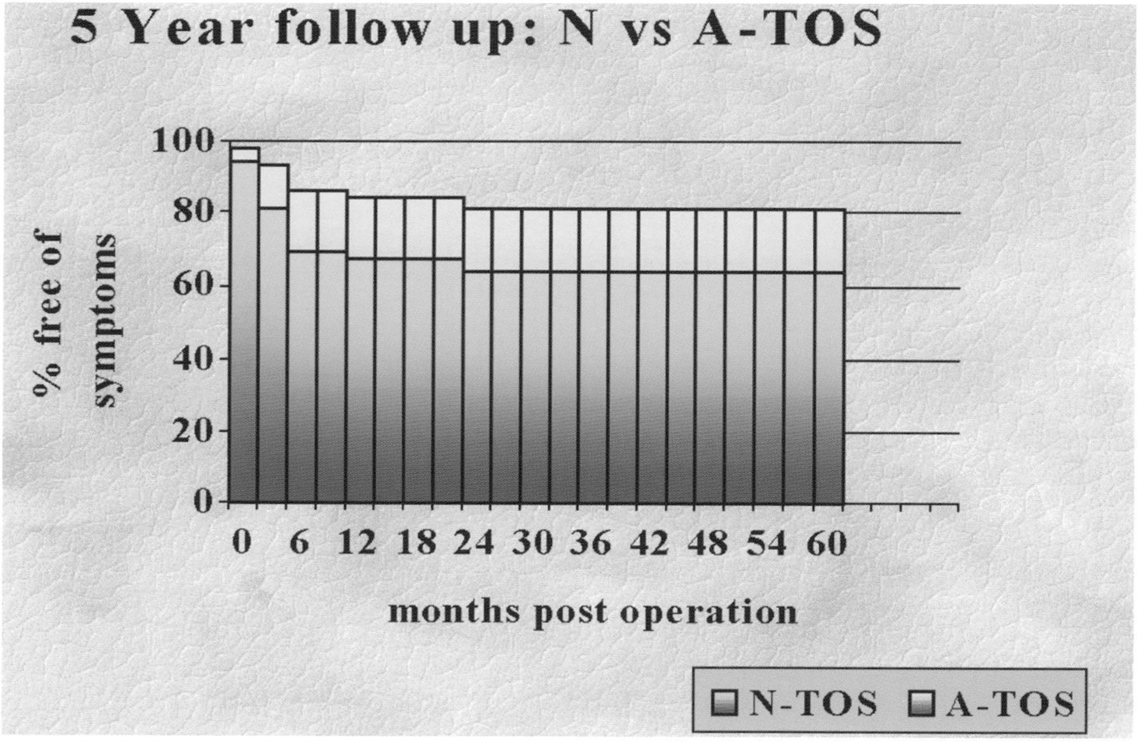

Figure 7. Outcome following decompression for A-TOS and N-TOS in 132 patients. Note initial failures within 6 months followed by durable relief of symptoms.

Surgical tips

For transaxillary first rib resection, please refer to reference [1]. For supraclavicular resection, the patient is positioned as for carotid endarterectomy, with an inflatable empty 500ml saline bag between the shoulders. The scalene fat pad is reflected cranially so that the plexus can be wrapped in it at the end of the operation. The anterior scalene muscle is detached from the scalene tubercle and resected, protecting the phrenic nerve. Nerve stimulation is useful until experience is gained. The artery is controlled with slings and mobilised by dividing the transverse cervical artery.

The plexus is then dissected free; beware the suprascapular nerve which has a variable course and the long thoracic nerve which is tiny. The cervical rib is then dissected free. The author uses Kerrison's neurosurgical cutters to divide the neck of the rib and nibblers to divide the distal end. The scalene tubercle is then nibbled back. A check is made for residual costoclavicular compression and, if present, the first rib is removed. The anterior costochondral junction is resected via a small infraclavicular incision to avoid damage to the subclavian vein which cannot be seen from above. Haemostasis should be meticulous.

Results of surgery

Most series report success in 75-80% of cases, defined as relief of primary symptoms. Life-table analysis of patients from Exeter was done using a structured questionnaire administered by a doctor not involved in their management (Figure 7). Recurrence was always within 6 months with a durable result afterwards.

Key points

- A careful history and physical examination should distinguish between the various types of thoracic outlet syndrome.
- There should be a clear indication for surgical intervention agreed by a multidisciplinary team and the patient.
- Careful pre-operative counselling is important as there are significant risks from surgery and this is an active area for litigation.
- In expert hands, surgical treatment of thoracic outlet syndrome has good results: consideration should be given to tertiary referral.

References

1. Roos DB. Thoracic outlet syndrome is underdiagnosed. *Muscle Nerve* 1999; 22: 126-9.
2. Wilbourne AJ. Thoracic outlet syndrome is overdiagnosed. *Muscle Nerve* 1999: 22; 130-6.
3. Kothari MG, Macintosh K, Heistand M, Logigian M. Medial antebrachial cutaneous sensory studies in the evaluation of neurogenic thoracic outlet syndrome. *Muscle Nerve* 1998: 21; 647-9.
4. Novak C Conservative management of thoracic outlet syndrome. *Thorac Cardiovasc Surg* 1996; 8: 201-7.
5. Thompson JF. Transaxillary first rib resection. In: *Vascular and Endovascular Techniques*. Greenhalgh RM, Ed. WB Saunders, New York, 2001.
6. Jordan SE Ahn SS, Freischlag J, Gelabert HA, Machleder HI. Selective botulinum chemodenervation of the scalene muscles for treatment of neurogenic thoracic outlet syndrome. *Ann Vasc Surg* 2000; 14: 365-9.
7. Axelrod DA, Proctor MC, Geisser ME, *et al.* Outcomes after surgery for thoracic outlet syndrome. *J Vasc Surg* 2001; 33: 1220-5.

Case vignette

Digital emboli caused by congenital scalene band

John F Thompson MS FRCS (Ed) FRCS, Consultant Surgeon, Royal Devon and Exeter Hospital, Exeter, UK

A 46-year-old woman presented with left arm digital emboli and rest pain. An angiogram showed a small subclavian artery with a localised stenosis and post-stenotic dilatation, with no evidence of atherosclerosis elsewhere (Figure 1). This was thought to be in an unusual site for atherosclerosis (not at the subclavian origin) and well above the first rib. On re-questioning, she confessed to a long history of early arm fatigue. The provisional diagnosis was made of a congenital scalene band.

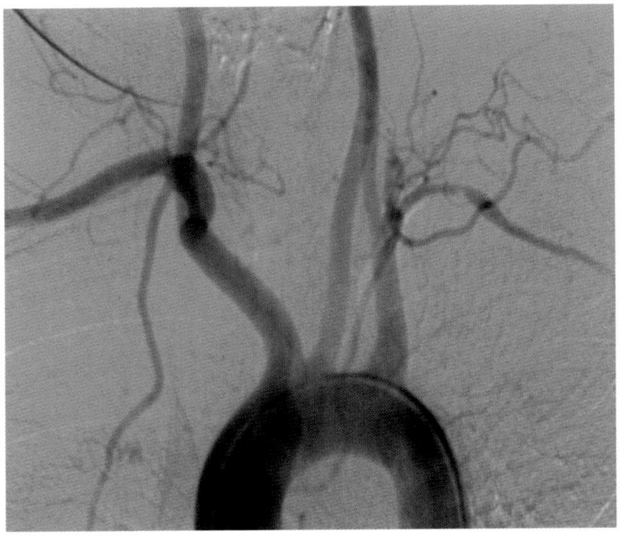

Figure 1.

At operation a relatively common variant of the scalenus medius was found (Figure 2). The scalene fat pad has been reflected and the phrenic nerve is just out of sight on the left. The artery is slung and the tight interscalene groove where it was wedged is evident. The anterior border of the scalene muscle is inserted as a fused tendon with the posterior border of scalenus medius in a similar fashion to many cervical ribs. Pre-operative duplex imaging had been negative for thoracic outlet syndrome because arm elevation lifted the artery out of the cleft. The muscle was resected and a short length of artery excised. An end-to-end anastomosis was possible due to the stretching of the artery in its pathological course.

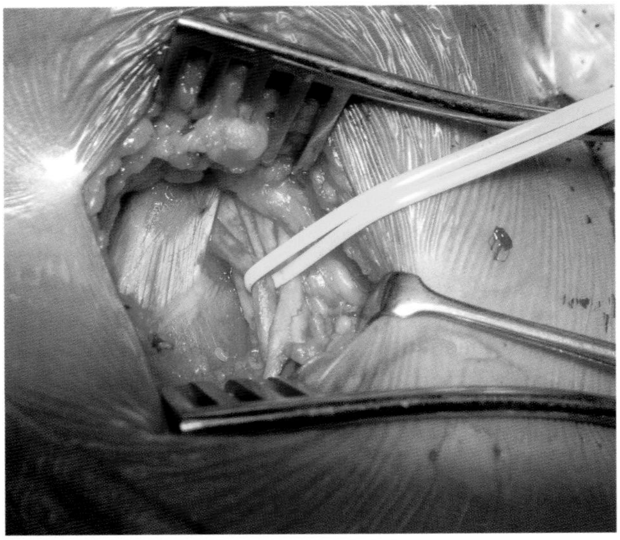

Figure 2.

Chapter 20

Paget Schroetter syndrome

John F Thompson MS FRCS (Ed) FRCS, Consultant Surgeon
Royal Devon and Exeter Hospitals, Exeter, UK

Introduction

Acute axillo-subclavian vein thrombosis in otherwise fit individuals was described by Ludwig von Schroetter in 1884 and by Sir James Paget the following year. The condition is relatively rare but important, as it results in chronic disabling upper limb swelling in up to 50% of patients, most of whom are young and active [1]. Approximately 10% present with pulmonary embolus and there have been fatalities. Most cases remain undiagnosed as they are managed in primary care or medical settings. The popularity of sport and commercial fitness centres has undoubtedly contributed to an increased incidence.

Careful patient selection for active treatment and a logical multidisciplinary approach is rewarded by normal arm function and a return to sporting activity.

Definition

Catheter-related and paraneoplastic thrombosis are the most common causes of upper limb venous thrombosis [2]. In Paget Schroetter syndrome (PSS), the underlying mechanism is primary costoclavicular compression as the subclavian vein exits the thorax over the first rib. The hypertrophied subclavius muscle narrows this space, which is bordered posteriorly by the anterior scalene muscle. Repeated trauma due to exercise forms a fibrous sheath around the vein. The final contribution is a constant valve at that point which acts as a focus for thrombus formation.

The bony anatomy is almost always normal (in contrast to other variants of the thoracic outlet syndromes). Likewise, patients are often extremely fit; blood tests including thrombophilia screens are usually normal and the only thrombotic risk factor may be the contraceptive pill, which can be recommenced after successful treatment. The dominant limb is affected more frequently. Swimming, tennis and gym work are common causes, followed by repetitive occupational exposure (e.g. strimming) or carrying heavy loads over the shoulder.

Clinical presentation

The history should include the factors outlined above as well as any specific points that may preclude lysis or surgery on the chest wall. The patient presents with a tense swollen arm including the deltoid region. There is usually a history of previous "herald" episodes which resolve spontaneously and may have been forgotten.

On examination the superficial veins are dilated and the limb has a suffused purple/pink hue. The dilated veins do not empty when the limb is elevated above the level of the heart. Assuming the "surrender" position often results in disappearance of the radial pulse, indicating costoclavicular compression, but patients seldom report prior symptoms of ischaemia or ulnar neuralgia.

If a patient does not fit the classical picture, there should be a high index of suspicion for occult malignancy or an alternative diagnosis; appropriate investigation (usually cross-sectional imaging of the thorax) should be requested.

Investigation

A chest X-ray is done to exclude malignancy and to show bony anomalies. Ventilation/perfusion scanning or CT angiography should be ordered to exclude pulmonary embolism if there is low pleuritic pain or haemoptysis. D-dimer levels are usually raised, but other blood tests are less helpful. A blood group and antibody screen should be requested.

Duplex imaging is both sensitive (94%) and specific (96%) in making the diagnosis of axillary vein thrombosis. The vein is examined for the presence of thrombus and for compression during provocative manoeuvres. The normal enhancement of flow on deep inspiration may be lost. The contralateral side may display similar features. Arterial compression during arm elevation is a useful surrogate marker, and indicates thoracic outlet compression.

MRI is seldom helpful but may demonstrate arterial compression. An absent venous flow void can sometimes be seen, but the best specific investigation is contrast venography.

The technique of venography is important. A diagnostic venogram can be done with a good sized cannula in the antecubital fossa coupled with an upper arm tourniquet to drive contrast into the deep veins, but the best approach is to catheterise the basilic or brachial vein under ultrasound guidance. The catheter is then advanced into the thrombus to see if it is soft for lysis. Positional views are taken.

Management

It is useful to discuss the management options with the patient before the diagnosis is confirmed at venography, so that a lysis catheter can be left *in situ*, if approved. The key issues in deciding whether or not to use lysis are as follows:

- Anticoagulation (for 3 months) is needed as a minimum treatment to prevent pulmonary embolus.
- A majority of thromboses will eventually resolve clinically, with the development of collateral veins over several months.
- Disabling swelling persists in 33-85% of patients.
- There is no way of predicting which patients will get persisting symptoms.

With this in mind, the following guidance for treatment can be offered.

- In older patients who will accept reduced activity or whose non-dominant arm is affected, the safest option is warfarin for 3 months.
- Younger competitive, sporting types or musicians may demand more of their arm in the future and may accept the risks of lysis.
- Lysis alone is followed by a high rate of rethrombosis.
- Lysis followed by surgery should be offered as a package (Figure 1).

Consent to lysis should include the risk of bleeding, a theoretical risk of embolism and the mandatory warning of stroke. This is estimated at 1% but there is no report of stroke following upper limb venous lysis in young patients in the literature.

Thrombolysis

Locally directed lysis with tissue plasminogen activator (t-PA) is highly effective if the clot is less than about 4 weeks old. The author has had success with older clot which is presumably in a state of turnover rather than chronically adherent. A side-hole catheter is embedded in the thrombus and a bolus dose of 5mg t-PA is injected followed by infusion of 0.5-

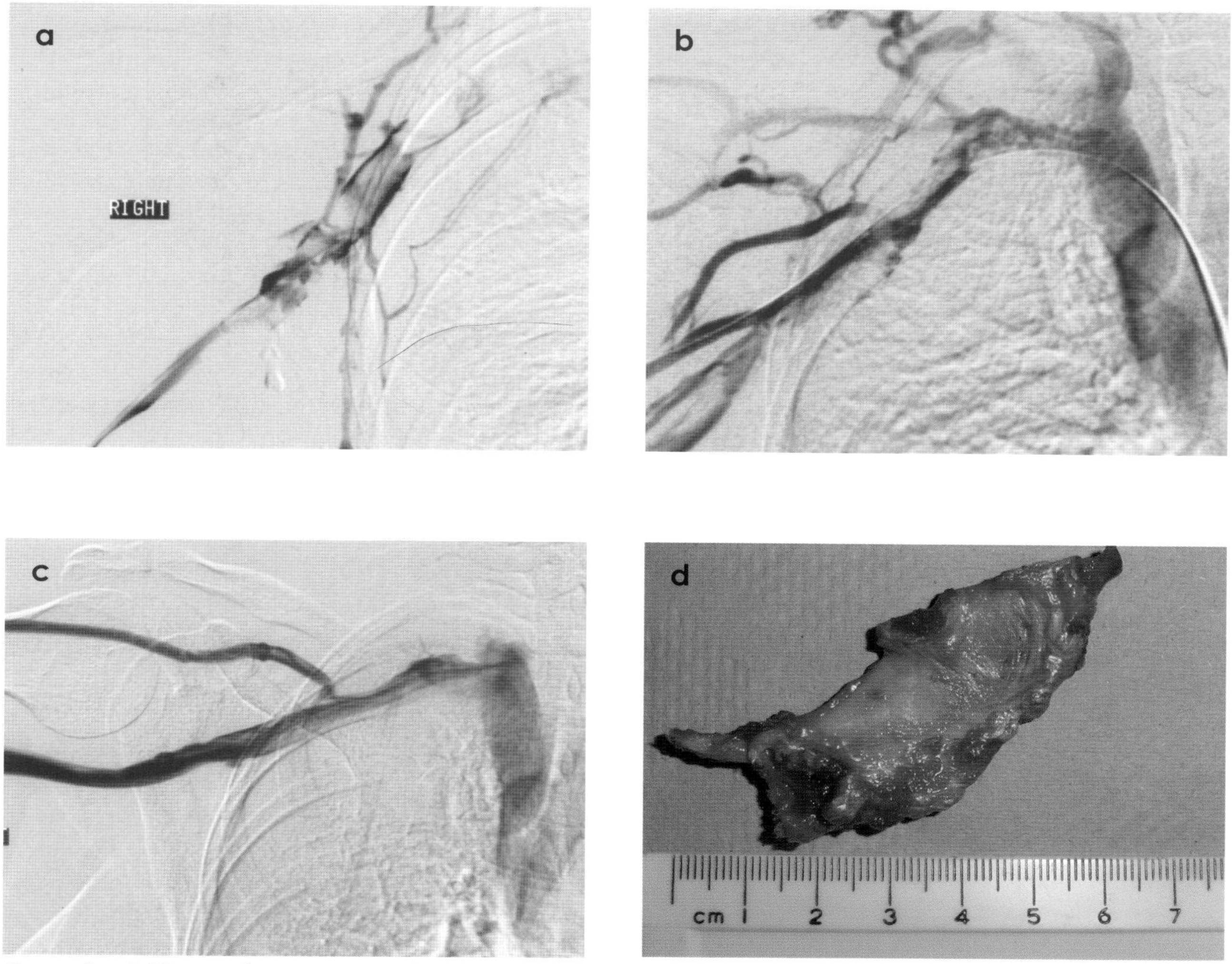

Figure 1. a) Diagnostic venogram showing axillary/subclavian vein thrombus in a woman who had been vacuuming vigorously in her job as a professional cleaner. b) After lysis, but pre-operative venogram showing residual thrombus but patent subclavian vein. c) Three weeks after transaxillary first rib resection and venolysis; stressed view showing rapid free flow in the vein and no collateral filling. Venoplasty was not needed. d) Resected mid-section of right first rib showing area worn smooth by subclavian vessels and T1 nerve root. Note the bone spicule posteriorly - great care must be taken when removing this initial specimen!

1.0mg/h, usually overnight. Heparin, 250IU/h, is infused through the 5 FG angiographic sheath to discourage pericatheter thrombosis or re-thrombosis and aspirin 75mg is given routinely.

Decompression surgery

After successful reopening of the axillary/subclavian vein, decompression surgery should be planned for the next available elective operating list in view of the risk of rethrombosis or even fatal pulmonary embolism [3]. Early surgery also yields better functional results. The patient can be anticoagulated, pending operation, using either intravenous heparin infusion or therapeutic subcutaneous low molecular weight heparin in the interim. The injection is best given in the evenings so that the peak of anti-factor Xa activity is past, well before the morning list.

Patients should be counselled about possible neurovascular injury (<2.0%), phrenic nerve palsy

(<0.5%), anaesthesia in the intercostobrachial nerve distribution, and the possible need for chest drainage, thoracotomy and blood transfusion.

The best approach is a transaxillary first rib resection and circumferential venolysis. The technique is described in detail elsewhere [4], but there are several tips specific to the treatment of PSS.

- Surgeons who undertake these operations should be properly trained and perform them regularly. This is an unforgiving area patrolled by lawyers.
- Experienced nursing staff and a good assistant are vital. The team must be trained and prepared to deal with serious intrathoracic bleeding by thoracotomy or median sternotomy in an emergency. The anaesthetic is usually easy, but can degenerate rapidly.
- Big mistakes are indeed made through small holes; a balance must be struck between access and cosmesis.
- Each anatomical step of the dissection must be completed before moving on to the next. Cutting corners usually results in bleeding or an inability to perform the next move properly.
- Take great care when removing the rib as bone splinters can tear vessels or nerves. It is sometimes safer to remove the middle section of the rib and then nibble back the stump under direct vision.
- The subclavius tendon takes origin from a surprisingly large area on the upper surface of the first rib and costal cartilage. This must be divided with either scissors or a scalpel; the vein lies immediately behind.
- Once the rib has been removed the wound should be packed for 5 minutes to achieve haemostasis, and checked again. Patients are prone to ooze afterwards.
- The operation is completed by freeing the whole vein of its "rind". Start the dissection in the normal axillary vein and work medially to the innominate vein.
- The pleura should be opened routinely. If a haemothorax occurs it is better to drain this with an intercostal drain than to have haematoma around the neurovascular bundle.

Postoperative venoplasty

Postoperative venography should be performed 2-3 weeks after decompression, before scar tissue forms. In some cases the vein is wide open and no further action is required. In others there is a residual stenosis at the site of the thrombosis and the valve. Venoplasty is performed with an 8-10mm balloon with high inflation pressures. A cutting balloon is sometimes required. Patients are then either kept on postoperative oral anticoagulation or simply an antiplatelet agent for 3 months at the discretion of the surgical team. Recently, on-table venoplasty at the time of rib resection has been reported - this would appear to be a good idea if high quality imaging facilities are available in theatre [5].

Stents should NOT be employed in these young patients as they tend to fracture if the rib is not resected, or to cause late thrombosis.

Late presentation

Patients presenting with an established axillary vein thrombosis often have symptoms related to arterial or neurological thoracic outlet syndrome. Where there is doubt, invasive pressure measurements can be done with an occlusive arm tourniquet and during the Roos manoeuvre (see Chapter 19, Thoracic outlet syndrome). Raised venous pressure can then be correlated (or not) with the appearance of symptoms. It may be reasonable to proceed with transaxillary rib resection, which does not compromise collateral drainage, in these patients.

A-V fistula

Patients with incapacitating venous hypertension present a special difficulty. Venous bypass operations have had mixed success in the past. The author performs a brachial artery to cephalic vein 8mm fistula under local anaesthetic. This drives the formation of an impressive collateral circulation, but does not lead to painful venous hypertension as seen in patients with central venous occlusion due to catheter thromboses. The fistula is disconnected several months later and the arm returns to normal.

Key points

- Treatment of Paget Schroetter syndrome involves close co-operation between surgeon, radiologist and the patient.
- Teams should be properly trained and experienced.
- Timing of interventions is moving towards a "one-stop" approach.
- Selection of the right patient for the right procedure is essential.

References

1. Kahn SN, Stansby G. Paget Schroetter syndrome. *Phlebology* 2003 18: 2-11.
2. Prandoni P, Bernardi E, Marchiori A, *et al.* The long-term clinical course of acute deep vein thrombosis of the arm: prospective cohort study. *BMJ* 2004; 329: 484-5.
3. Bliss S, Weinberger S, Meier M, Saint S. Clinical problem-solving. The unusual suspect. *N Engl J Med* 2002; 347: 1876-81.
4. Thompson JF. Transaxillary first rib resection. In: *Vascular and endovascular techniques.* Greenhalgh RM, Ed. WB Saunders, New York, 2001.
5. Schneider DB, Dimuzio PJ, Martin ND, *et al.* Combination treatment of venous thoracic outlet syndrome: open surgical decompression and intraoperative angioplasty. *J Vasc Surg* 2004; 40: 599-603.

Case vignette

Embolic arm ischaemia due to primary axillary artery aneurysm

Frank CT Smith BSc MD FRCS FRCS (Ed) FRCS (Glas), Consultant Senior Lecturer, Bristol Royal Infirmary, UK

A 65-year-old man presented with acute left arm ischaemia and digital necrosis (Figure 1). Examination revealed a pulsatile mass palpable above the clavicle and in the left axilla. Selective angiography revealed a primary axillary artery aneurysm containing thrombus (Figure 2), the source of the embolus. Brachial embolectomy and exclusion bypass of the aneurysm using reversed long saphenous vein, tunnelled beneath the clavicle, was undertaken (Figure 3). Revascularisation was confirmed by completion angiography (Figure 4).

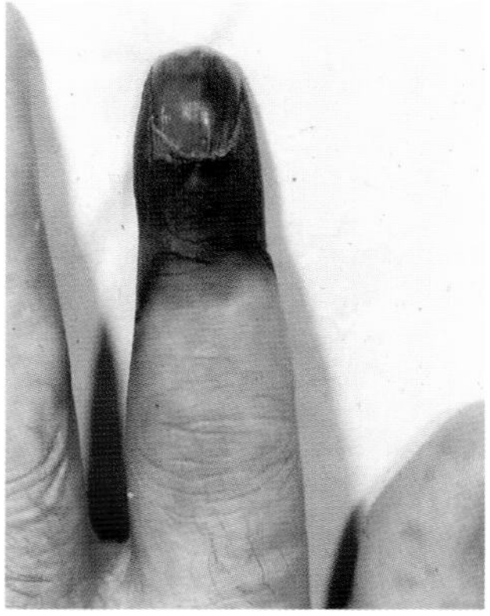

Figure 1.

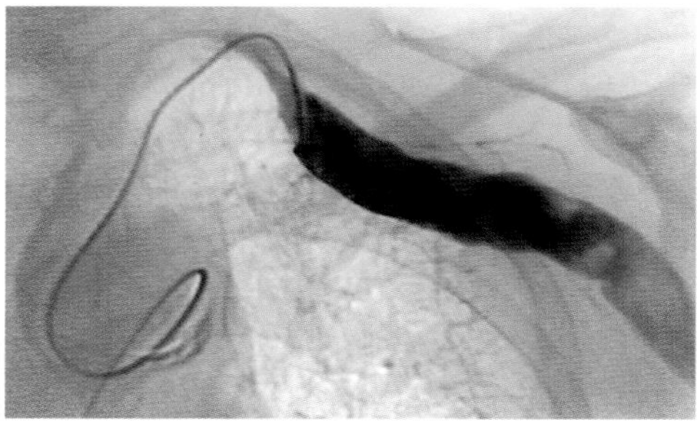

Figure 2.

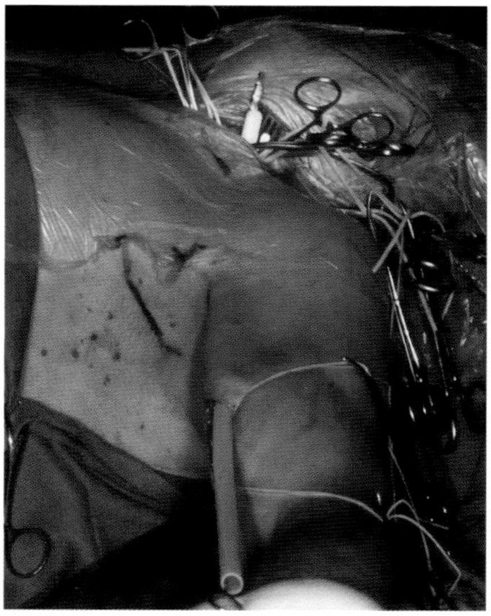

Figure 3.

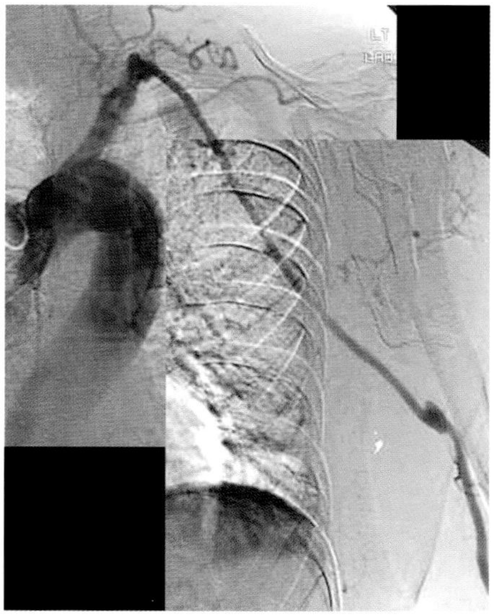

Figure 4.

Chapter 21

Subclavian steal syndrome

Mark Scriven BSc (Hons), MB ChB MD FRCS, Consultant Vascular Surgeon
John Henderson MB ChB MRCP FRCR, Consultant Interventional Radiologist
Birmingham Heartlands Hospital, Birmingham, UK

Introduction

Subclavian steal occurs when reversed blood flow in the vertebral artery deprives the posterior intracranial circulation of blood to favour the ipsilateral arm instead. This phenomenon occurs in the presence of several vascular lesions, singularly or in combination, including stenosis or occlusion of the ipsilateral subclavian or innominate artery proximal to the origin of the vertebral artery (Figure 1). When symptomatic, this haemodynamic phenomenon is an important cause of syncope and upper limb ischaemia. In the symptomatic patient this phenomenon is termed the subclavian steal syndrome (SSS). Similarly, anginal symptoms can occur when blood is "stolen" from the coronary circulation via the left internal mammary artery to supply the arm in individuals who have previously undergone coronary artery bypass grafting (CABG) based on the left internal mammary artery (LIMA). This has been termed the coronary-subclavian steal syndrome (see vignette on page 148).

Aetiopathology

Subclavian steal syndrome is a rare condition, but is more common in caucasians because of their increased incidence of atherosclerosis. The precise prevalence remains unknown, but the condition accounts for 1-2% of extracranial carotid artery procedures in selected units [1]. The incidence of SSS demonstrates a geographical variation. In the USA, the Joint Study of Extracranial Arterial Occlusion demonstrated the angiographic incidence of steal to be 2.5% of which only 5.3% had neurological symptoms. In Europe, the incidence of radiological steal is 1.3% of which, similarly, only 5% have symptoms. The underlying pathology in Europe and America is usually atherosclerosis, unlike the Far East where up to 36% of patients with SSS have Takayasu's disease. Atherosclerotic SSS generally affects patients older than 55 years with a male: female ratio of 2:1, and is commoner on the left side by a factor of 2-3 times. However, in the Far East where the aetiology includes Takayasu's arteritis the male:female ratio is reversed and the age of presentation is typically less than 30 years of age (see Chapter 5, Takayasu's arteritis).

Symptomatic steal, as opposed to the radiological demonstration of reversed blood flow in the vertebral artery, is associated with concomitant lesions in the contralateral vertebral and one, or both carotid arteries in 35-85% of subjects. Some clinicians recommend treating the carotid rather than the subclavian lesion to obtain relief of symptoms,

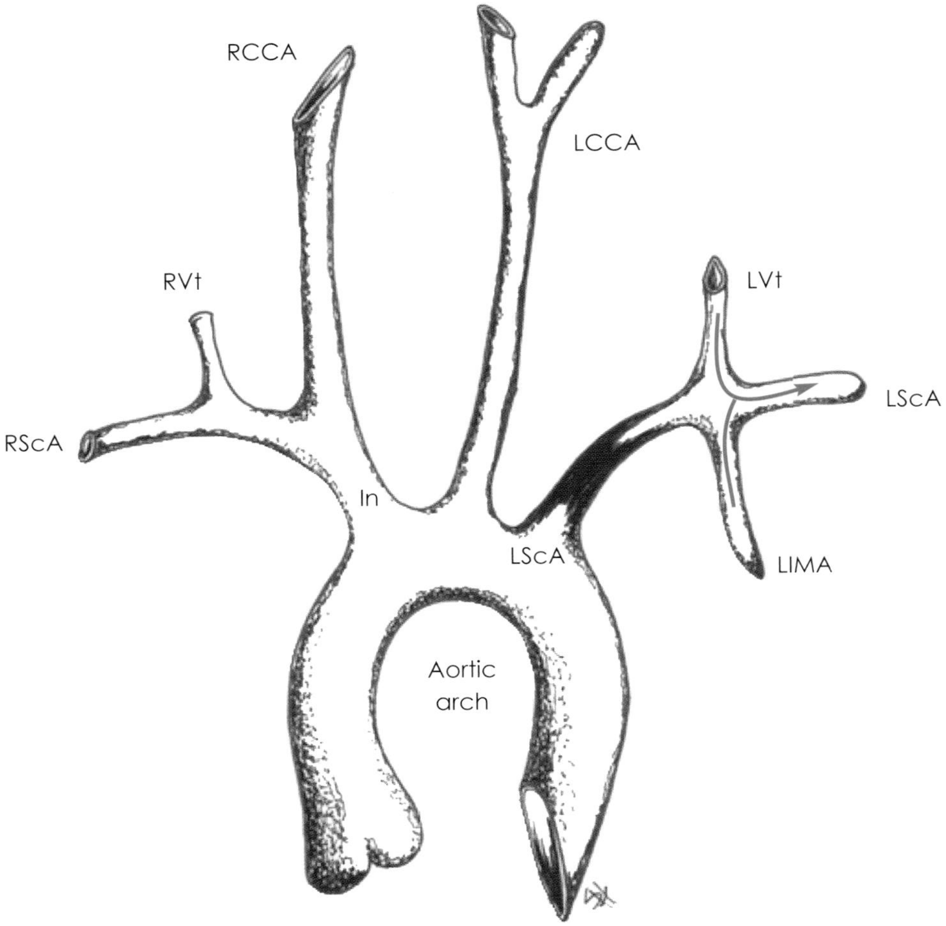

Figure 1. Subclavian steal syndrome. Reversed flow in the vertebral artery on arm exercise. Diagrammatic representation of left (L) and right (R) common carotid (CCA), vertebral (Vt), subclavian (ScA), innominate (In) and left internal mammary (LIMA) arteries.

presumably because extensive disease in multiple vessels results in global cerebral hypoperfusion.

Historical background

Harrison in 1829 and Smyth in 1864 [2] described atherosclerotic occlusive lesions of the innominate and subclavian arteries. Contorni [3] radiologically identified reversed blood flow in the vertebral artery of a patient with an asymptomatic subclavian artery occlusion in 1960. In 1961, Reivich *et al* first used the term subclavian steal syndrome (SSS) [4].

Various open and endovascular surgical options are available to relieve the symptoms of SSS. Initial treatments involved transthoracic procedures, and the full range of vascular surgical techniques has been employed at some time to revascularise the subclavian artery. Sources of arterial inflow have included the aortic arch, great vessels, contralateral upper limb and the lower limb using a femoro-axillary artery bypass in the opposite manner to the more familiar axillo-femoral conduit [2].

Clinical presentation

Clinical history

Patients with SSS may be classified into four groups based on symptomatology [5]:

- asymptomatic;
- upper limb symptoms;
- cerebellar symptoms and non-cerebral hemispheric symptoms (vertebrobasilar insufficiency); and
- symptoms of associated extracranial carotid artery stenoses.

Patients with an isolated subclavian occlusion rarely describe symptoms because of the rich anastomosis of collateral vessels supplying the head, neck and shoulder. However, when present, neurological symptoms include dizziness, vertigo, impaired balance, light-headedness, syncopal attacks, visual disturbances and hemiparesis/hemisensory dysfunction [4]. The classical association between neurological symptoms and arm exercise is present in only a small number of patients. Arm symptoms include fatigue, pain during use of the arm (arm claudication), paraesthesia, coolness and a sensation of heaviness. Chronic arm ischaemia is much less common than leg ischaemia. Arm symptoms are often due to repeated episodes of micro-embolisation from the subclavian lesion rather than reduced flow across it. It is also important to identify concomitant carotid territory symptoms such as transient ischaemic attacks and amaurosis fugax, suggestive of a symptomatic carotid stenosis, which should also be considered for treatment, either sequentially or synchronously.

The analogous condition, coronary-subclavian steal syndrome appeared in the literature in the early 1970s. It presents with recurrent myocardial ischaemia following coronary artery bypass grafting. This is usually brought on by arm exercise when flow in the internal mammary artery conduit is reduced or reversed to supply blood to the arm. The incidence of subclavian artery stenosis in patients undergoing coronary artery bypass grafting is 0.5-1.1%, and the incidence of coronary-subclavian steal syndrome is reported as up to 3.4% occurring 2-31 years following CABG. Thus, patients being prepared for CABG where a LIMA graft is anticipated, need full assessment of left subclavian artery patency.

Physical examination

This involves a full clinical assessment, focusing on the arms and extracranial carotid arteries. Subclavian steal (unless bilateral) may be suspected if the characters of the left and right radial pulses are asymmetric (more commonly the left side is affected) and associated with a differential blood pressure measurement in each arm. Typically, a difference in systolic pressure of 40-50mmHg is apparent, but pressure differences ranging from 20-140mmHg have been described. Although unrelated to the degree of stenosis or occlusion, the presence of a supra/infraclavicular (subclavian) or carotid bruit should be conventionally sought as an indicator of an underlying arterial abnormality.

Investigation

A clinical diagnosis of SSS is confirmed by appropriate imaging. Although contrast angiography has been considered the gold standard, there are a number of alternative methods. Non-invasive techniques include ultrasound imaging, CT and MRI specifically, magnetic resonance angiography (MRA). In many instances these non-invasive methods allow the diagnosis to be confirmed as an outpatient, with traditional catheter angiography being used for absolute confirmation and as a prelude to open or endovascular treatment.

Non-invasive imaging techniques

Ultrasound scanning

Duplex ultrasound imaging is the usual first-line method in most centres, giving useful information about anatomy and haemodynamics. In fact, the subclavian steal phenomenon is often diagnosed incidentally during imaging of the carotid and vertebral arteries. However, this technique can be

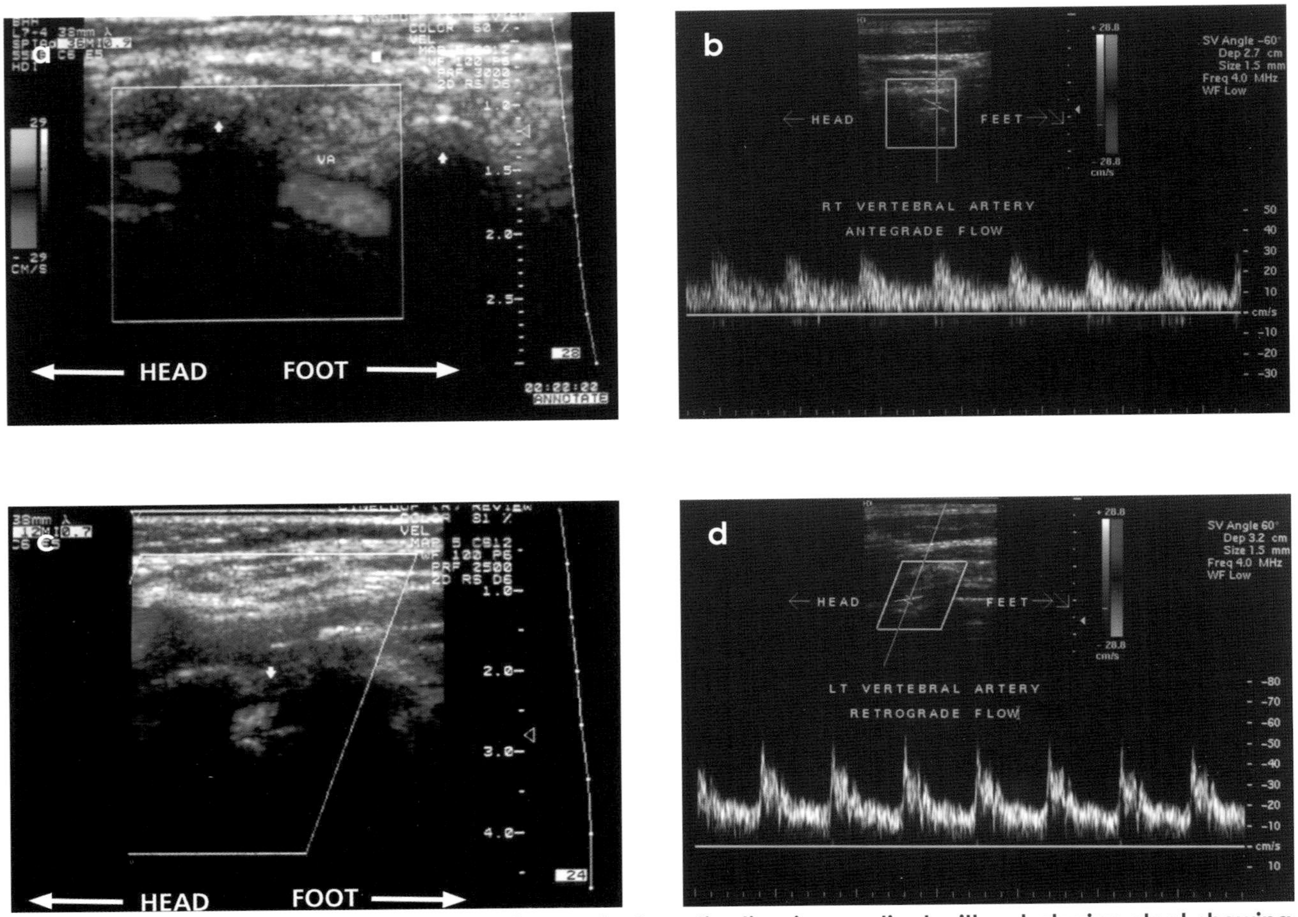

Figure 2. a & c) Colour duplex and b) & d) Doppler investigation in a patient with subclavian steal showing reversal of flow in the left vertebral artery. Note the Doppler beam has been angled towards the head in figures c & d, hence reversed flow is towards the probe.

compromised by the overlying bony structures (clavicle, ribs, and sternum). The duplex signs suggestive of a steal phenomenon include a decrease in the midsystolic vertebral artery flow velocity. This decrease is exaggerated with the degree of steal until the direction of initially diastolic, then both diastolic and systolic flow is reversed. This reversed blood flow, in the left vertebral artery for example, is associated with normal cephalad flow in the contralateral (right) vertebral artery (Figure 2). It must be remembered, however, that even continuous total reversal of flow in the vertebral artery does not indicate the presence of neurological symptoms. Reversed flow in the vertebral artery may be enhanced by imaging this vessel during a period of reactive hyperaemia induced by arm exercise. The presence of a proximal subclavian artery stenosis or occlusion can be inferred from changes in the spectral waveform detected in the distal subclavian, axillary or brachial arteries, typically loss of the usual triphasic pattern. Similarly, compensatory flow may be evident in the remaining extracranial arteries in the presence of steal syndrome. Despite severe proximal left subclavian artery occlusive disease, flow reversal in the ipsilateral vertebral artery may be absent in 6% of subjects when the left vertebral artery originates directly from the aortic arch. This anatomical variant may be difficult to image directly with duplex because of the encroaching bony structures, but is clearly apparent during angiography.

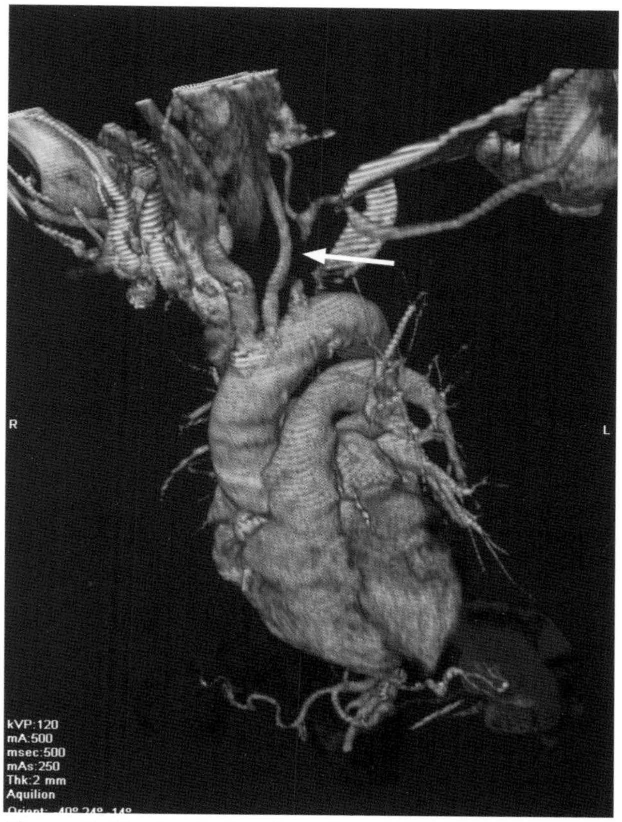

Figure 3. 3D shaded surface image from a multi-slice CT acquisition showing a proximal left subclavian artery occlusion (arrow).

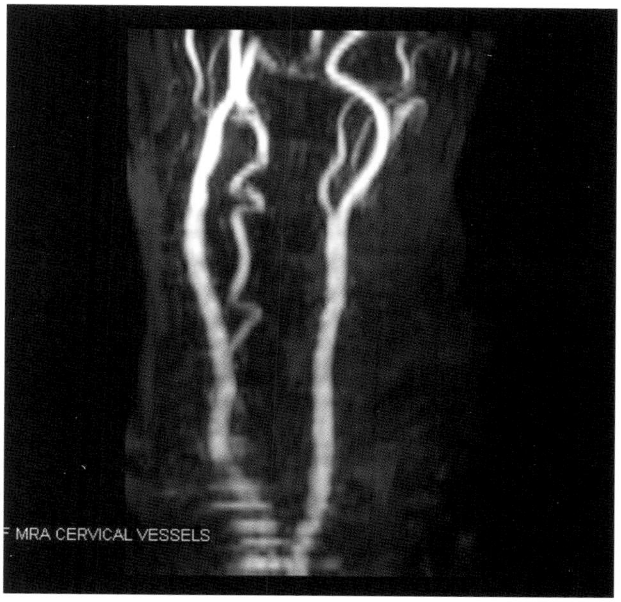

Figure 4. 2D time-of-flight magnetic resonance angiography showing apparent occlusion of the left vertebral artery.

Transcranial Doppler (TCD)

Examination of the basilar artery and circle of Willis with TCD can characterise flow dynamics in the collateral vessels. The demonstration of reversed flow in the basilar artery is often associated with neurological symptoms, especially if accompanied by carotid artery disease.

Computed tomography (CT)

CT angiography can delineate the anatomy of the aortic arch vessels along with complex soft tissue anatomy and adjacent bony structures. Vessel identification is greatly improved with the advent of multidetector CT, as the rapid acquisition of images ensures a high concentration of contrast medium. Simultaneous software developments allow image manipulation and three-dimensional reconstruction can provide information about the degree and location of occlusive disease (Figure 3). The route of intravenous contrast delivery may be important. In SSS, visualisation of the arch vessels and left subclavian origin is improved by delivery from the right arm, thus removing any potential artefact due to dense contrast in the left subclavian or brachiocephalic veins. CT angiography, however, requires exposure to ionising radiation and unlike conventional angiography does not facilitate intervention.

Magnetic resonance imaging (MRI)

MRI is a rapidly developing technique in most units with expanding clinical applications. Time-of-flight MR angiography uses the principle of flow-related enhancement and may be performed either as a two-dimensional (2D TOF MRA) or 3-dimensional (3D TOF MRA) technique. In particular, 2D TOF MRA is often used as a quick method of imaging the cervical carotid and vertebral arteries. Whilst it is generally reliable in demonstrating anatomy and vessel patency, it can overestimate the degree of arterial narrowing and is less reliable in tortuous vessels and in the presence of turbulent or reversed blood flow (Figure 4). If SSS is suspected, placement of an inferior saturation band rather than the usual superior saturation band, is necessary to allow visualisation of reversed flow in the vertebral artery (Figure 5). Techniques such as 2D TOF MRA are not readily applicable to the arch and great vessels by virtue of

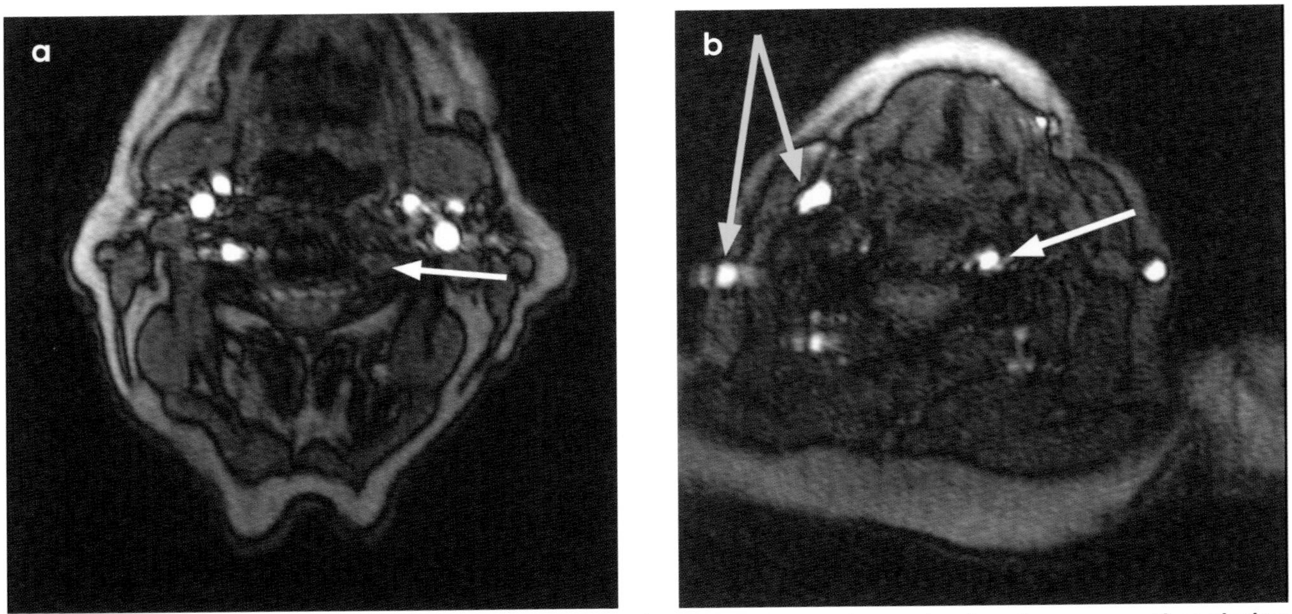

Figure 5. a) Single image from 2D time-of-flight magnetic resonance angiography showing apparent occlusion of the left vertebral artery. b) Substitution of an inferior saturation band reveals flow in the left vertebral artery (white arrow) and adjacent neck veins (yellow arrows).

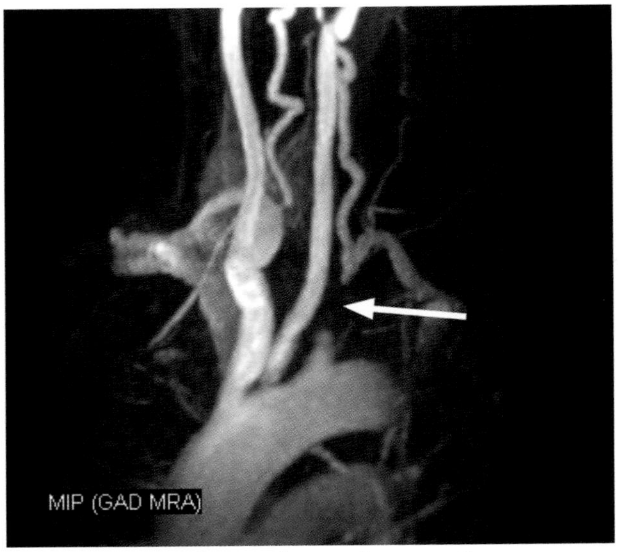

Figure 6. Gadolinium-enhanced magnetic resonance angiography of the aortic arch showing a proximal left subclavian artery occlusion (arrow).

the relatively large area, complex anatomy and complex flow patterns. Imaging the arterial tree with gadolinium enhancement is less susceptible to artefacts from complex anatomy and flow patterns and can cope with larger anatomical areas (Figure 6). Subtraction techniques provide high resolution, high contrast vascular imaging. MRA, however, remains a technique which some patients cannot tolerate (claustrophobia) or cannot undergo because of comorbidity (pacemakers, cerebral aneurysm clips, etc.).

Invasive imaging

Contrast angiography

Conventional digital subtraction angiography (DSA) is the traditional method of imaging the arterial tree. Arch aortography is a relatively low-risk procedure often performed as a day-case procedure. It reliably delineates the arch anatomy and any anatomical variants (Figure 7) without interference from overlying bony structures. In the case of SSS, it demonstrates the subclavian lesion and the filling of the ipsilateral vertebral artery is increasingly delayed with greater degrees of flow reversal. It is important to examine angiographic images in real time as it may be possible to see the vertebral artery on the side of the lesion filling retrogradely in the delayed images and the other vertebral filling antegradely (Figure 8). This temporal information is not readily available with either CT or MR imaging.

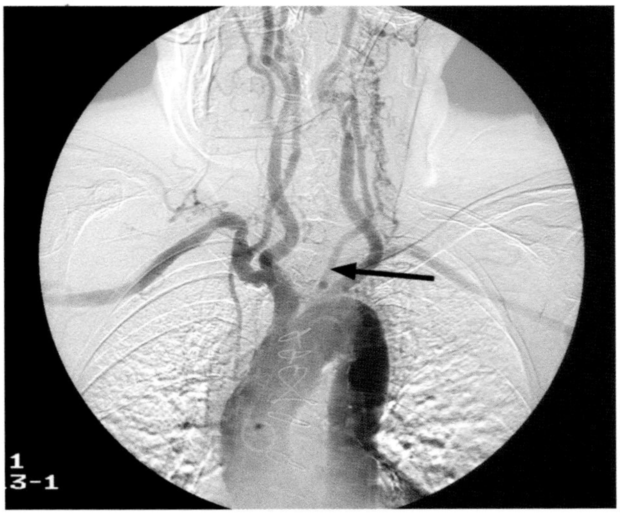

Figure 7. Arch aortogram showing anatomical variant: left vertebral artery arises directly from the aorta (arrow).

Contrast angiography carries the well known but low risk of complications: vessel damage, embolisation, exposure to ionising radiation and risk of contrast nephropathy and allergic reactions. Despite these drawbacks, DSA is invaluable in planning therapeutic strategies, especially endovascular procedures. One important advantage of angiography is the option to allow intervention in addition to diagnosis at the same sitting.

Treatment

The indications for intervention in SSS include vertebrobasilar insufficiency, arm ischaemia and more recently, myocardial ischaemia in patients with a left internal mammary artery coronary bypass graft and subclavian lesion. Several surgical or endovascular options are available.

Surgical treatment

If the ipsilateral common carotid artery is normal, then reconstruction should be based on this vessel. The options are carotid-subclavian artery bypass or, less commonly, subclavian artery transposition. Either method is appropriate to treat vertebrobasilar insufficiency or arm ischaemia, but subclavian artery transposition is not indicated for treatment of myocardial ischaemia due to coronary-subclavian steal syndrome.

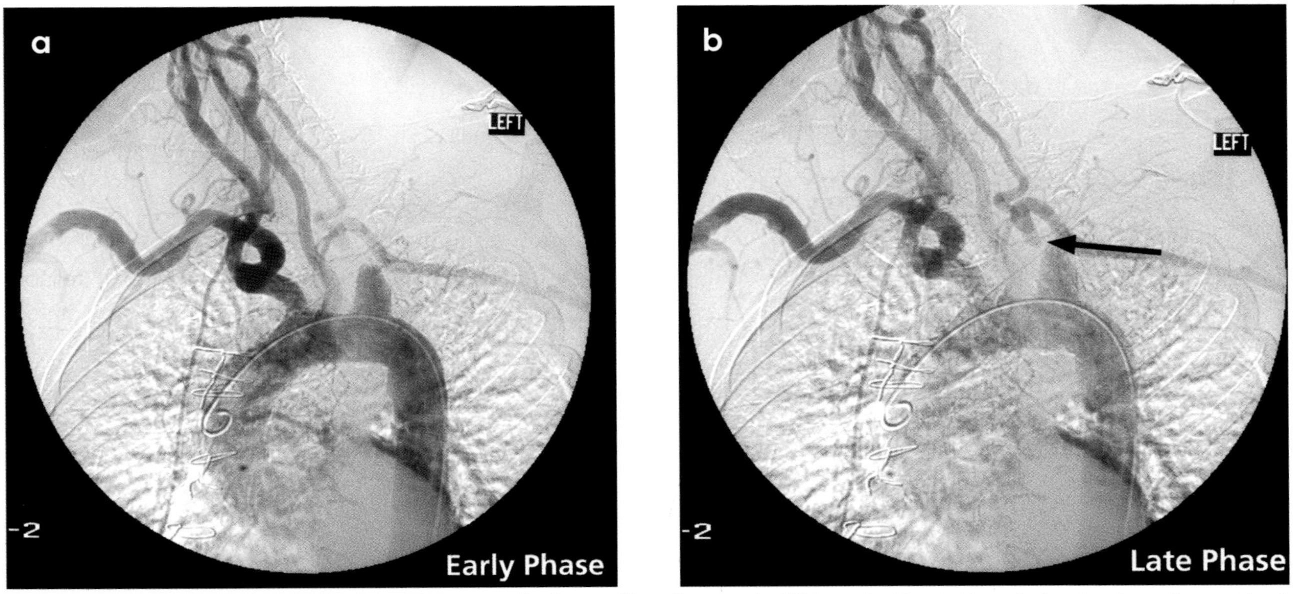

Figure 8. Proximal left subclavian artery occlusion with retrograde filling via the left vertebral artery (arrow) a) Early phase. b) Late phase.

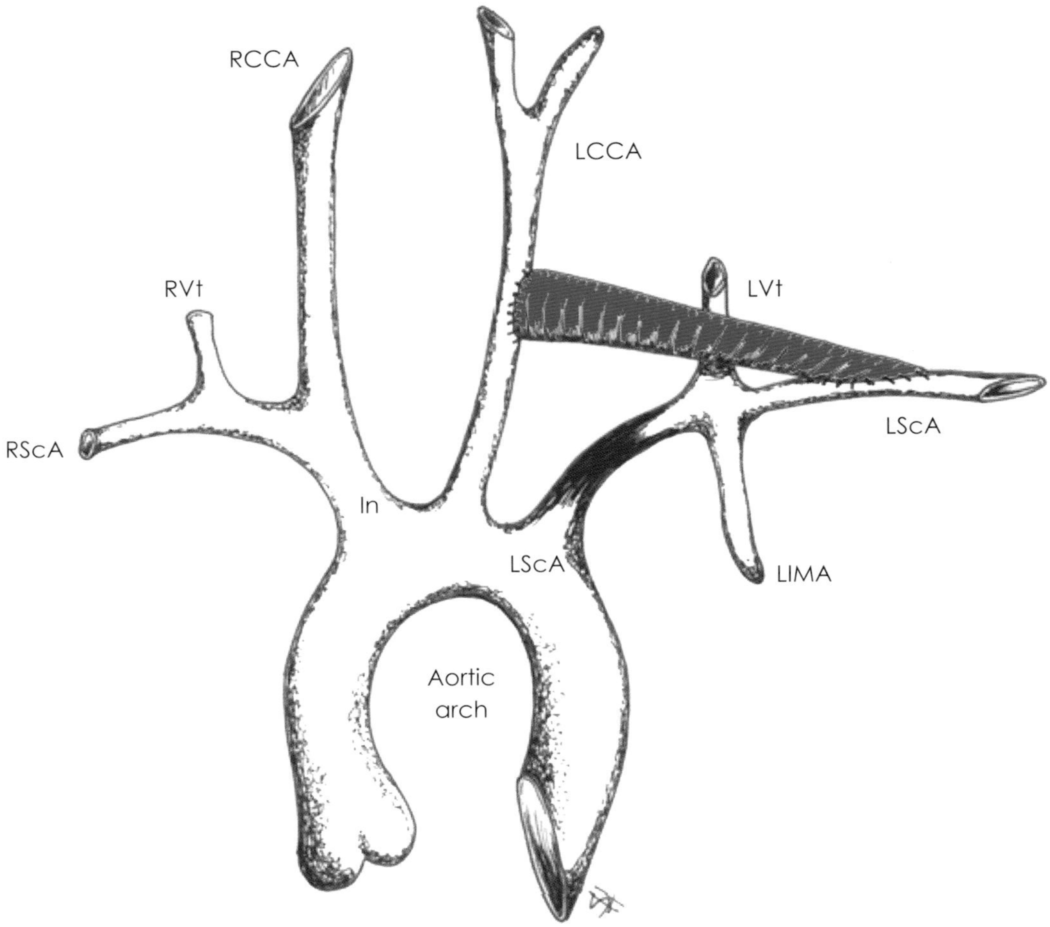

Figure 9. Diagrammatic representation of carotid-subclavian bypass. Graft inserted between left common carotid artery (CCA) and left subclavian artery (ScA).

Carotid-subclavian artery bypass (Figure 9)

A general anaesthetic is employed with the patient supine and a sandbag between the scapulae, with a head ring to support the head and neck. The neck is extended and the head turned away from the side of the lesion. A transverse supraclavicular incision is made and the subclavian artery is dissected having divided the scalenus anterior muscle, preserving the phrenic nerve and thoracic duct. The subclavian, vertebral, internal mammary arteries and thyrocervical trunk are controlled. In the medial part of the wound, deep to the internal jugular vein the common carotid artery (CCA) is dissected and controlled, protecting the vagus nerve. After systemic heparinisation, an arteriotomy is made on the lateral wall of the CCA and a short, 6-10mm diameter (depending on the size of the subclavian artery) prosthetic graft is anastomosed end-to-side to the CCA, tunnelled beneath the jugular vein and anastomosed end-to-side to the subclavian artery distal to the origin of the vertebral artery. Patency is superior if a prosthetic material is used: PTFE 95%, dacron 84% vs. saphenous vein 65%, over 3-5 years [6]. If the subclavian lesion was a source of emboli then the subclavian artery may be ligated proximal to the vertebral artery to prevent further embolisation.

In the absence of CCA stenosis proximal to the CCA arteriotomy, steal down the internal carotid artery is unlikely as a complication of carotid-subclavian

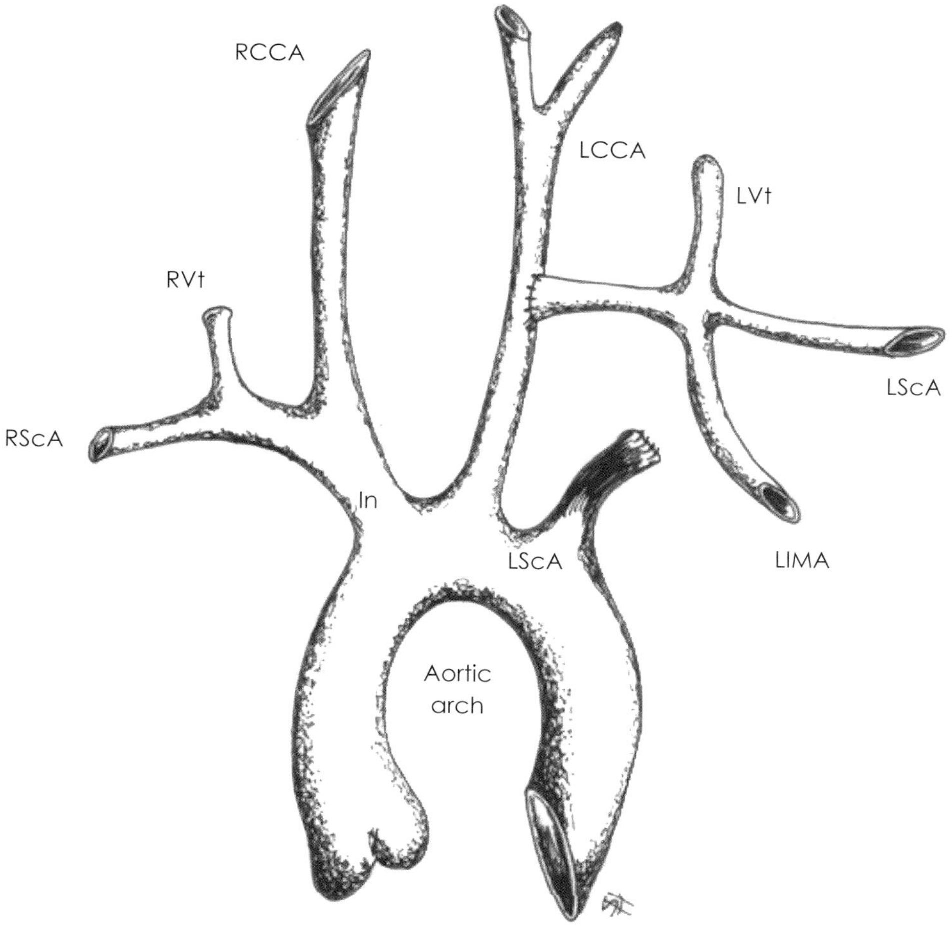

Figure 10. Diagrammatic representation of subclavian artery transposition procedure. Common carotid (CCA), vertebral (Vt), subclavian (ScA) and left internal mammary arteries (LIMA) marked.

bypass (carotid-subclavian steal syndrome). In patients with significant carotid bifurcation disease, carotid endarterectomy alone may improve cerebral perfusion without revascularising the vertebral artery. A carotid shunt will be required during the procedure.

A review of 124 procedures by Vitti [7], demonstrated that the primary graft patency was 94% and symptom-free survival at 10 years was 87%. This was associated with an operative mortality of 0.8% and a zero stroke rate. One potential cause of peri-operative stroke is embolisation from a thrombosed bypass graft. This should be managed with full anticoagulation and re-operation. Other reported major complications include thoracic duct injury (lymphatic fistula or chylothorax), sympathetic (Horner's syndrome), phrenic or cranial nerve injury and graft infection.

Subclavian artery transposition (Figure 10)

First reported by Parrott in 1964, this procedure does not require a prosthetic bypass and involves only one anastomosis. It does however, necessitate dissection of the subclavian artery proximal to the origins of both vertebral and internal mammary arteries. Transposition is reported to be superior to carotid-subclavian bypass in terms of patency (up to 100% at 10 years) and with equal safety (0% stroke, 1.4% mortality).

The patient is positioned and prepared in the same manner as for carotid-subclavian bypass, and the operative approach is similar. The subclavian artery requires more extensive proximal dissection to allow its division between the lesion and the origin of the vertebral artery, leaving enough length for the subsequent anastomosis. The proximal stump is oversewn and the distal subclavian artery is anastomosed to the side of the CCA passing behind the phrenic nerve.

Endovascular treatment

Balloon angioplasty with, or without the use of a concomitant endoluminal stent has been used to treat both atherosclerotic and Takayasu lesions of the subclavian artery. Bachman and Kim [8] reported the first subclavian artery angioplasty for steal in 1980. Further reports demonstrated the safety and efficacy of this procedure. In a review of 12 cases of subclavian artery angioplasty, all had symptoms of arm ischaemia and five additionally described vertebrobasilar symptoms. Five occlusions and seven stenoses were treated with success in 11/12 procedures [9]; eight patients remained symptom-free at follow-up (1 month-6 years) and three improved. Results of subclavian artery angioplasty alone demonstrate initial technical success rates of 83-100% and patency ranging from 43% for occlusions to 100% for stenoses at late follow-up periods. Unfortunately, although the number of complications is smaller, these results do not compare well with surgical patency. The addition of an intravascular stent improves initial success rates depending on the lesion treated, with primary patency rates of 84% at 35 months follow-up [10]. The number of complications described by Sullivan [10] in 66 subclavian artery angioplasties with stents was low: one embolisation to the arm requiring embolectomy; one embolisation to a LIMA coronary graft treated by thrombolysis; and two inadvertently covered vertebral arteries with no reported symptoms. Transient ischaemic attack was recorded in only one series and involved one procedure in 69; this may be accounted for by the observed delay in return of reversed to antegrade flow in the vertebral artery following angioplasty.

Many interventionists would demonstrate anatomy by angiography via the transfemoral route, but attempt endovascular treatment via the brachial/axillary route. The left arm retrograde approach is particularly useful when dealing with occlusive disease. Access can be achieved easily despite the absence of arm pulses using ultrasound-guided puncture techniques. The shorter route from the brachial/axillary access site to the site of the lesion allows finer catheter and wire manipulation and more control for the placement of a stent. Furthermore, the reversed flow down the left vertebral artery gives a degree of protection from any potential posterior circulation embolisation. Once access is established and angiography performed, the patient is systemically heparinised and a hydrophillic guide wire is used to cross the lesion. The lesion is predilated under roadmapping guidance to an appropriate size (4-10mm), and then a suitably sized stent is deployed and completion imaging performed. A variety of stents have been used including balloon and self-expanding stents (especially if the lesion is long). All patients should be on antiplatelet therapy postoperatively as part of best medical therapy.

Key points

- **Subclavian steal syndrome is often asymptomatic and can be managed conservatively.**
- **Recurrence of angina after CABG using a left internal mammary artery graft should prompt further investigation of the great vessels, especially the left subclavian artery.**
- **Imaging is achieved using non-invasive techniques (duplex, CT and MRA); catheter angiography is reserved for endovascular intervention.**
- **Endovascular treatment with angioplasty and stent deployment is effective but surgical revascularisation has better patency and remains the treatment of choice in fit patients.**
- **All patients should have additional best medical therapy.**

References

1. Delaney CP, Couse NF, Mehigan D, *et al.* Investigation and management of subclavian steal syndrome. *Br J Surg* 1994; 81: 1093-5.
2. Williams II, SJ. Chronic upper extremity ischaemia: current concepts in management. *Surg Clin North Am* 1986; 66: 355-75.
3. Contorni L. Il circolo collaterale vertebro-vetrebrale nell obliterazione dell'arteria succlavia alla sua origine. *Minerva Chir* 1960; 15: 268.
4. Reivich M, Holling HE, Roberts B, *et al.* Reversal of blood flow through the vertebral artery and its effects on cerebral circulation. *N Engl J Med* 1961; 265: 818-85.
5. Al-Khaffal H, Kalra M, Farrell A, *et al.* The "subclavian steal" syndrome. *Vasc Surg* 2000; 34: 5-10.
6. Law MM, Colburn MD, Moore WS, *et al.* Carotid-subclavian bypass for brachiocephalic occlusive disease: choice of conduit and long-term follow-up. *Stroke* 1995; 26: 1565-71.
7. Vitti MJ, Thompson BW, Read RC, *et al.* Carotid subclavian bypass: a twenty-two year experience. *J Vasc Surg* 1994; 20: 411-8.
8. Bachman MD, Kim RM. Transluminal dilatation for subclavian steal syndrome. *Am J Radiol* 1980; 135: 995-6.
9. Nicholson AA, Kennan NM, Sheridan WG, *et al.* Percutaneous transluminal angioplasty of the subclavian artery. *Ann R Coll Surg Eng* 1991; 71: 46-52.
10. Sullivan TM, Gray BH, Bacharach JM, *et al.* Angioplasty and primary stenting of the subclavian, innominate, and common carotid arteries in 83 patients. *J Vasc Surg* 1998; 28: 1059-65.

Case vignette Coronary-subclavian steal syndrome

Christopher P Gibbons MA DPhil MCh FRCS, Consultant Surgeon, Morriston Hospital, Swansea, UK

A 65-year-old woman with a history of Type 2 diabetes, ischaemic heart disease and hypertension was referred for a vascular opinion because of increasing angina and left arm claudication with absent pulses in the left arm. She had undergone coronary artery bypass grafts including a left internal mammary artery (LIMA) graft 4 years previously. Angiography (Figure 1) showed an occlusion at the origin (a) of the left subclavian artery (b) and reversed flow in the LIMA graft (c) indicating a coronary-subclavian steal syndrome. Angioplasty failed to recannalise the occlusion. A dacron bypass (Figure 2) (b) was taken from the left carotid (a) to the subclavian artery (c). An internal jugular venous aneurysm (d) was also found but left alone. The operation relieved her arm claudication and improved her angina.

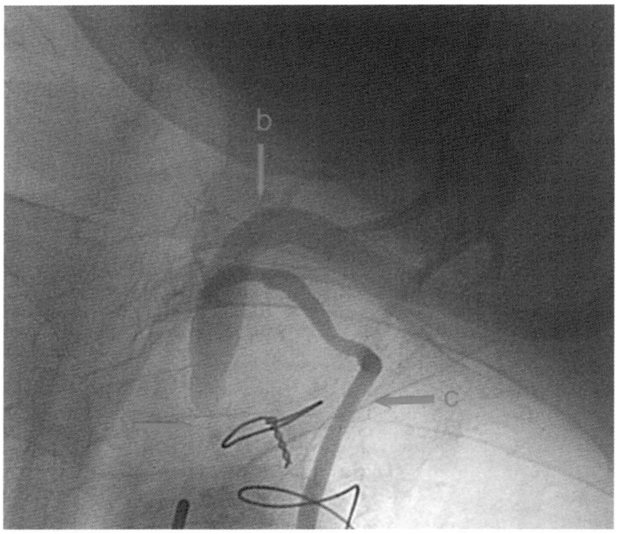

Figure 1.

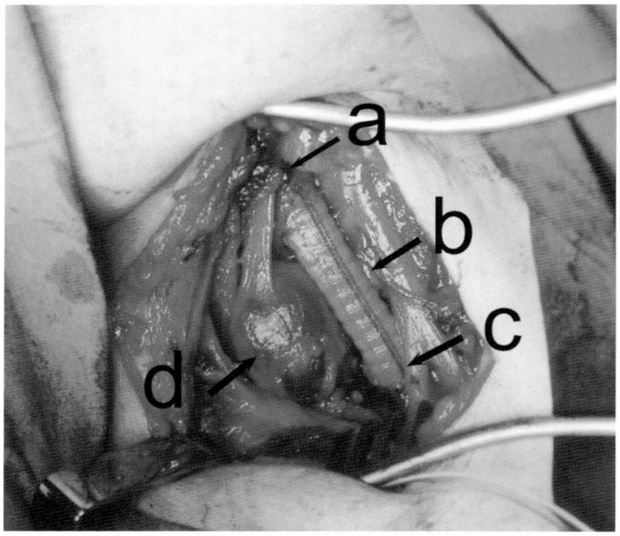

Figure 2.

Chapter 22

Acute arm ischaemia

Jonothan J Earnshaw DM FRCS, Consultant Vascular Surgeon
Gloucestershire Royal Hospital, Gloucester, UK

Introduction

Compared with acute leg ischaemia, acute arm ischaemia is less common and less likely to lead to limb amputation or death [1]. A recent review suggested it accounted for 17% of cases of acute limb ischaemia [2]. Acute arm ischaemia usually occurs in elderly patients with other associated cardiac diseases. Because it is perceived as less dangerous, and there are genuine risks from surgical embolectomy, acute arm ischaemia is often treated conservatively, simply by anticoagulation. Although the arm is not usually threatened, routine use of heparin can risk subsequent disability from forearm claudication [1,3]. Occasionally, acute arm ischaemia can lead to major disability and even amputation (Figure 1). The vascular surgeon has to determine when the ischaemia is dangerous and requires intervention, yet there is little available research to help aid the decision.

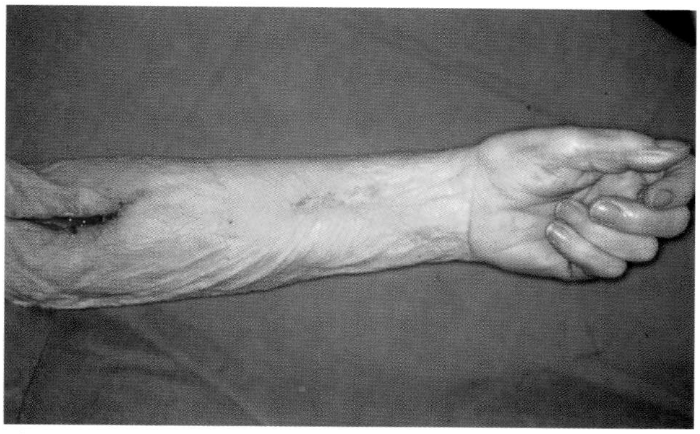

Figure 1. Failed embolectomy, which resulted in wound dehiscence, ischaemic necrosis of the extensor muscle compartment, flexion contracture of the fingers, and a useless, painful arm.

Aetiopathology

Acute arm ischaemia is usually due to embolism. Atherosclerotic disease of the peripheral upper limb arteries is rare, although arteritis is a possibility (see Chapter 4, Major vessel arteritis including lupus). Atherosclerosis does affect the aortic arch and proximal arm vessels, where the disease is often subclinical and asymptomatic. Trauma is a relatively common cause as the extremity is exposed to injury; in reviews it accounts for 15-45% of cases of acute arm ischaemia [2]. The most worrying is supracondylar fracture of the humerus in children, where failure to recognise the condition and apply corrective treatment can be catastrophic. As with all traumatic ischaemia, surgical intervention is required urgently and there are standard procedures that should be followed, including no delay for arteriography and early arterial revascularisation with fracture fixation later. In some hospitals, iatrogenic damage to the brachial artery is common, particularly when brachial puncture is employed for cardiac catheterisation. Another catastrophic traumatic cause of arm ischaemia is inadvertent puncture of the brachial artery by injecting drug users. If any significant volume of particulate matter is injected into the artery, limb salvage is very unlikely (Figure 2).

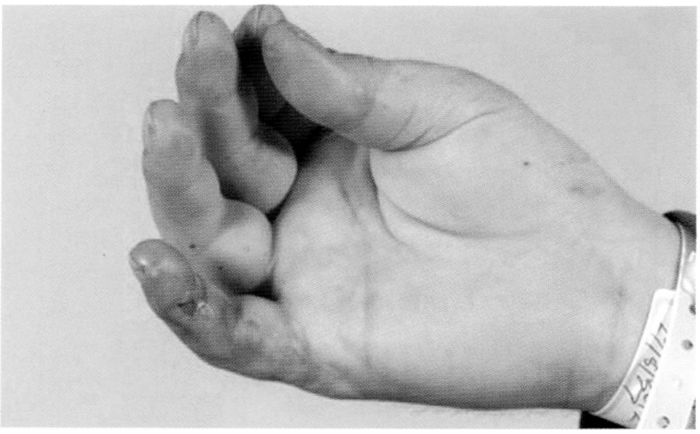

Figure 2. Digital necrosis in an intravenous drug user who accidentally injected heroin into the digital artery, instead of a vein he had been using at the base of his little finger.

Approximately 75% of emboli in the arm come from a cardiac source, either the right atrium in patients with atrial fibrillation, or mural thrombus from acute myocardial infarction. Occasionally, athero-embolus can be dislodged from a proximal source such as a subclavian artery stenosis, where platelet thrombus has accumulated. In thoracic outlet syndrome, the axillary artery is trapped between the first rib and the clavicle, and in extreme cases it can be damaged, resulting in a significant stenosis (see Chapter 19, Thoracic outlet syndrome). Other rare causes of ischaemia include graft occlusion, though bypass grafts are seldom required in the arm. Arm ischaemia is one late result from anastomotic complications at the top end of an axillobifemoral graft.

The severity of the ischaemia is partly dependent on the level of occlusion; the more proximal the occluded artery, the more severe the ischaemia. Subclavian and axillary artery occlusions are most limb-threatening. Fortunately, the most common site of occlusion is at the brachial bifurcation. There are numerous collateral arteries around the elbow, which is the reason that the ischaemia is often not so severe for occlusions at this level. The more proximal the occlusion, the less likely it is to be caused by an embolus.

Diagnosis and investigation

Compared with leg ischaemia, patients with acute arm ischaemia are more likely to be female, and tend to be older (mean age 67 years vs. 64 years) [2]. Clinical examination is usually all that is required to make the diagnosis. The patients classically complain of a painful hand that is white and cold. They usually present quickly; late, missed ischaemia is rare in the arm. Loss of peripheral pulses usually makes the diagnosis easy and the level of the occlusion can be determined accurately by examination. If necessary, the diagnosis can be confirmed with duplex imaging, or occasionally angiography (Figure 3).

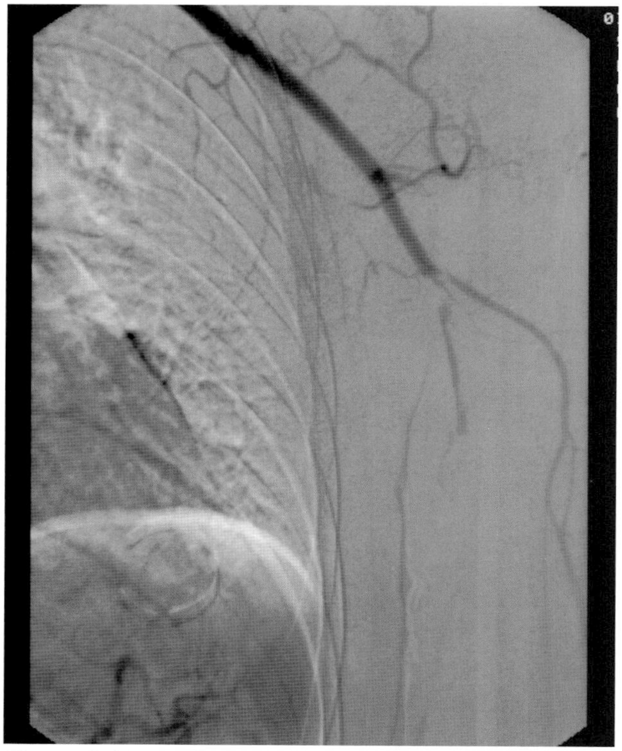

Figure 3. Upper limb angiogram done in a 34-year-old man with acute arm ischaemia, showing normal proximal arm vessels and an embolus in the upper brachial artery.

As with leg ischaemia, management should depend on an assessment of the severity of the ischaemia. Severe ischaemia, including loss of sensation or motor function in the hand, and tender forearm muscles is a strong indication that intervention should be urgent. The lack of an arterial signal at the wrist using hand-held Doppler is also a sign that collateral blood supply is poor. Patients with normal sensation and motor function and audible Doppler signals at the wrist can probably be observed without intervention and treated simply with anticoagulation to see whether there is spontaneous improvement.

All patients, including those who do not have a revascularisation procedure, and those who improve spontaneously, should later be investigated to search for the source of the embolus, otherwise, untreated, they risk recurrent embolism. Investigation may include duplex imaging of the proximal arm arteries to look for a source of athero-embolism, and echocardiography to look for intracardiac thrombus. If a decision is made initially that a patient should be anticoagulated permanently, it is questionable whether or not the search for cardiac thrombus is worthwhile.

Management

It is easy to forget that much has changed in the treatment of acute arterial ischaemia following the description of the embolectomy catheter by Thomas Fogarty in 1963. As recently as 50 years ago, the only possible treatments were warming, vasodilators, anticoagulation, stellate ganglion block, cervical sympathectomy, and only rarely, direct surgical exploration.

In modern times, in the acute situation, anticoagulation with heparin is important first aid. An intravenous infusion, adequately monitored, is the most flexible, though use of therapeutic low molecular weight heparin is increasing. Anticoagulation prevents secondary thrombosis that can lead to limb deterioration. The role of anticoagulation in the long term is less certain and depends on the cause of the ischaemia. As most patients have cardiac emboli, there is a significant potential for a recurrence and long-term anticoagulation should be beneficial. There is no scientific evidence for this, though anticoagulation is effective in reducing the late risk after embolic occlusion in the legs. Many patients with arm ischaemia are old and frail, and the risks of anticoagulation with warfarin may outweigh the benefits. The author occasionally uses a combination of aspirin and clopidogrel in these patients; their combined antiplatelet effect is profound without requiring anticoagulant monitoring.

Patients with critical arm ischaemia require urgent revascularisation. This can be done either surgically with brachial embolectomy or radiologically using thrombolysis.

Brachial embolectomy (Figure 4)

This operation should normally be undertaken under local anaesthetic in a fully monitored patient in a well equipped operating theatre [4]. It is helpful to have an anaesthetist present to monitor observations and control administration of intravenous fluids, and to give a small amount of sedation if required. Low-dose intravenous propofol is a very suitable sedative. An oblique skin incision is made over the brachial artery, which is controlled with rubber slings. Historically, a lazy-S incision is described for this procedure, but this heals poorly, and there remains the flexibility to extend an oblique incision if further exposure is needed (Figure 4b). It is important to make a transverse arteriotomy in the brachial artery to avoid narrowing when the arteriotomy is closed. A size three Fogarty embolectomy catheter may be passed proximally and a size two catheter passed distally. Some authors have suggested that the proximal radial and ulnar arteries should be dissected out individually (as for the femoral arteries in the groin). This, however, increases the complexity of the operation, particularly if done under local anaesthetic, and revascularisation of either of these vessels is adequate to salvage the arm. Failure to establish arterial inflow may require a more complex procedure with bypass of the axillary artery using reversed long saphenous vein. The transverse arteriotomy is best repaired with interrupted 6/0 or 7/0 polypropylene sutures (Figure 4c). Intra-operative angiography may be used to check the completeness of embolectomy, and there is some evidence that this can improve the chance of a successful outcome [5].

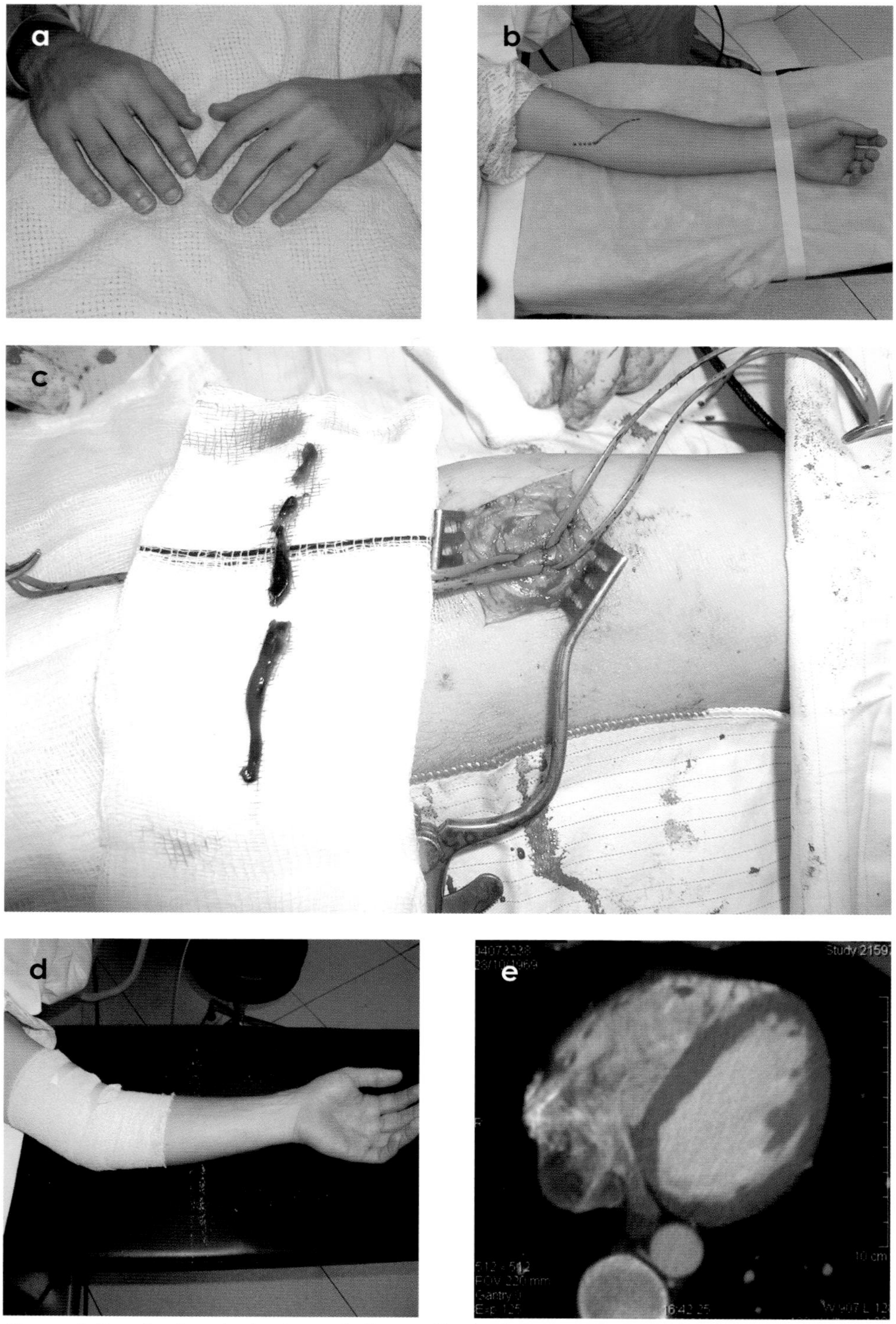

Figure 4. Surgical embolectomy in the patient whose angiogram is depicted in Figure 3. a) Ischaemic left hand of six hour's duration. b) Position on operating table with oblique incision marked and dotted line showing potential extension. c) After successful embolectomy with embolus shown and arterial repair with prolene sutures. d) Pulses restored, and crepe bandage positioned over subcuticular suture repair to prevent haematoma. e) CT of the heart shows thrombus in the left ventricle that caused the embolus. The patient was anticoagulated.

Thrombolysis

As experience with endovascular procedures grows, it is becoming possible to reopen an occluded brachial artery using techniques such as aspiration embolectomy or thrombolysis. Aspiration embolectomy is done using a 7Fr percutaneous catheter to aspirate or debulk an occlusion; additional thrombolysis may be required to remove residual clot. Intra-arterial thrombolysis is used less commonly in the arm than in the leg for two reasons. First, there is less risk to limb and life in acute arm ischaemia. Thrombolysis carries a small risk of significant bleeding complications: approximately 8% risk of major haemorrhage and 2% risk of stroke [6]. For an ischaemic leg where there is a significant risk of amputation, the risks of thrombolysis are better justified. Also, there is the specific danger of "whirlpool embolism", whereby the fact that there is a distal occlusion causes thrombus as it breaks up to wash back up the arm arteries and enter the vertebral or carotid arteries and cause an embolic stroke. Each situation should be treated on individual merits, and thrombolysis using low-dose intra-arterial tissue plasminogen activator may be particularly indicated for distal occlusions that are out of reach of an embolectomy catheter. It is also possible to use thrombolysis during embolectomy to deal with residual distal occlusions.

Other revascularisation procedures

When investigation reveals an isolated stenosis or short occlusion of the proximal limb arteries, treatment with balloon angioplasty, with or without stenting, is usually an option (Figure 5). It must not be forgotten that the procedure carries a small risk of major complications such as stroke [7]. It should be done by an experienced radiologist after informed consent. Occasionally, there is a long occlusion of the limb arteries that requires surgical bypass. Few surgeons have great experience with upper limb revascularisation surgery and the interventions should be tailored to the individual. Reversed saphenous vein is the usual conduit employed [8].

Occasionally, after revascularisation of a severely ischaemic arm, a fasciotomy is required to prevent compartment syndrome, rhabdomyolisis and acute

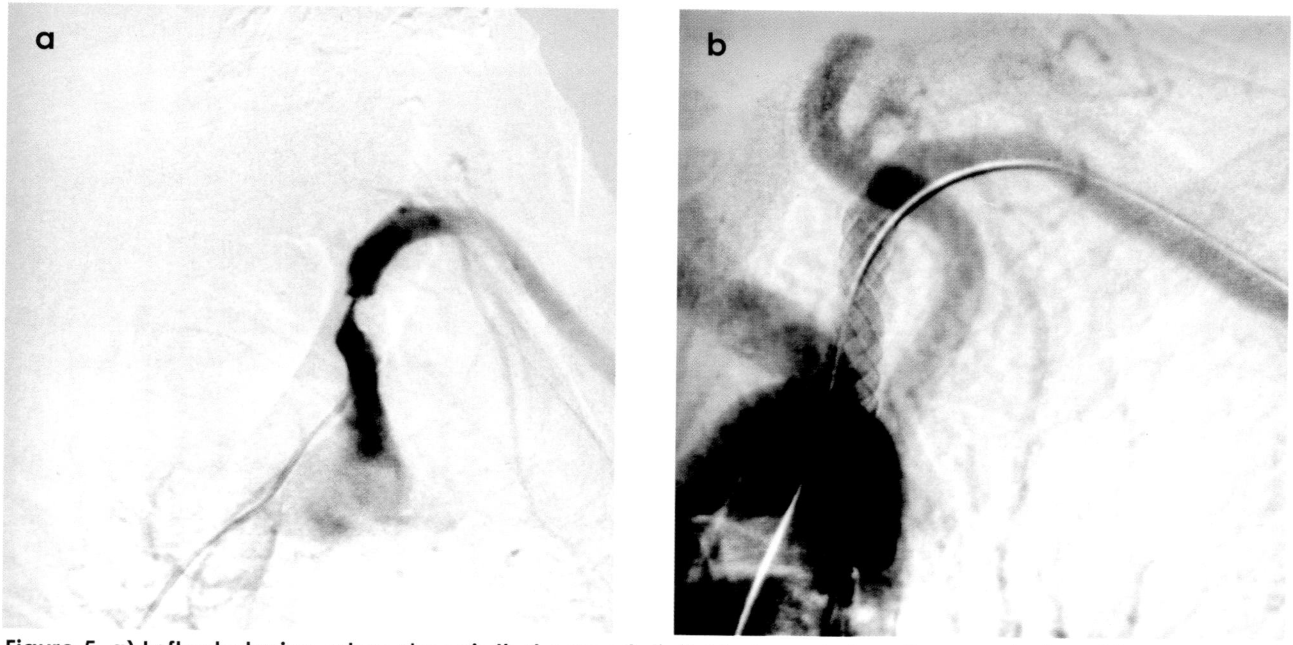

Figure 5. a) Left subclavian artery stenosis that caused digital ischaemia by athero-embolism. b) After balloon angioplasty with stenting, the circulation is restored.

Table 1. Case report: a fatal episode of acute arm ischaemia.
An 80-year-old man was admitted as an emergency with an ischaemic arm. Apparently he had fallen over at home (his wife was in hospital having a hip replacement) and lain on the arm for 12 hours before he was found. The arm was profoundly ischaemic, with mottled discolouration to the elbow and no brachial or axillary pulse. A brachial embolectomy was done under local anaesthetic, and the pulses at the wrist were restored. He was transferred for monitoring to the high dependency unit, but developed acute renal failure due to myoglobinuria from a revascularisation syndrome. He had a raised troponin level suggesting acute myocardial infarction as a possible cause for collapse, and also possible brachial embolus. Despite active intervention he died 48 hours later. A fasciotomy was considered at the time of operation, but it was decided to await the development of any postoperative swelling.

renal failure (Table 1). This is done simply by making separate longitudinal incisions over the flexor and extensor muscle compartments and then leaving the wounds open to heal by secondary intention or skin grafting [9]. The arm is elevated postoperatively.

Outcome and complications

The true outcome after acute arm ischaemia is unknown, since many episodes are treated conservatively on medical wards. Most clinical series are reported by vascular surgeons who have treated their patients actively, where only 9-30% of episodes are treated by anticoagulation alone [2]. Most series describe few late sequelae after conservative treatment, but in the report by Savelyev *et al*, 75% had functional impairment [3]. Galbraith reported that 50% had late forearm claudication [1]. The true natural history of acute arm ischaemia remains a mystery.

Brachial embolectomy is generally a safe and effective procedure, particularly when done under local anaesthetic by an experienced surgeon. A successful embolectomy will usually return an arm completely to normal. The rate of failed revascularisation is low and the most significant complications relate to wound infection or haematoma, particularly in the presence of continued anticoagulation [10,11]. Amputation is required in only a very small number of patients and death is usually secondary to other medical problems rather than the ischaemic arm (Table 1).

Digital ischaemia

A relatively common variant of upper limb ischaemia involves the digits alone. Acute ischaemia of a single finger is generally thought to be an embolic problem. It often presents as an emergency with severe pain and purple discolouration of the digit (Figure 6). Initial treatment is anticoagulation; in Gloucester, a consecutive series of patients with digital ischaemia were investigated using duplex imaging or angiography, and also echocardiography. In the series, if the wrist pulses were present, no

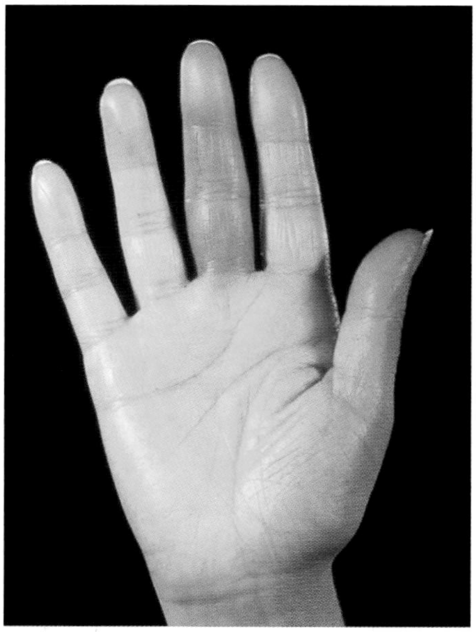

Figure 6. Acutely ischaemic middle finger due to digital embolus.

proximal source for a digital embolus was found. In this situation it is very hard to recommend long-term anticoagulation. Less frequent causes of digital ischaemia include arteritic conditions such as secondary Raynaud's disease, where the risk of local amputation is significant.

Patients with digital ischaemia present with a very painful digit with purple discolouration. If there is sufficient arterial inflow, and wrist pulses are present, the finger usually recovers, sometimes simply shedding a small amount of skin at the tip. However, a significant patch of gangrene can develop at the tip of the finger that requires local amputation. A combination of treatments is required for these patients including analgesia, antiplatelet agents and vasodilators such as nifedipine; rarely, a cervical sympathectomy is useful. Anticoagulation may be reserved for the identification of an obvious cause of embolism. When vasospasm is contributory, an intravenous infusion of iloprost, a synthetic prostanoid, can be valuable. Occasionally, a revascularisation procedure will be required to get the fingers to heal. This may be done with an angioplasty if the proximal inflow vessels are involved, or a vascular reconstruction as described above.

Key points

- **Acute arm ischaemia carries less risk to life and limb than acute leg ischaemia.**
- **Conservative treatment with anticoagulation alone risks late functional sequelae such as forearm claudication.**
- **Urgent intervention should be considered if there is a neurosensory deficit in the hand or no Doppler signals at the wrist.**
- **Brachial embolectomy done under local anaesthetic by an experienced surgeon has a high chance of restoring the circulation at low risk.**

References

1. Galbraith K, Collin J, Morris P, Wood RF. Recent experience with arterial embolism of the limbs in a vascular unit. *Ann R Coll Surg Engl* 1985; 67: 30-3.
2. Eyers P, Earnshaw JJ. Acute non-traumatic arm ischaemia. *Br J Surg* 1998; 85: 1340-6.
3. Savelyev VS, Zatevakhin II, Stepanov NV. Artery embolism of the upper limbs. *Surgery* 1977; 81: 367-75.
4. Thompson JF, Kinsella DC. Vascular disorders of the upper limb. In: *Vascular and Endovascular Surgery*. Beard JD, Gaines PA, Eds. WB Saunders, 2001: 199-217.
5. Ebner H, Zaraca F, Randone B. The role of intra-operative angiography in arterial thromboembolectomy for non-traumatic upper limb ischaemia. *Chir Ital* 2004; 56: 345-50.
6. Earnshaw JJ, Whitman B, Foy C on behalf of the Thrombolysis Study Group. National Audit of Thrombolysis for Acute Leg Ischemia (NATALI): clinical factors associated with outcome. *J Vasc Surg* 2004; 39: 1018-25.
7. Marshall C, Ives C, Jackson R, Rose J, Stansby G. Subclavian angioplasty: what are the risks and do we consent our patients adequately? *Br J Surg* 2003; 90: A505-6.
8. McCarthy WJ, Flinn WR, Yao JST, Williams LR, Bergan JJ. Result of bypass grafting for upper limb ischemia. *J Vasc Surg* 1986; 3: 741-6.
9. Varma S, Padberg F Jr, Hobson RW III, Duran WN. Metabolic and systemic consequences of acute limb ischaemia and reperfusion. In: *Comprehensive Vascular and Endovascular Surgery*. Hallett JW, Mills JL, Earnshaw JJ, Reekers JA, Eds. Mosby 2004; 18: 235-46.
10. Hernandez-Richter T, Angele MK, Helmberger T, Jauch KW, Lauterjung L, Schildberg FW. Acute ischaemia of the upper extremity: long-term results following thromboembolectomy with the Fogarty catheter. *Langenbecks Arch Surg* 2001; 386: 261-6.
11. Licht PB, Balezantis T, Wolft J-F, *et al.* Long-term outcome following thromboembolectomy in the upper extremity. *Eur J Vasc Endovasc Surg* 2004; 28: 508-12.

Case vignette

An unsuitable case for interventional radiology

John F Thompson MS FRCS (Ed) FRCS, Consultant Surgeon, Royal Devon and Exeter Hospitals, Exeter, UK

A 64-year-old female smoker presented with a 1-week history of right upper limb ischaemia. She had absent radial pulses, a blood pressure of only 100/60mmHg in the left arm and a systolic pressure of 80mmHg on the right. There was incipient gangrene of the fingers of the right hand (Figure 1). Duplex imaging revealed a moderate carotid stenosis with retrograde flow in the left vertebral artery due to subclavian steal.

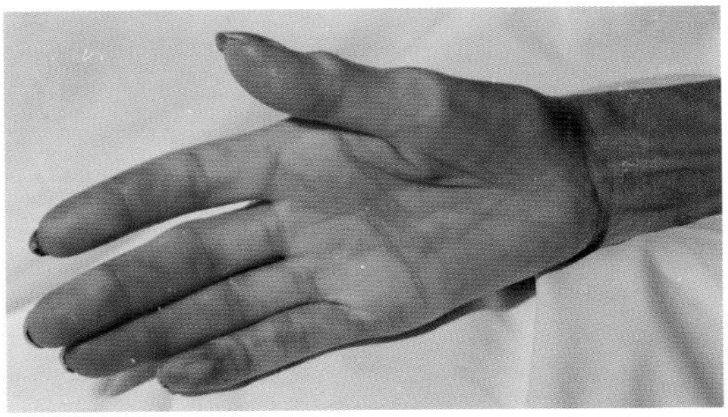

Figure 1. Severe ischaemia of the right hand caused by digital emboli with proximal subclavian stenosis.

Selective angiography (Figure 2) confirmed the stenosis and demonstrated loose thrombus above it. It was felt that endovascular treatment could be dangerous and that even the passage of a guide wire would carry a serious risk of brainstem embolism.

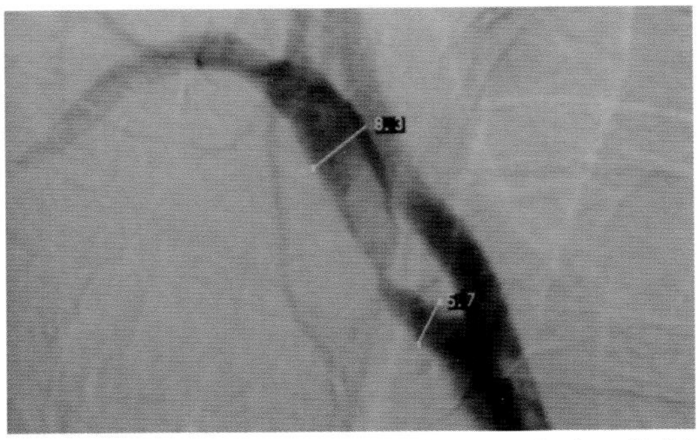

Figure 2. Arch angiogram demonstrates tight stenosis in proximal subclavian artery with much loose thrombus.

Therefore, the right subclavian and common carotid arteries were approached via a short vertical incision between the heads of the sternomastoid muscle (Figure 3). This approach provides good exposure, avoids the thoracic duct on the left, the phrenic nerve and division of the supraclavicular nerves which can lead to allodynia. The vertebral artery was controlled before dividing the subclavian artery, which was swung up and anastomosed end-to-side to the common carotid artery (Figure 4). The vertebral and distal carotid arteries were back bled before flushing the reconstruction into the arm. She made a good recovery with a bounding radial pulse.

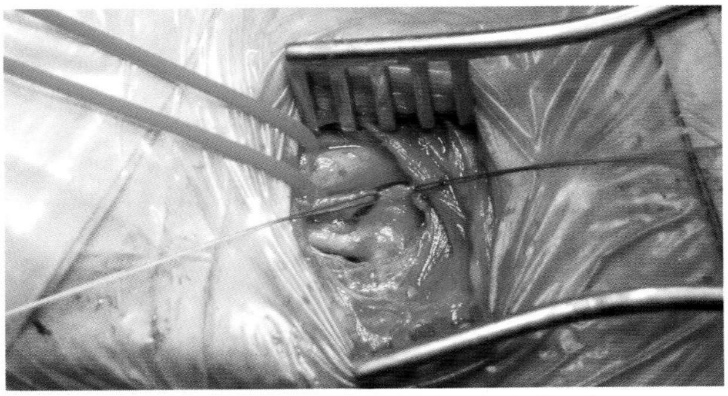

Figure 3. Division of the vertebral vein is the key move in exposure of the first part of the subclavian artery.

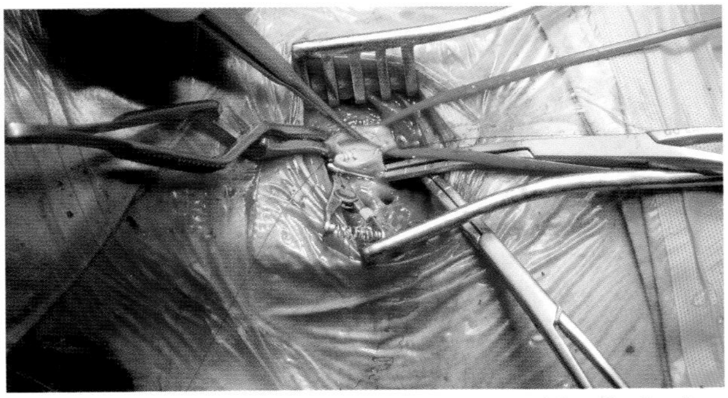

Figure 4. Posterior aspect of the carotid-subclavian anastomosis in progress.

Chapter 23

Aneurysm of an aberrant right subclavian artery

Matt Thompson MD FRCS, Professor of Vascular Surgery
Rob Morgan FRCR, Consultant Vascular Radiologist
Graham Munneke FRCR, Specialist Registrar, Vascular Radiology
Tom Loosemore MS FRCS, Consultant Vascular Surgeon
St. George's Hospital, London, UK

Introduction

An aberrant right subclavian artery (ARSA) arising from the left aortic arch is the most common congenital aortic arch anomaly, occurring in 0.5% of the population. It arises as the fourth branch from the proximal descending aorta and passes behind the oesophagus in 80% of cases. Most patients with ARSA are asymptomatic but in some, compression of the oesophagus leads to "dysphagia lusoria". A dilatation of the origin of the aberrant right subclavian artery is very rare and was described by Kommerell [1].

Aneurysms of the ARSA are associated with distal embolism, oesophageal and tracheal compression and rupture. A review of the literature by Austin and Wolfe [1] included 31 patients. Rupture of the aneurysm occurred in six, all of whom died. Patients in this series suffered rupture in aneurysms as small as 4cm in diameter. As a result, it is generally accepted that the presence of an aneurysm of the ARSA is an indication for surgery, whether symptomatic or not [2]. Techniques for open operative repair vary but are all associated with considerable morbidity and mortality, up to 30% [2].

Case report

A 74-year-old man presented with a history suggestive of vertebrobasilar ischaemia and a previous episode of an ischaemic right hand, whist on warfarin for atrial fibrillation. A carotid duplex scan suggested an aneurysmal brachiocephalic artery. CT demonstrated an aneurysmal (4cm) aberrant right subclavian artery arising as the fourth branch from the aortic arch and passing behind the oesophagus (Figure 1). The aneurysm contained significant thrombus and was considered to be the cause of his cerebral and upper limb symptoms. Angiography demonstrated that the left common carotid artery, left subclavian artery and aberrant right subclavian artery all arose from the aortic arch in very close proximity (Figure 2).

Cardiothoracic review indicated that conventional replacement of the aortic arch or aneurysm resection was contra-indicated due to significant medical comorbidity. The position of the aberrant right subclavian artery offered the possibility of an endovascular approach to reconstruct the aortic arch and then to cover the origin of the aneurysmal vessel with an endograft. By using supraclavicular extra-anatomic bypass grafts, the aim was to derive the blood supply to both subclavian arteries and the left

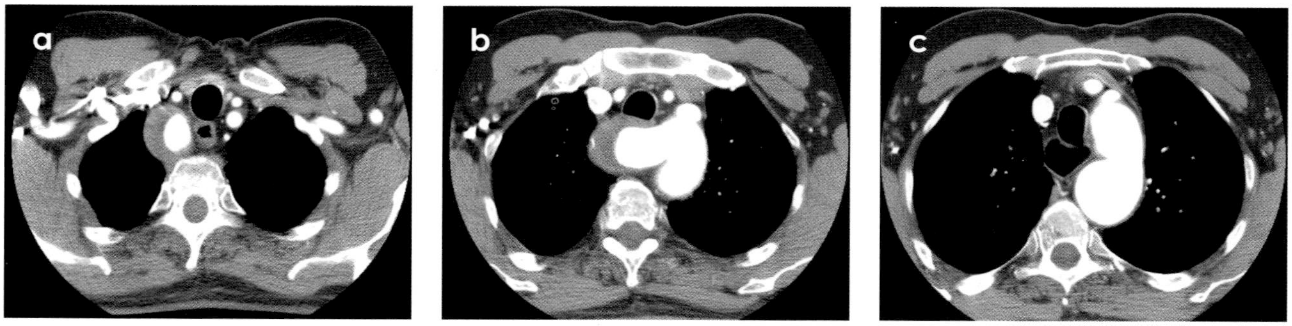

Figure 1. a) CT demonstrating an aberrant right subclavian artery aneurysm with luminal thrombus. b) The aneurysm passes posteriorly from left to right behind the oesophagus. c) The left subclavian artery and left common carotid arise in close proximity from the top of the arch.

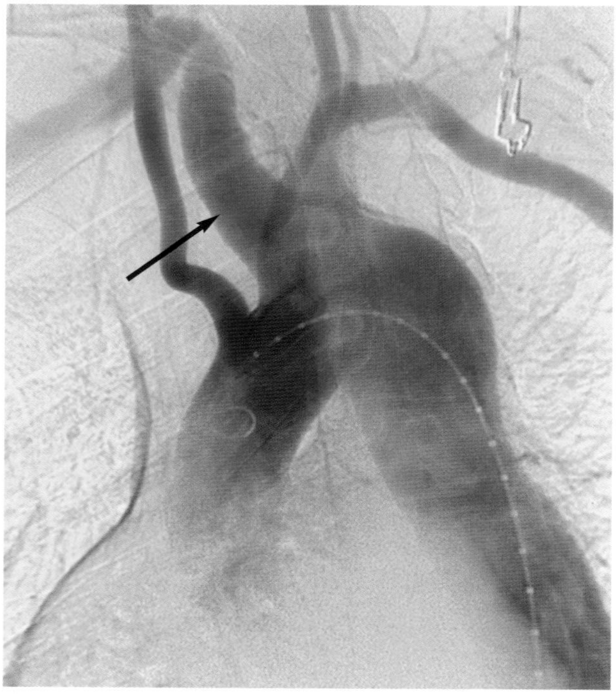

Figure 2. Angiogram demonstrating aberrant right subclavian artery aneurysm (arrow).

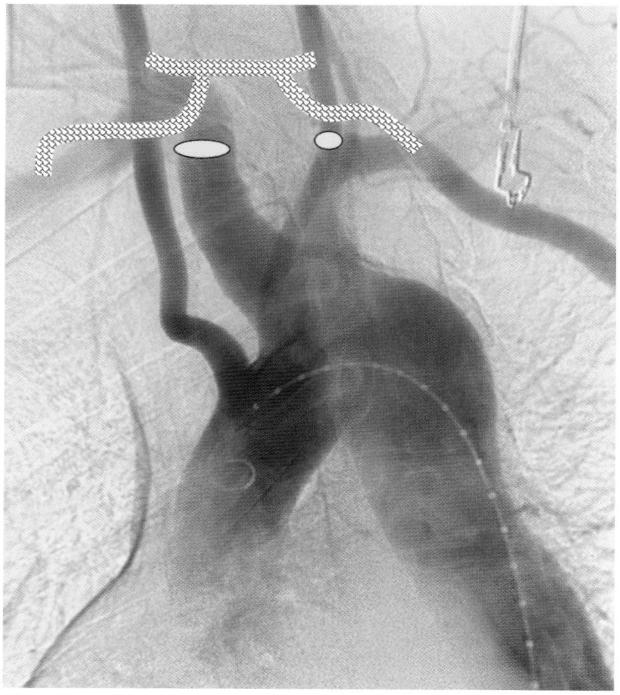

Figure 3. Schematic plan of extracranial reconstruction. Carotid-carotid bypass with bilateral carotid-subclavian bypass was planned with ligation of the left proximal carotid artery and distal right subclavian artery.

common carotid from the right common carotid artery (Figure 3).

Supraclavicular incisions were used to expose the subclavian and carotid arteries bilaterally. With bilateral TCD monitoring, a right to left carotid-carotid bypass was performed using 8mm ePTFE, tunnelled beneath the strap muscles anteriorly (Figure 4). Similar grafts were then anastomosed (end-to-side) to both subclavian arteries, and then either end of the carotid crossover. The left common carotid artery was then ligated in the root of the neck.

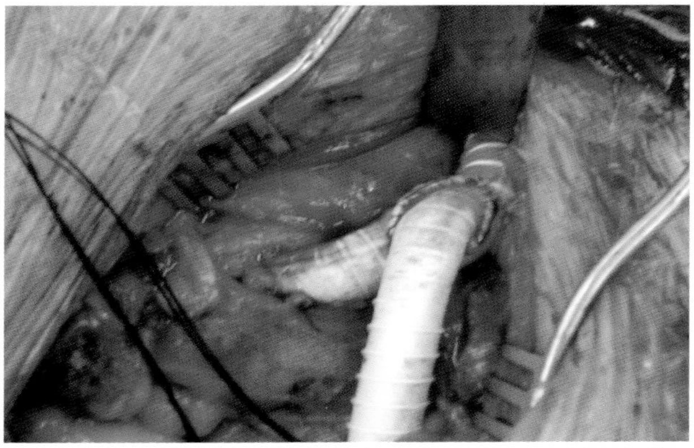

Figure 4. Carotid-carotid bypass showing the proximal extent of carotid-subclavian bypass.

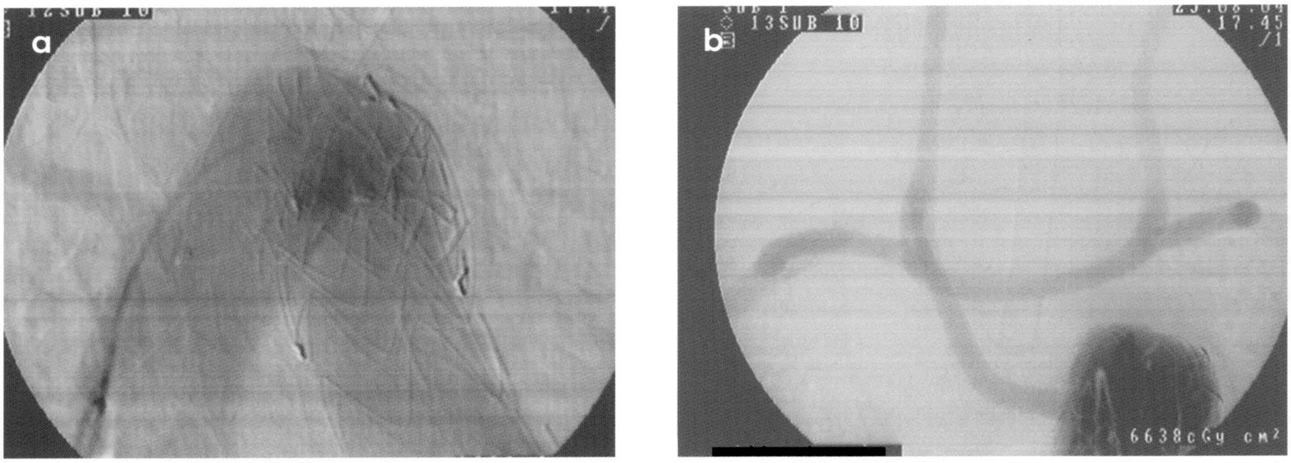

Figure 5. Angiograms after deployment of the Talent graft just distal to the right carotid artery showing: a) exclusion of the subclavian aneurysm; and b) patency of the bypass grafts.

Following completion of the extracranial bypass, a 34mm Talent thoracic endograft was deployed just distal to the origin of the right common carotid artery through a right femoral arteriotomy. A second device of the same dimensions was deployed distally to ensure good stent overlap and cover of the right subclavian artery origin. Completion angiography demonstrated patency of the crossover grafts (Figure 5). The distal right subclavian artery was then ligated to exclude the aneurysm completely. The patient made an uneventful postoperative recovery and was discharged after 6 days.

CT 6 weeks postoperatively revealed complete thrombosis of the aneurysm and good flow through the bypass grafts. The patient remains well and has had no further neurological events.

Discussion

As conventional surgery was contra-indicated in the present patient, an endovascular approach was considered. The two options were a covered stent-graft within the aneurysm itself [3,4] or exclusion of inflow and outflow. As there was no neck to the aneurysm the only possibility was the option employed in the case report.

Several case studies describing the technique of vessel transposition and bypass of the supra-aortic branches have recently been published, and allow an expansion of the indications for thoracic endografting [5,6]. The procedure is usually performed to allow intentional coverage of the left subclavian or left common carotid artery with an endograft. Experience has suggested that it is usually safe to cover the left subclavian artery origin in the presence of a patent right vertebral artery [6,7].

These bypass procedures are increasingly useful to create an adequate proximal fixation site over the left carotid artery, where an aneurysm or dissection affects the distal aortic arch. The carotid-carotid bypass may be tunnelled in front of, or behind the oesophagus, and is usually straightforward to perform. The carotid-subclavian bypass lies better if the proximal anastomosis is to the proximal portion of the carotid crossover, rather than to the carotid artery itself. The patency of these supra-aortic bypasses is not documented in any great detail for this particular indication, but good patency rates are reported for occlusive disease [8-10]. Carotid and subclavian reconstructions are likely to become increasingly common with the increase in thoracic endografting.

Key points

- **Aberrant right subclavian artery is the most common congenital abnormality of the aortic arch.**
- **Endovascular repair of the aortic arch is possible with increasing use of extracranial great vessel bypass.**
- **Covering the origin of the left subclavian artery is usually safe.**

References

1. Austin EH, Wolfe WG. Aneurysm of aberrant subclavian artery with a review of the literature. *J Vasc Surg* 1985; 2: 571-7.
2. Kieffer E, Bahnini A, Koskas F. Aberrant subclavian artery: surgical treatment in thirty-three adult patients. *J Vasc Surg* 1994; 19: 100-9.
3. Davidian M, Kee ST, Kato N, *et al.* Aneurysm of an aberrant right subclavian artery: treatment with PTFE covered stentgraft. *J Vasc Surg* 1998; 28: 335-9.
4. Puech-Leao P, Orra HA. Endovascular repair of an innominate artery true aneurysm. *J Endovasc Ther* 2001; 8: 429-32.
5. O'Neill-Kerr D, Shaw D, Gordon M, *et al.* Carotid-carotid bypass prior to endoluminal exclusion in a patient with acute type B aortic dissection. *Cardiovasc Intervent Radiol* 2004; 27: 182-5.
6. Tiesenhausen K, Hausegger KA, Oberwalder P, *et al.* Left subclavian artery management in endovascular repair of thoracic aortic aneurysms and aortic dissections. *J Card Surg* 2003; 18: 429-35.
7. Hausegger KA, Oberwalder P, Tiesenhausen K, *et al.* Intentional left subclavian artery occlusion by thoracic aortic stent-grafts without surgical transposition. *J Endovasc Ther* 2001; 8: 472-6.
8. Abou-Zamzam AM, Jr., Moneta GL, Edwards JM, *et al.* Extrathoracic arterial grafts performed for carotid artery occlusive disease not amenable to endarterectomy. *Arch Surg* 1999; 134: 952-6.
9. Owens LV, Tinsley EA, Jr., Criado E, *et al.* Extrathoracic reconstruction of arterial occlusive disease involving the supraaortic trunks. *J Vasc Surg* 1995; 22: 217-21.
10. Perler BA, Williams GM. Carotid-subclavian bypass - a decade of experience. *J Vasc Surg* 1990; 12: 716-22.

Chapter 24

Abdominal aortic aneurysm with horseshoe kidney

Peter Lamont MD FRCS, Consultant Vascular Surgeon
Bristol Royal Infirmary, Bristol, UK

Introduction

Although it is rare to find a horseshoe kidney during surgery for abdominal aortic aneurysm (AAA), it is still common enough that most vascular surgeons will encounter a few such patients during their career. Horseshoe kidney is rare enough in itself, with an estimated incidence of around 0.25% of the population [1]. It occurs twice as often in men as in women and if that is put together with the male preponderance of AAA then the very high male:female ratio of 13:1 for horseshoe kidney with an AAA is perhaps not surprising [2]. Up until 2001, only 176 cases had been described in the world literature, 134 elective and 42 ruptured [2]. In one large series of 1650 aortic procedures, horseshoe kidney was found in 10 patients (0.6%) [3].

In utero, at around the 5th week of gestation, the kidneys lie in the pelvis from where they rotate medially as they ascend into their normal position in the loin. If the kidneys' precursors, the metanephric masses, come into contact then they may fuse, usually at the lower poles. If this happens then medial rotation of the kidney is prevented and the ureters remain anterior to the kidney (Figure 1). When the horseshoe kidneys ascend towards the loins, the isthmus connecting the lower poles together catches under the inferior mesenteric artery and prevents full ascent (Figure 2). This isthmus usually contains renal parenchyma, although in around 2% of cases it is just a fibrous band [2]. The kidneys lie low because of their arrested ascent and they may also be asymmetrical, distorting the position of the collecting system on one side so that sometimes it lies partially within the isthmus and leads to a risk of urinary fistula if the isthmus is divided.

Renal artery anomalies are very common with horseshoe kidneys, occurring in nearly three quarters of the patients with horseshoe kidney and AAA [1]. The commonest anomalies are accessory renal arteries to either the isthmus from the aneurysm above it (Figure 3) or to the lower pole of the kidney from the common iliac artery below it. In such patients, the two main renal arteries are normally placed above the neck of the aneurysm. Rarely, one or both of the main renal arteries may be either missing or arise distally from the AAA itself (Figure 4). It is important to be aware of the potential for these anomalies when operating on such patients.

Diagnosis

Very few patients (around 4%) report a history of problems relating to their horseshoe kidney, although hydronephrosis, calculi or recurrent urinary tract

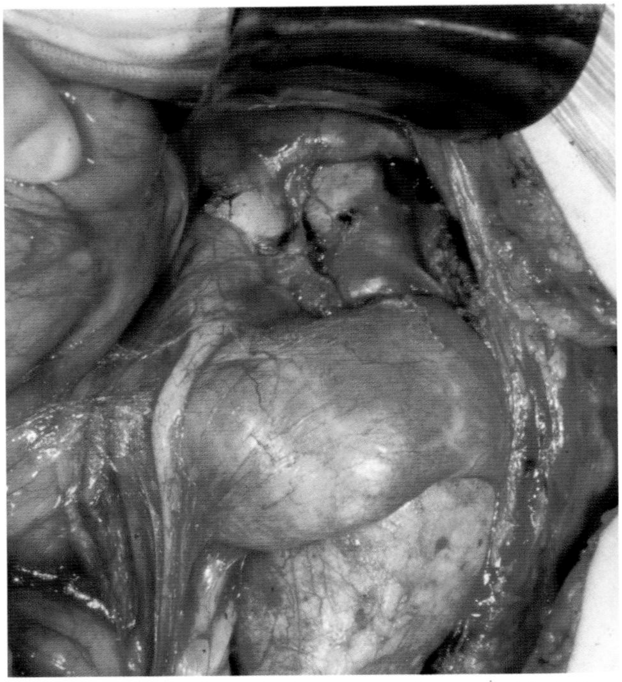

Figure 1. Horseshoe kidney covering an AAA. The right ureter can be seen lying anterior to the kidney. The neck of an AAA is at the top of the picture.

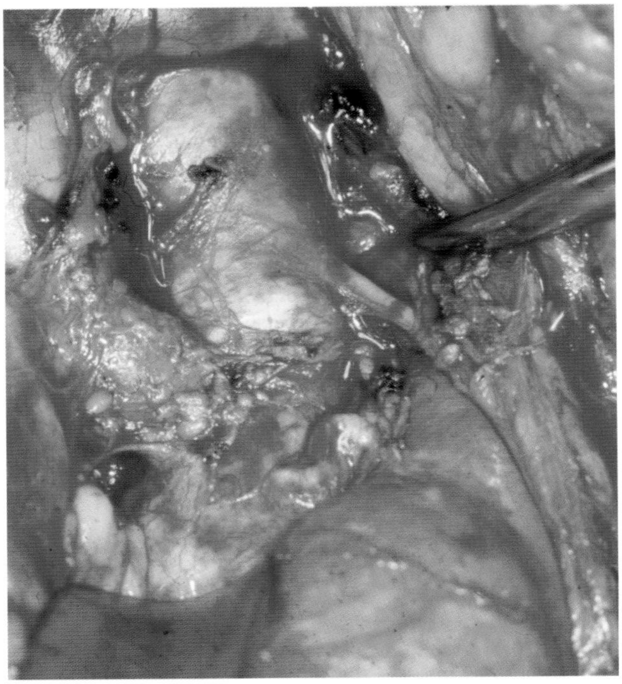

Figure 2. The isthmus of the horseshoe kidney is trapped in the angle between the inferior mesenteric artery and the aorta, preventing full ascent of the kidney in utero. The neck of an AAA is at the top of the picture.

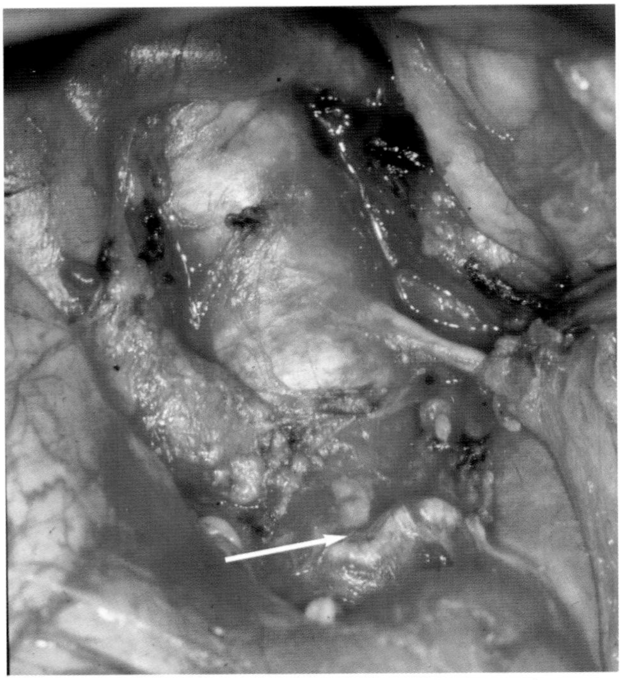

Figure 3. A midline accessory renal artery is seen arising from the anterior surface of an abdominal aortic aneurysm and supplying the renal isthmus (arrow). The left renal vein is seen at the top of the picture and the inferior mesenteric artery arises above and to the (patient's) left of the isthmus.

infections may have brought the condition to light in the past [2]. An elevated serum creatinine or urea may be present in a minority of patients but is rather non-specific. The horseshoe kidney is most commonly found incidentally whilst imaging the AAA (Figure 5). Although ultrasound is often used to monitor aneurysm size, it cannot be relied upon to pick up a horseshoe kidney. In one series from the Cleveland Clinic, ultrasound used in the late 1970s picked up only 5/13 (38%) horseshoe kidneys found at surgery for AAA, whereas CT introduced in the early 1980s at the same centre found 9/10 of them [1]. Intravenous pyelography (IVP) is also an accurate way to image horseshoe kidneys, although it is rarely part of the standard work-up for AAA. Angiography is increasingly used in the work-up for endovascular repair of AAA, and reveals a horseshoe kidney, if present. It is more useful once a horseshoe kidney has been identified and information on the commonly associated arterial anomalies can be obtained, either by conventional intra-arterial contrast, or by CT angiography (Figure 4).

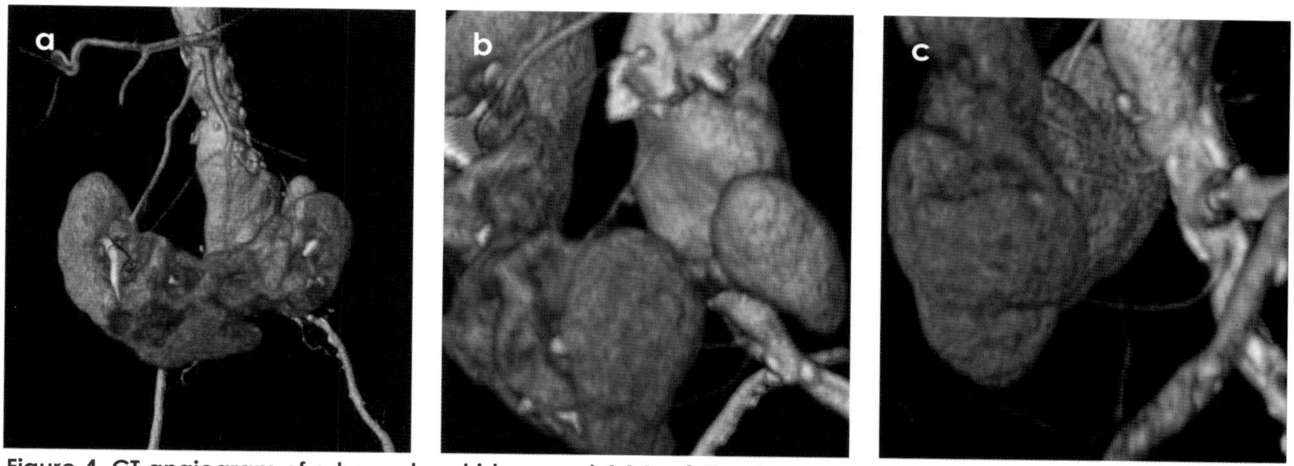

Figure 4. CT angiogram of a horseshoe kidney and AAA. a) The right renal artery arises just below the superior mesenteric artery. b) The left renal artery is small and arises from the AAA sac. c) There are three accessory left renal arteries arising from the distal AAA sac. Courtesy of Mr. SD Parvin.

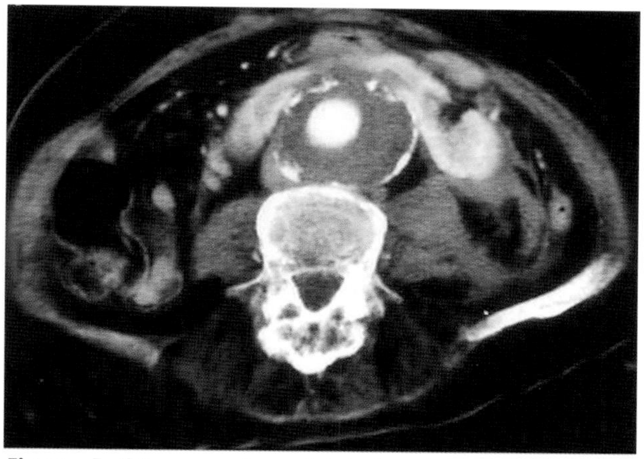

Figure 5. CT scan of an AAA showing an incidental horseshoe kidney. Courtesy of Mr. F Smith.

Surgical and endovascular options

Surgical repair of an AAA in the presence of a horseshoe kidney has always been considered a technical challenge, with both transperitoneal and retroperitoneal approaches described. More recently, experience has been growing with the use of endovascular stent repair, where the need to preserve accessory renal arteries has been challenged.

Open transperitoneal repair

The main issue surrounding open transperitoneal repair is whether or not to divide the renal isthmus to improve access to the AAA. Generally speaking it is usually possible to dissect the isthmus off the front of the AAA sac and leave it intact, simply tunnelling the aortic graft beneath it (Figure 6). Division of the isthmus to improve access can be done safely in the small percentage of patients where the isthmus is a fibrous band, but there are dangers in dividing renal parenchyma. Division of an abnormally sited collecting system can result in urinary fistula, with consequent risk of infection to the aortic graft. Postoperative haemorrhage from the divided renal tissue has also been described [2]. Postoperative renal insufficiency appears commoner after division of the isthmus during transperitoneal repair, occurring in 4/31 (13%) of such patients after elective surgery compared to only 1/84 (1%) where the isthmus was preserved, based on an analysis of all reported cases in the literature [2]. The number of divided renal arteries originating from the aneurysm does not appear to influence postoperative renal function [2]. The need for postoperative dialysis is related to pre-operative renal function; O'Hara *et al* described a series of 19 patients where 3/6 with pre-operative renal impairment had postoperative dialysis compared to 0/13 patients with normal renal function before surgery (p=0.02) [1].

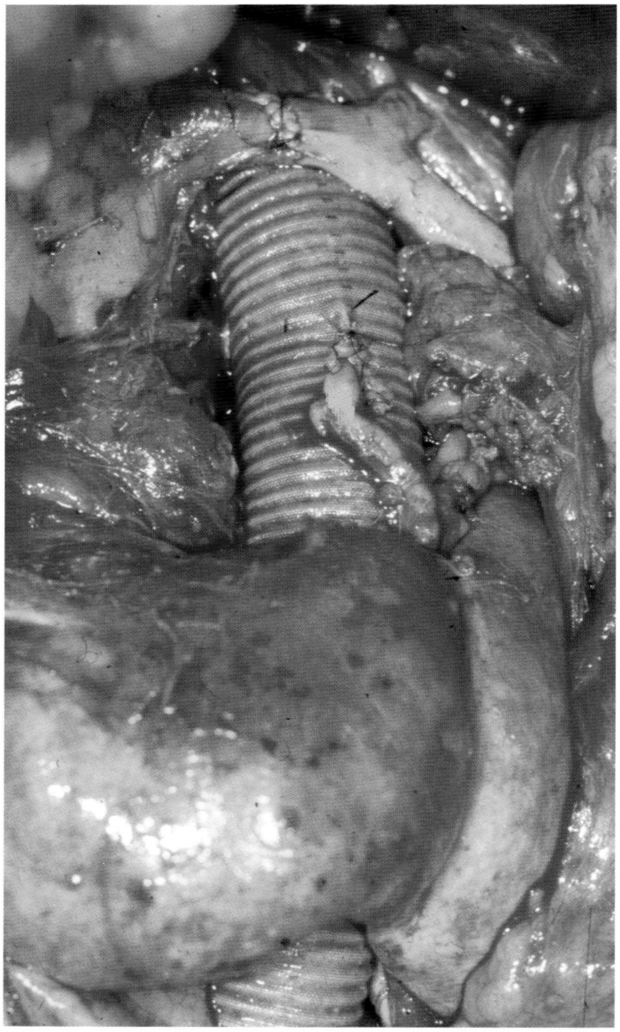

Figure 6. The AAA has been repaired with a dacron graft tunnelled underneath the isthmus of a horseshoe kidney. A midline accessory renal artery has been re-implanted into the graft because the isthmus remained ischaemic on clamp release. The left renal vein was divided to improve access to the neck of the aneurysm and has also been repaired.

The one benefit of open repair is that the kidney is easily visible and it is possible to re-implant an accessory renal artery onto the graft when part of the kidney remains ischaemic on release of the aortic clamps (Figure 6). Open transperitoneal repair is also advisable to give the best access for ruptured AAA even though the isthmus is likely to be divided in up to 50% of such patients [2].

Open retroperitoneal repair

Although only described in ten elective patients to date, the retroperitoneal approach through a left flank incision does allow access to the aorta behind a horseshoe kidney and has been advocated as the open approach of choice [2]. It avoids any interference with the isthmus, ureters and accessory vessels, although access to the right common iliac artery can be more difficult and may require a separate right iliac incision. In all published cases, any accessory renal arteries have been oversewn or divided without re-implantation and this has not appeared to cause problems in the small number of procedures described [1].

Endovascular repair

Over the past 6 years, several reports of endovascular repair of AAA in the presence of horseshoe kidney have emerged, with promising results [4,5,6]. In 1999, the Mount Sinai Medical Centre in Cleveland reported on 12 out of 24 patients with anomalous renal arteries who had undergone endovascular AAA repair where one or more of the anomalous renal artery origins were covered and excluded by the stent [7]. The excluded arteries were all less than 3mm in diameter and the patients had normal pre-operative renal function. Only one of these patients had an associated horseshoe kidney, but all had a good outcome. Small segmental renal infarcts occurred in half of the patients on postoperative CT, but only one patient had a transient rise in serum creatinine.

The other potential risk of endovascular repair is that a covered accessory renal artery may fail to thrombose, creating a type II endoleak. Although experience of this complication is very limited, at least one case has successfully been treated by wire coil embolisation of the accessory renal artery without deterioration in renal function (Thompson MM, personal communication).

In view of these promising results, endovascular repair is increasingly being considered as the treatment of choice where the AAA morphology is suitable and where there are two normally positioned renal arteries above the aneurysm neck. Where pre-operative renal function is normal, any additional accessory renal artery origins can safely be covered by the endoluminal stent.

Key points

- Horseshoe kidney occurs in 0.6% patients with AAA, with a 13:1 male:female preponderance.
- CT is the best imaging method for pre-operative diagnosis, but can still miss 10% of cases.
- Pre-operative arteriography or CT angiography is needed to delineate accessory or anomalous renal arteries, which occur in 75% of patients.
- Accessory renal arteries can be divided or excluded safely provided there are two normal main renal arteries and pre-operative renal function is normal.
- Division of the renal isthmus should be avoided if possible and retroperitoneal or endovascular repair are favoured over transperitoneal repair to prevent problems with access caused by the isthmus.

References

1. O'Hara PJ, Hakaim AG, Hertzer NR, *et al.* Surgical management of aortic aneurysm and coexistent horseshoe kidney: review of a 31-year experience. *J Vasc Surg* 1993; 17: 940-7.
2. Stroosma OB, Kootstra G, Schurink GWH. Management of aortic aneurysm in the presence of a horseshoe kidney. *Br J Surg* 2001; 88; 500-9.
3. Faggioli G, Freyrie A, Pilato A, *et al.* Renal anomalies in aortic surgery: contemporary results. *Surgery* 2003; 133: 641-6.
4. Loftus IK, Thompson MM, Fishwick G, *et al.* Endovascular repair of aortic aneurysm in the presence of horseshoe kidney. *J Endovasc Surg* 1998; 5: 278-81.
5. Jackson RW, Fay DM, Wyatt MG, Rose JD. The renal impact of aortic stent-grafting in patients with a horseshoe kidney. *Cardiovasc Intervent Radiol* 2004; 27: 632-6.
6. Ruppert V, Umscheid T, Rieger J, *et al.* Endovascular aneurysm repair: treatment of choice for abdominal aortic aneurysm coincident with horseshoe kidney? Three case reports and review of literature. *J Vasc Surg* 2004; 40: 367-70.
7. Kaplan DB, Kwon CC, Marin ML, Hollier LH. Endovascular repair of abdominal aortic aneurysms in patients with congenital renal vascular anomalies. *J Vasc Surg* 1999; 30: 407-15.

Case vignette

Peripheral vascular manifestations of meningococcal septicaemia

Frank CT Smith BSc MD FRCS FRCS (Ed) FRCS (Glas), Consultant Senior Lecturer, Bristol Royal Infirmary, UK

Patient 1. A 42-year-old tourist to the UK developed a flu-like illness accompanied by fever, malaise and lethargy. She was admitted with circulatory collapse secondary to meningococcal septicaemia. Intravenous antibiotics and respiratory support were provided, but she developed disseminated intravascular coagulation. Five days after admission all limb extremities were gangrenous, requiring peripheral amputations. Figure 1 illustrates necrosis of the hand with larval infestation. The patient eventually succumbed to multisystem organ failure.

Patient 2. (Figure 2) A 19-year-old university student was admitted to ICU following a short flu-like illness with fever, malaise, arthralgia and neck stiffness. The patient rapidly developed a coalescent petechial rash affecting hands and feet. Meningococcal septicaemia was diagnosed and treated. Digital necrosis occurred, but the acute phase of the disease responded to antibiotics and late minor debridement of necrotic tissue sufficed.

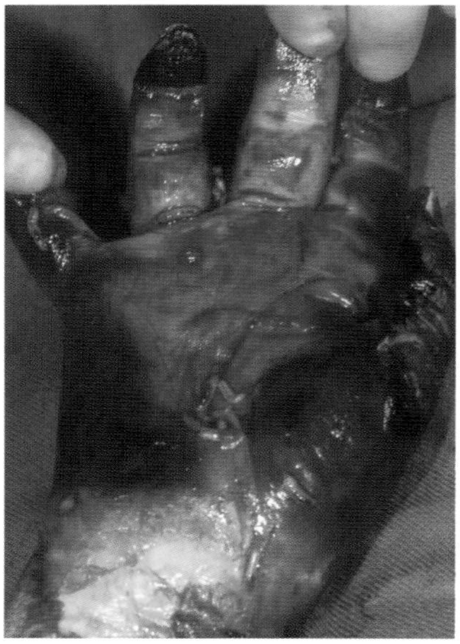

Figure 1.

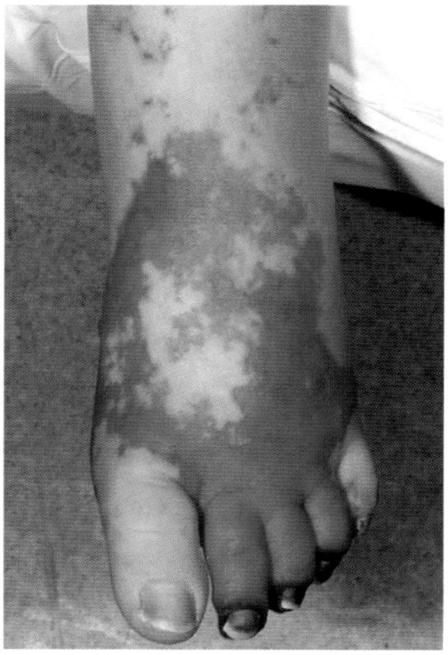

Figure 2.

Chapter 25

Aortocaval fistula

Michael Horrocks MS FRCS, Professor of Surgery
James Metcalfe MRCS, Clinical Research Fellow, Vascular Surgery
Royal United Hospital, Bath, UK

Introduction

Aortocaval fistula (ACF), though uncommon, is a well recognised and documented condition. ACF complicates fewer than 1% of all abdominal aortic aneurysms (AAA) and 2-4% of ruptured aortic aneurysms [1,2]. Rupture of an atherosclerotic AAA into the inferior vena cava (IVC) accounts for about 80% of ACF [3]. Other causes include trauma and rare diseases such as syphilis, bacterial infections, Marfan's syndrome and Ehlers-Danlos syndrome.

The mortality from ACF due to AAA is 40-50%, which is the same as the mortality from ruptured aortic aneurysm without a fistula [4].

Historical perspective

ACF complicating AAA was first reported in 1831 by James Syme [5]. In 1938, Lehman attempted the first repair of an ACF in a patient with syphilitic aneurysm, but the patient died within 15 hours [6]. It was not until 1954 that Cooley carried out the first successful repair of a spontaneous ACF [7].

Clinical considerations

Due to its most common aetiology the vast majority of ACF occur in the infrarenal abdominal aorta. ACF can be considerable in size and can involve both the bifurcation and common iliac arteries.

Most patients present with a palpable AAA, abdominal bruit and high output cardiac failure. Presentation with angina, renal failure or pelvic venous congestion has also been described. Formation of a fistula may be asymptomatic and its presence may only be recognised during elective surgery for a repair of an AAA. In one reported series, 78% of patients presented with abdominal pain, 61% had a bruit and 56% had a pulsatile abdominal mass [8]. A pathognomic finding is that the bruit is equally loud during systole and diastole. Other signs and symptoms depend on whether or not the aneurysm has ruptured, and whether or not the IVC is compressed by the aneurysm [9]. If compression is significant, there may be distal truncal and leg signs comprising of cyanosis, oedema and haematuria. If there is no compression, systemic pressure will be transmitted in both directions, and high output cardiac failure can occur secondary to this shunting.

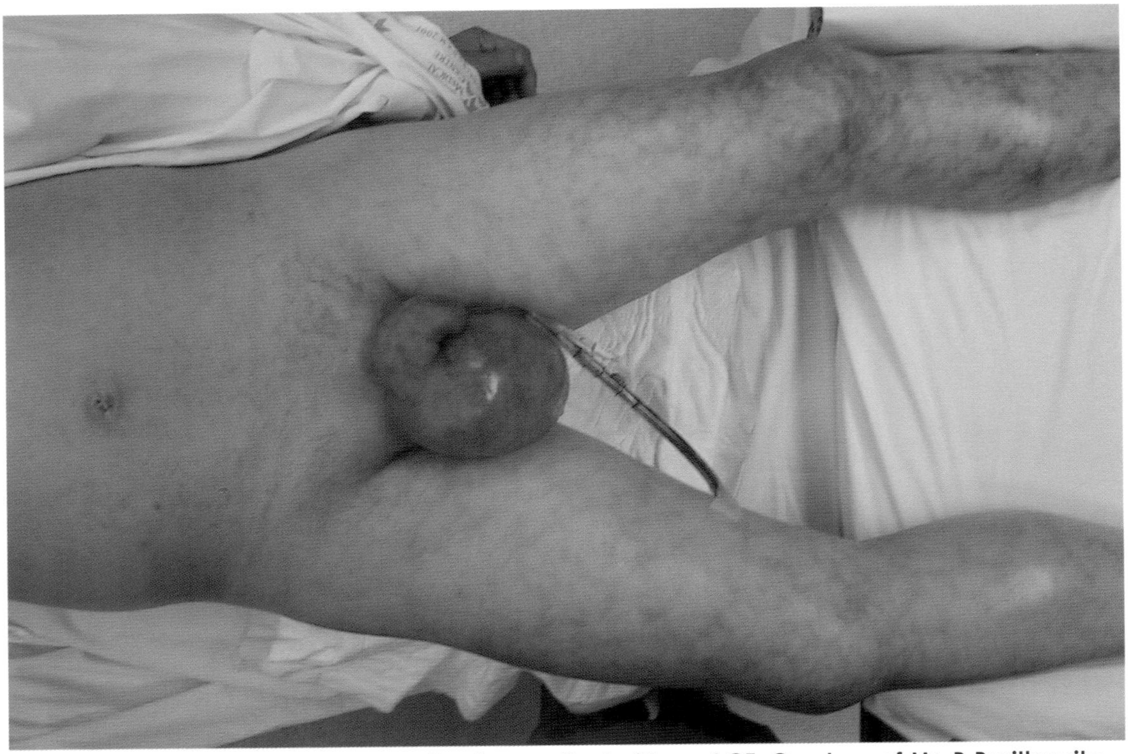

Figure 1. Lower limb venous congestion in a patient with an ACF. Courtesy of Mr. B Braithwaite.

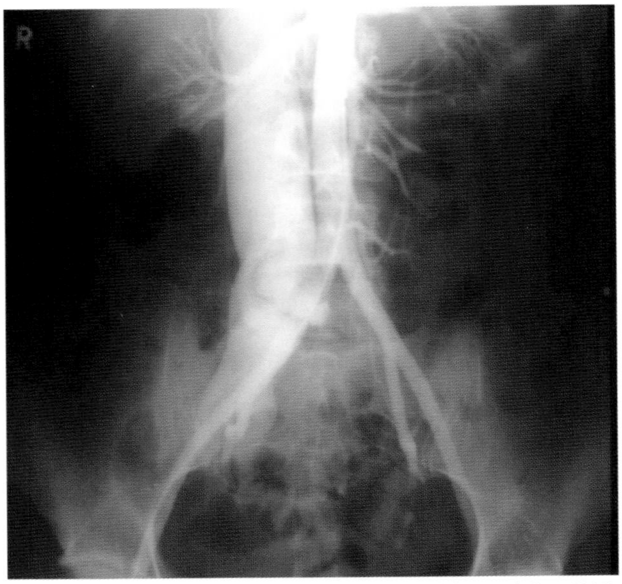

Figure 2. Angiogram showing early filling of the IVC and right common iliac vein in a patient who developed leg swelling and high output cardiac failure some while after open lumbar discectomy. Although the exact site of the ACF is not seen, it appears to be in the vicinity of the aortic bifurcation. Courtesy of Mr. A McL Jenkins.

Hepatic and renal function is often impaired secondary to venous congestion and increased splanchnic venous pressure. A high central venous pressure reading in a person with a suspected leaking AAA may give a clue to the existence of an ACF. A clinical clue is seen when a patient who is shocked with a clinical diagnosis of leaking AAA, looks blue and cyanosed, with distended neck and peripheral veins (Figure 1).

Clinical management

The diagnosis of ACF should be confirmed with imaging in all patients who are haemodynamically stable. Aortography remains the most accurate technique for establishing the diagnosis, but its role remains controversial because of the small but definite risk, and the potential waste of time associated with the procedure (Figure 2). Advances in non-invasive radiological imaging can demonstrate the anatomy in sufficient detail. Ultrasound examination may show a jet of aortic blood flow into

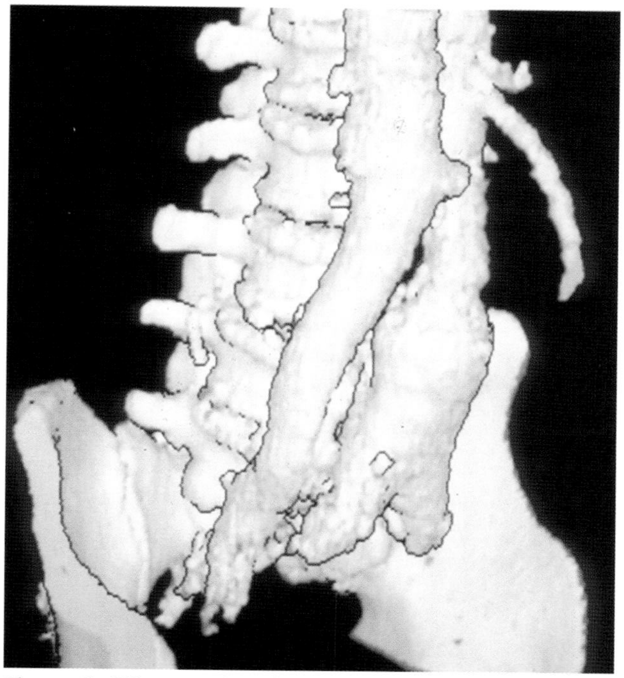

Figure 3. CT reconstruction of an ACF. Courtesy of Mr. C Soong and Mr. L Lau. Reproduced with permission from the Society for Vascular Surgery and the American Association for Vascular Surgery, © 2001 [12].

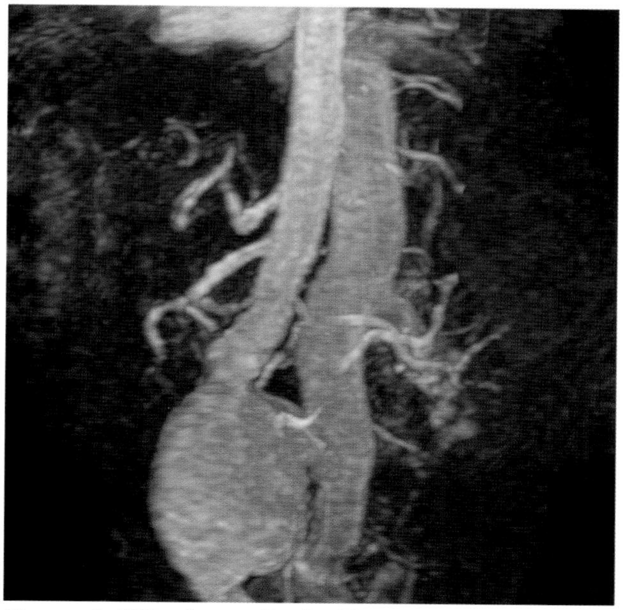

Figure 4. MRI of a patient with an aortic aneurysm and an ACF. Courtesy of Ms. F Meyer.

the IVC but the diagnosis is often missed when ultrasound is used alone. The precise site of the fistula can be identified by CT and is characterised by IVC effacement, loss of the fat plane with early synchronous and equivalent enhancement of the IVC and aorta, often associated with dilatation of the IVC and pelvic veins (Figure 3) [10]. CT not only informs the surgeon of the extent of the aneurysm but also yields information with regard to the venous anatomy. MRI is an alternative (Figure 4).

In spite of the continuing developments in diagnostic techniques, it is not unusual for the diagnosis of ACF only to be made at the time of surgery for repair of an AAA.

Principles of treatment

Correction of ACF is indicated in all patients [8]. The mortality from open repair is greatly increased in patients with cardiovascular decompensation. When an ACF is present, however, the technical complexity of the surgery is increased, and precautions must be taken to prevent thrombus, atherosclerotic debris or air from entering the IVC.

Operative technique

At elective operation it may be possible to control the iliac veins below and the IVC above the fistula using clamps and slings. This avoids excessive blood loss when the fistula is opened and facilitates its closure. The aorta is controlled in the usual way. In an emergency, or when the diagnosis is only made during aneurysm repair, caval bleeding can be massive, and expeditious control is usually possible with digital compression or a sponge stick above and below the fistula. As in all aortic surgery, the use of red cell salvage is helpful, as blood loss can be considerable.

The fistula is closed from within the aneurysm sac by rapid suturing using a large running suture (e.g. 0 Nylon), with good-sized bites into the adjacent aneurysm wall. It is not usually possible to identify the edges of the IVC separate from the aortic wall. IVC occlusion from over-enthusiastic suturing does not

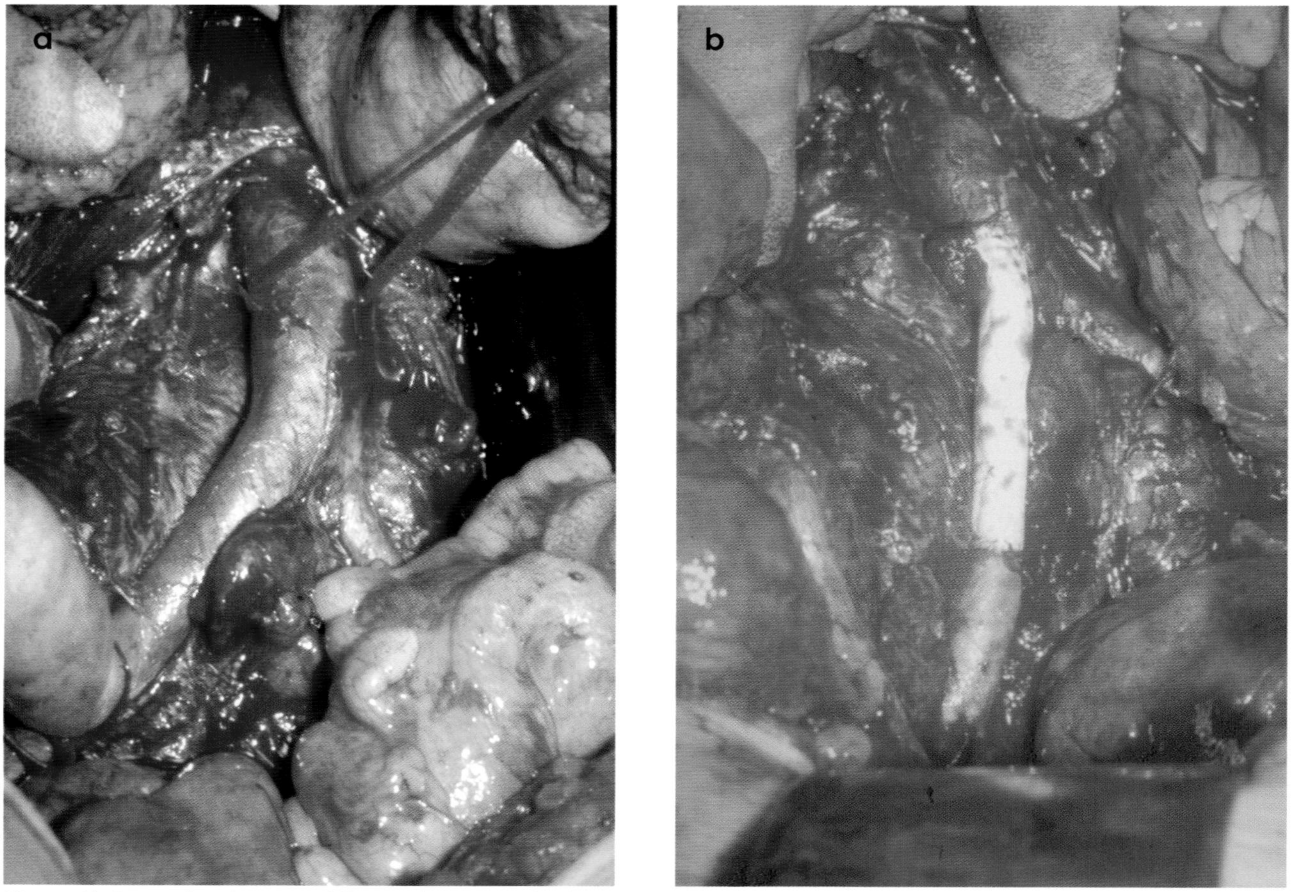

Figure 5. Operative image of the patient seen in Figure 2. a) The ACF arises between the proximal right common iliac artery and the bifurcation of the IVC. The inflammatory tissue at the aortic bifurcation can be seen adjacent to the right common iliac artery. The distal aorta has been controlled. b) Following resection of the right common iliac artery and suture repair of the underlying defect in the right common iliac vein/distal IVC, an interposition PTFE graft has been used to reconstruct the right common iliac artery to minimise the risk of recurrent fistula. Courtesy of Mr. A McL Jenkins.

seem to be a clinical problem. Repair of the fistula should be completed before any venous clamps are removed, distal first. A venous leak into the aneurysm can then be sutured directly from within the aneurysm sac. A tube dacron graft is used to restore arterial continuity in the normal way.

Traumatic ACF can be managed in a similar fashion, but if the track is chronic, it may be necessary to replace the arterial segment with a graft to prevent recurrent fistula formation (Figure 5).

Physiological consequences of surgical closure of ACF

On cross-clamping the aorta, there is typically a significant drop in central venous pressure; following an initial rise in arterial blood pressure this usually falls off in line with the central venous pressure. The anaesthetist should be warned that the central venous pressure must be maintained by generous intravenous fluid infusion, and that inotropic support may be required.

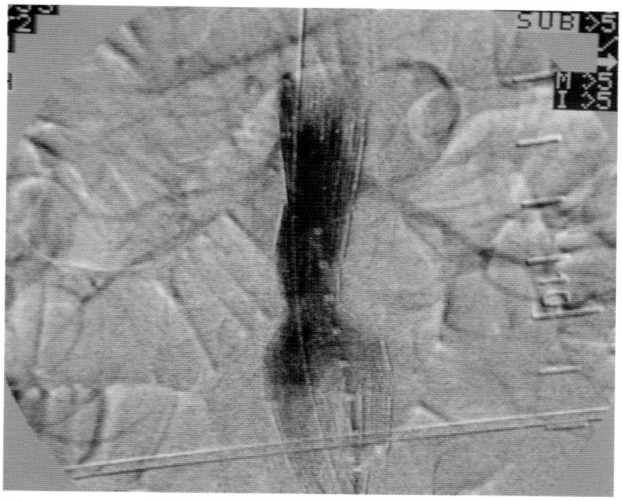

Figure 6. Completion angiogram after endovascular stent repair of an ACF. Courtesy of Mr. B Braithwaite.

Endovascular option

An alternative, particularly for patients with significant comorbidity, is treatment by an endovascular approach, though the long-term results of endograft exclusion of ACF remain unclear. Boudghene *et al* reported successful treatment of ACF using percutaneous stent grafts in an experimental study in which the ACF was created percutaneously in eight sheep. They subsequently went on to perform endovascular stent graft repair of a spontaneous ACF complicating an AAA. Such treatment is not without technical problems, including haemodynamic changes and endoleaks [11]. CT allows assessment of the aorto-iliac anatomy for suitability, and follows the same procedure as standard endovascular stent graft repair of an AAA (Figure 6). Early postoperative CT is recommended after stent graft repair of ACF as the consequences of endoleak are far greater. Recognition of endoleak may be difficult in these patients, and careful follow-up is required.

As after open repair, endovascular repair of ACF results in a sudden and dramatic fall in cardiac output, with a drop in central venous pressure. The patient may then develop severe systemic hypertension due to a sudden increase in systemic vascular resistance; glyceryl trinitrate infusion and other vasodilator agents may be required [12].

After both types of ACF repair, a brisk diuresis may ensue because of improved renal perfusion and reduced venous resistance. This requires careful fluid balance and close monitoring of serum electrolytes with appropriate fluid replacement over the recovery. There are no long-term data on the outcome of endovascular repair of ACF.

Acknowledgement

The authors would like to thank Mr. B Braithwaite, Queen's Medical Centre, Nottingham, Mr. A McL Jenkins, Royal Infirmary, Edinburgh, Mr. C Soong and Mr. L Lau, City Hospital, Belfast and Ms. Felicity Meyer, Norfolk and Norwich University Hospital, Norwich for kindly providing the Figures.

Key points

- Correction of aortocaval fistula is indicated in all patients.
- The clinical diagnosis should be confirmed with imaging, usually CT in all haemodynamically stable patients.
- The anaesthetist should be aware that the physiological response to correction of an aortocaval fistula can be profound.
- In spite of the developments in diagnostic techniques, most aortocaval fistulae are discovered only at operation for the repair of a ruptured abdominal aortic aneurysm.

References

1. Baker WH, Sharzer LA, Ehrenhaft JL. Aortocaval fistula as a complication of abdominal aortic aneurysm. *Surgery* 1973; 72: 933-8.
2. Alexander JJ, Imbembo AL. Aortocaval fistula. *Surgery* 1989; 102: 1-12.
3. Duppler DH, Herbert WE, Dillihurst RC, Ray FS. Primary arteriovenous fistulas of the abdomen. *Arch Surg* 1985; 120: 786-90.
4. Neurinhaus HP, Javid H. The distinct syndrome of spontaneous abdominal aortocaval fistula. *Am J Med* 1968; 44: 464-72.
5. Syme J. Case of spontaneous varicose aneurysm. *Edinburgh Medical and Surgical Journal* 1831; 36: 104-5.
6. Lehman EP. Spontaneous arteriovenous fistula between the abdominal aorta and the inferior vena cava: case report. *Ann Surg* 1938; 108: 694-700.
7. Cooley DA. Discussion of paper by Javid and Coll: resection of ruptured aneurysm of abdominal aorta. *Ann Surg* 1955; 142: 623.
8. Davies PM, Gloviczki P, Cherry KJ Jr., *et al.* Aortocaval and ilio-iliac arteriovenous fistulae. *Am J Surg* 1998; 176: 115-8.
9. Phipps RF. Spontaneous aortocaval fistula. *Br J Hosp Med* 1988; 17: 390-3.
10. Rosenthal D, Atkins CP. Diagnosis of aortocaval fistula by computed tomography. *Ann Vasc Surg* 1998; 12: 86-7.
11. Boudghene F, Sapoval M, Bonneau M, Bigot JM. Aortocaval fistulae: a percutaneous model and treatment with stent grafts in sheep. *Circulation* 1996; 94: 108-12.
12. Lau LL, O'Reilly MJ, Johnston LC, Lee B. Endovascular stent-graft repair of primary aortocaval fistula with an abdominal aorto-iliac aneurysm. *J Vasc Surg* 2001; 33: 425-8.

Chapter 26

Aorto-enteric fistula

Marcus J Brooks MD FRCS, Specialist Registrar, Vascular Surgery
John HN Wolfe MD FRCS, Consultant Vascular Surgeon
St. Mary's Hospital, London, UK

Introduction

The commonest form of aorto-enteric fistula (AEF) is an aortoduodenal fistula between the third part of the duodenum and the proximal anastamosis of an infrarenal aortic graft. The incidence of such secondary fistulae is between 0.3-2% of all aortic procedures. Primary AEF are rare, with fewer than 250 cases reported in the literature. Eighty percent of primary fistulae develop secondary to an atherosclerotic aneurysm, with inflammatory aneurysms at greatest risk. The causes of aorto-enteric fistula are shown in Figure 1.

Carcinomas reported as causing aorto-enteric fistulae include pancreatic, colonic, metastatic squamous cell, renal and lymphoma.

History

Death from a primary AEF was first reported by Sir Astley Cooper in 1822. The first secondary fistula was reported in 1953 by Brock. In 1957, Haberer reported the successful repair of a secondary fistula by simple suture. The first report of removal of an infected aortic prosthesis and aortic stump closure with an extra-anatomic reconstruction was by Spanos in 1976. In the 1980s, a more conservative approach was adopted with the use of an *in situ* replacement covered by antibiotics. *In situ* replacement of the aorta has subsequently been described using prosthetic grafts (PTFE and dacron), aortic homografts and superficial femoral vein autografts. Recently, cases have been reported of AEF complicating endovascular aortic procedures (20 at the time of writing).

Pathophysiology

AEF develop as a result of disruption of the intestinal wall with communication to the aortic lumen. In the case of secondary fistulae the main sites of bowel disruption are duodenum (60%), jejunum (30%) and colon (5%). In the absence of infection, mechanical stress is believed to cause the fistula. The duodenum is closely apposed to the proximal anastomosis in most aortic repairs. Failure to separate the graft and intestine by not closing the aneurysm sac and peritoneum, an over-long aortic graft and excessive anterior suture material or knots have all been proposed as aetiological factors in AEF formation. High levels of proteolytic enzymes (metalloproteases) in the aortic wall may also play a part in local tissue destruction. Secondary fistulae

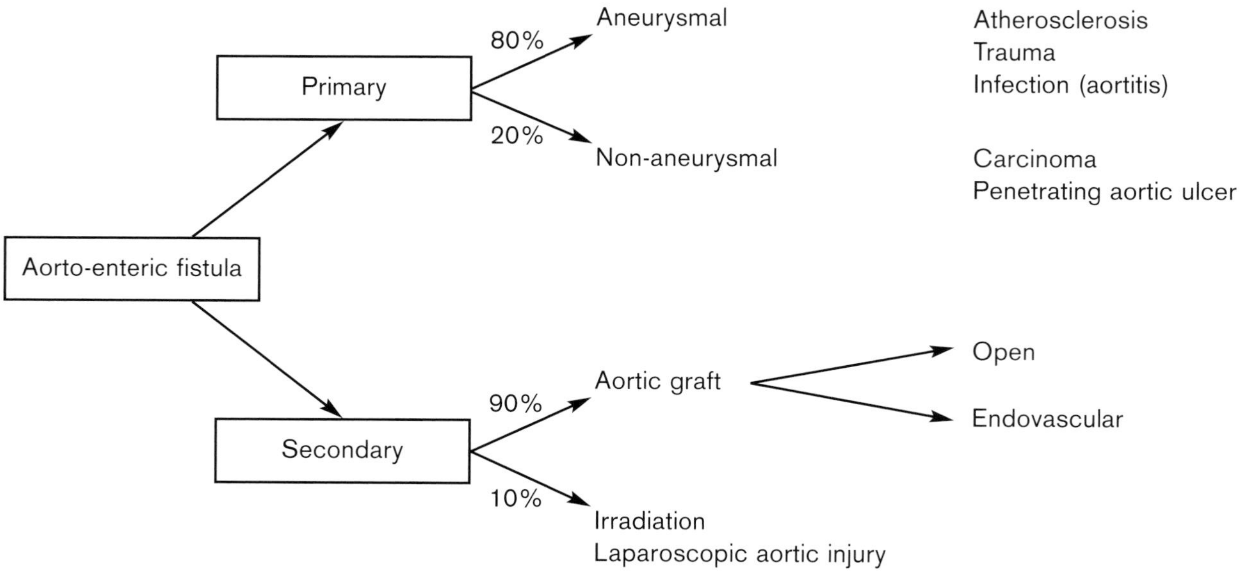

Figure 1. The aetiology of primary and secondary aorto-enteric fistula.

developing after endovascular repair appear to relate to excessive neck angulation or erosion of the stent through the aortic wall.

The most commonly identified organisms in primary fistulae are *Staphylococcus aureus*, *Enterobacter cloacae*, *Candida albicans* and *Staphylococcus epidermidis*. Less common organisms are *Salmonella*, *Klebsiella*, *Tuberculosis* and *Syphilis*. Staphylococci are thought to be implanted at the time of surgery. Methicillin-resistant *Staphylococcus aureus* (MRSA) is increasing in prevalence and has a poor prognosis.

Table 1. Clinical symptoms and signs of aorto-enteric fistula.
Haematemesis Rectal bleeding Abdominal or back pain Palpable aneurysm Unexplained fever with: • lower limb septic emboli • multicentric osteomyelitis • unilateral hypertrophic osteoarthropathy • pyogenic vertebral spondylitis Previous aortic procedure (secondary fistula)

Clinical presentation

The diagnosis of an AEF is dependent on a high index of suspicion and is complicated by the fact that patients may present to several different specialist teams. A primary AEF should be suspected in any patient presenting with a pulsatile abdominal mass and upper gastro-intestinal haemorrhage (although the cause is more likely to be gastric bleeding). A secondary AEF should be suspected in any patient presenting with upper gastro-intestinal haemorrhage who has had a previous aortic procedure. The common clinical features at presentation are listed in Table 1.

Patients who present with signs of systemic sepsis have a poor prognosis. Hypotension is not in itself a predictor of poor outcome as most patients respond to initial fluid resuscitation. The initial bleed is often minor and self-terminating (herald bleed). The interval between this bleed and death without intervention is variable; in one series 70% of patients survived 6 hours between first bleed and intervention or death [1]. In another series, 29% of patients survived more than 1 week between first bleed and death. Investigation and intervention must be tailored according to the patient's condition.

Clinical examination should include a search for signs of sepsis, abdominal examination for pulsation and epigastric tenderness and inspection for lower limb emboli. An abdominal bruit will occasionally be heard. Nasogastric tube insertion is useful to test for upper gastro-intestinal tract bleeding.

Investigation

In all patients with a suspected infected AEF, blood cultures should be taken and a full blood count and C-reactive protein level checked. Anaemia, thrombocythaemia and raised inflammatory markers are all indicative of chronic infection. It is not necessary to visualise the fistula; evidence of a peri-aortic infection and an upper gastro-intestinal bleed is sufficient evidence to warrant surgical exploration. The success rates of the main diagnostic modalities at diagnosing AEF are shown in Table 2.

Endoscopy

The first-line investigation of all patients with major gastro-intestinal haemorrhage is emergency upper gastro-intestinal endoscopy. If AEF is suspected, the third or fourth part of the duodenum may be seen using a paediatric colonoscope. The endoscopic findings of a fistula are erythema, granulation, adherent clot and even a visible graft or suture material. Endoscopy is often normal, but is useful in excluding other common causes of upper gastro-intestinal haemorrhage. Bleeding peptic ulcer remains the commonest cause, even in patients who have had an aneurysm repair.

Computed tomography (CT)

If endoscopy is not diagnostic and the patient is stable, a high resolution CT with intravenous contrast is the investigation of choice. The scan can be performed in a matter of minutes and provides invaluable information. Oral contrast should not be given, as this masks the diagnostic sign of contrast extravasation into the bowel lumen. The introduction of multi-array high-resolution spiral CT appears to coincide with improved diagnosis. The signs of an AEF on CT are loss of the fat pad between the aorta and duodenum, peri-graft fluid or gas, and extravasation of contrast into the bowel lumen (Figure 2). A CT will also show a true or false aneurysm at the aortic anastomosis and the extent of any graft infection. It should be remembered that peri-graft fluid may persist for up to 3 months after routine aortic surgery.

Table 2. Correct diagnosis of aorto-enteric fistula in published case series.

Author(s)	Year	CT	Endoscopy	Angiography
Champion *et al*	1982	-	5/11 (45%)	1/22 (5%)
Pick and Eidemille	1992	5/17 (29%)	8/28 (29%)	13/36 (36%)
Vorhoevre *et al*	1996	2/11 (18%)	3/17 (18%)	0/35 (0%)
Tareen *et al*	1996	-	-	2/15 (13%)
Burks *et al*	2001	6/7 (86%)	3/7 (43%)	2/6 (33%)
Dorigo *et al*	2003	18/29 (62%)	-	-

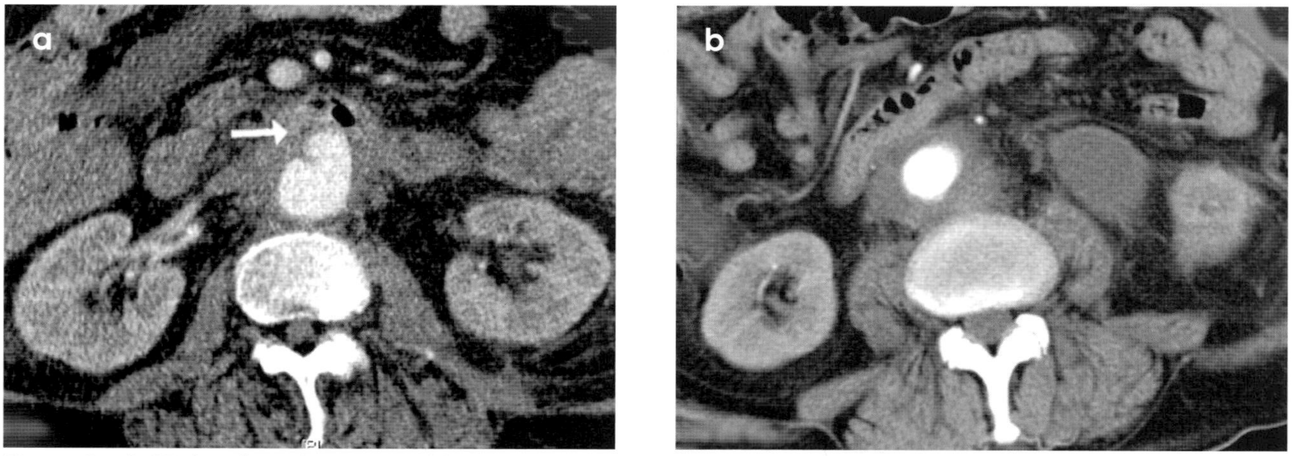

Figure 2. a) CT showing close apposition of the duodenum and the aorta with peri-aortic gas in a patient with a bleeding aorto-enteric fistula. b) CT showing loss of the normal peri-aortic fat pad and surrounding inflammation in a patient with an aorto-enteric fistula.

Angiography

Angiography used to be a first-line investigation for AEF, but is no longer necessary to define aortic anatomy as this can be done using CT reconstruction. An AEF will only be visualised if it is actively bleeding at the time of angiography. Flush aortography, not selective visceral cannulation, is used to demonstrate the fistula. Lateral views should be taken so contrast in the aorta does not obscure that in the fistula or duodenum. Angiography is occasionally useful in a stable patient, but is frequently negative.

Radionucleotide imaging

Nuclear medicine scans (Indium-111 and Technechium-99) are useful in diagnosing aortic graft infection if the patient is stable. A radionucleotide scan may also delineate the extent of graft infection. A labelled red cell scan may uncover bleeding into the duodenum alerting the clinician to the possibility of a primary fistula.

Management

The initial emergency management is to resuscitate the patient with intravenous fluid and blood, if necessary. The rate of bleeding and degree of diagnostic certainty determine subsequent investigation and speed of management. Most published case series report mortality approaching 100% for conservative management [1]. Deaths result from massive haemorrhage or overwhelming sepsis. The aim of surgical management is to prevent haemorrhage and excise all infected tissue (including all prosthetic material), while restoring perfusion to the pelvis and legs. Only rarely should part of an infected prosthetic graft be left *in situ* [2].

Graft excision, aortic stump closure and extra-anatomic bypass

This has become standard treatment for patients with AEF. In order to prevent recurrent sepsis, the communication with the gastro-intestinal tract is repaired, either by primary closure, or bowel resection and anastomosis (Figure 3). All infected tissue is excised and the lower limb arteries reconstructed using an extra-anatomic approach. Most surgeons employ an axillobifemoral graft (Table 3). Gentamicin-impregnated beads or swabs may also be placed into the bed of the infected graft.

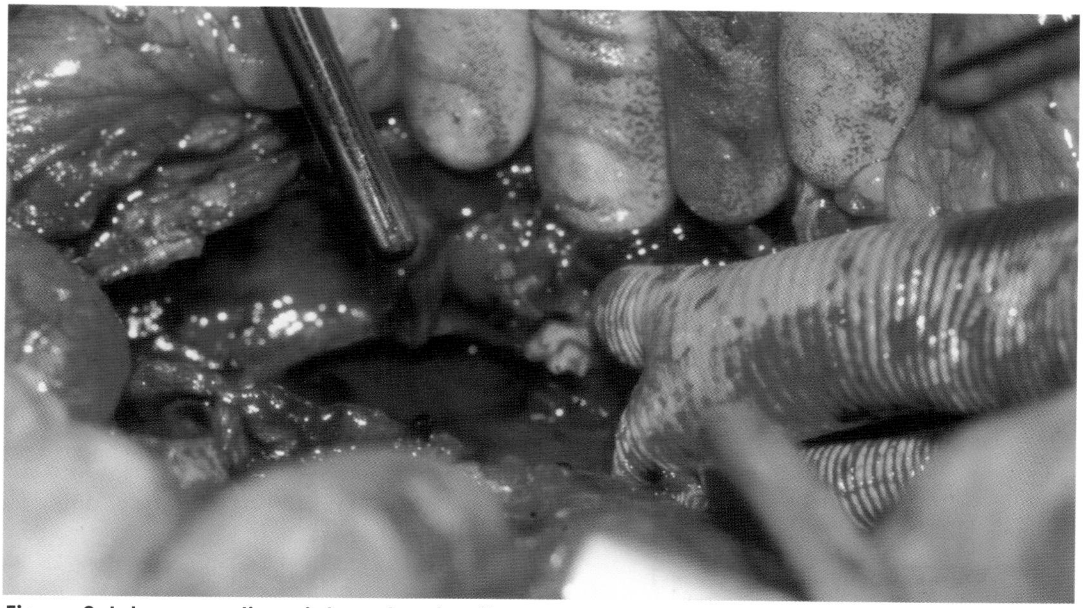

Figure 3. Intra-operative picture showing the aneurysm sac reopened and a large fistula into the duodenum.

The technical aspects of the procedure vary within case series. If a patient is actively bleeding, the AEF is exposed first. Usually the aortic defect is small and can be closed temporarily while bilateral axillofemoral bypass grafts are inserted. Controlled revascularisation of the legs allows the surgeon to concentrate on the potentially difficult intra-abdominal procedure with the knowledge that the legs are not at risk. These two procedures are usually combined during the same anaesthetic, but if a patient is stable, the two procedures can be staged; the axillofemoral grafts are inserted 24-48 hours before the AEF is exposed. If previous surgery involved the groins (aortobifemoral or aortobiprofunda), then the new graft should be anastamosed distally onto "virgin" profunda femoris or superficial femoral arteries.

Table 3. Published series reporting outcome of graft excision and extra-anatomic bypass for an infected aortic graft.

Author	Year	N[1]	30-day mortality (%)	Graft patency (%)	Follow-up (months)	Infection (%)
Jackson *et al*	2003	39 (39)	26	-	-	-
Dorigo *et al* [3]	2003	30 (30)	26	80 (30-day)	24	9
Yeager *et al* [4]	1999	60(16)	13	73 (5-yr)	41	10
Kuestner *et al*	1995	32 (32)	27	81 (5-yr)	50	15
Sharp *et al*	1994	27(8)	4	80 (3-yr)	-	0
Ricotta *et al*	1991	32 (8)	-	100 (5-yr)	34	0
Schmitt *et al*	1990	20 (9)	15	95 (5-yr)	44	0

[1] Number of patients with AEF in parentheses.

The 30-day mortality of this conventional technique is reported to be 25-90%, with a 5-25% amputation rate and 10-50% risk of aortic stump rupture. The extra-anatomic bypass has a good patency rate (>80% at 5 years), but up to 15% risk of late graft infection. Aortic stump rupture used to be the most lethal and frustrating complication after AEF repair. The risk of stump rupture can be minimised by taking wide aortic bites, including the anterior spinal ligament in the closure and avoiding excessive tension. By using these methods since 1983, this lethal complication has been avoided in the author's unit. It is essential that strict aseptic technique is maintained to avoid infecting the newly implanted graft and antibiotics are continued long-term postoperatively.

In situ graft replacement

After bowel repair and graft excision, prosthetic grafts, aortic homografts and superficial femoral vein autografts have all been used to revascularise the legs with the aim of shortening the procedure. In all cases the risk of placing a graft into an infected bed is that of recurrent graft sepsis. Despite the theoretical high risk of recurrent infection the results of selective *in situ* repair and extra-anatomic grafting appear comparable in the short term. If a prosthetic graft is used then it should be PTFE or rifampicin-soaked dacron, and omentum should be interposed between the graft and duodenum. Prolonged, if not life-long antibiotics should be given postoperatively.

Cadaveric aortic allografts have improved since the 1960s when they suffered from disintegration, early rupture and late aneurysmal dilatation. Allografts are presently only available for emergency use in a few major centres, worldwide. The largest published series of their use for *in situ* aortic replacement for graft infection, including aorto-enteric fistulae are shown in Table 4.

Kieffer's large series includes patients with fistulae to the duodenum (n=40), small intestine (n=12) and colon (n=6). There are no significant differences between these results and published results of extra-anatomic bypass. However, high graft re-intervention rates may offset mortality benefits arising from avoiding stump blowout.

Superficial femoral vein

The early results of using autogenous superficial femoropopliteal vein for the treatment of aortic graft infections presenting with systemic sepsis are no better than that of extra-anatomic bypass. Claggett reported 17 patients with an infected aortofemoral prosthesis in whom extra-anatomic bypass was not technically possible due to groin or thigh sepsis (including two patients with necrotising fasciitis). In these high-risk patients, early mortality and amputation rates were both 24% [7]. All grafts remained patent at 23 months The time required to harvest the superficial femoral vein restricts its use in an emergency.

Endovascular repair

Haemorrhage can be prevented or stopped by placing a stent graft across the neck of the AEF. The long-term risk is that the stent graft will become infected as it is in direct contact with the gut lumen. In

Table 4. Published series reporting outcome of graft excision and *in situ* homograft replacement for an infected aortic graft.

Author	Year	N[1]	30-day mortality (%)	Graft re-intervention (%)	Follow-up (months)
Kieffer *et al* [5]	2004	179 (58)	20	26	46
Chiesa *et al* [6]	-	68 (22)	16	14	30
Lesche *et al*	2001	28 (7)	20	17	35
Nevelsteen *et al*	1998	30 (7)	20	23	24

[1] Number of patients with AEF in parentheses.

separate published case reports of AEF managed using an endovascular approach (6 patients), none died acutely. Two developed recurrent sepsis at 5 months and 8 months postoperatively. In the only case series that included seven patients over 5 years, one patient died acutely of sepsis and there were three late deaths [8]. Endovascular fistula exclusion should therefore be reserved for patients with significant comorbidity in whom the risk of open surgery is unacceptable. It could perhaps be used in an emergency to stabilise a patient who is bleeding, so that definitive repair can be done later.

Conclusions

The outcome of patients with an AEF remains poor, due to late diagnosis. AEF must be considered early in any patient who has undergone open or endovascular aortic surgery, who presents with upper gastro-intestinal haemorrhage. Spiral CT is fast, sensitive and specific, making it the investigation of choice. If time allows, an experienced endoscopist can exclude other causes of haemorrhage and may actually be able to visualise the fistula. There is no evidence on which to base the ideal technique of aortic reconstruction. In all patients, prosthetic material should be removed completely and the area widely debrided with sufficient samples sent for bacterial culture. The timing and staging of the aortic reconstruction are dependent on the clinical condition of the patient. All open techniques are associated with early mortality rates of between 25-90% and amputation rates of 10-20%. Death after surgery usually results from sepsis-related multi-organ failure, aortic stump blowout or late graft infection. Endovascular fistula exclusion shows promising short-term results, but may not be durable.

Key points

- **The diagnosis of aorto-enteric fistula relies on a high index of suspicion.**
- **High resolution CT is the investigation of choice.**
- **Endovascular stent graft placement achieves short-term palliation.**
- **Definitive management necessitates surgical debridement, removal of all prosthetic material and arterial reconstruction using either an extra-anatomic or *in situ* technique.**

References

1. Sweeney MS, Gadacz IR. Primary aortoduodenal fistula; manifestations, diagnosis and treatment. *Surgery* 1984; 96: 492-7.
2. Hannon RJ, Wolfe JHN, Mansfied AO. Aortic prosthetic infection: 50 patients treated by radical or local surgery. *Br J Surg* 1995; 83: 654-8.
3. Dorigo W, Pulli R, Azas L, *et al.* Early and long-term results of conventional surgical treatment of secondary aorto-enteric fistula. *Eur J Vasc Endovasc Surg* 2003; 26: 512-8.
4. Yeager RA, Taylor LM, Moneta GL, *et al.* Improved results with conventional management of infrarenal aortic infection. *J Vasc Surg* 1999; 30: 76-83.
5. Kieffer E, Gomes D, Chiche L, *et al.* Allograft replacement for infrarenal aortic graft infection: early and late results in 179 patients. *J Vasc Surg* 2004; 39: 1009-17.
6. Chiesa R, Astore D, Frigerio S, *et al.* Vascular prosthetic graft infection: epidemiology, bacteriology, pathogenesis and treatment. *Acta Chir Belg* 2002; 102: 238-47.
7. Gordon LL, Hagino RT, Jackson MR, *et al.* Complex aortofemoral prosthetic infections: the role of autogenous superficial femoropopliteal vein reconstruction. *Arch Surg* 1999; 134: 615-20.
8. Burks JA, Jr., Faries PL, Gravereaux EC, *et al.* Endovascular repair of bleeding aortoenteric fistulas: a 5-year experience. *J Vasc Surg* 2001; 34: 1055-9.

Case vignette

An unusual case of rectal bleeding

Michael J Gough ChM FRCS, Consultant Vascular Surgeon, The General Infirmary at Leeds, Leeds, UK

A 69-year-old man underwent an anterior resection (2001) and aortic aneurysm repair (bifurcated graft to common iliac arteries) in 2003. One year later he developed rectal bleeding, anaemia and an *E. Coli* bacteraemia. CT was unhelpful but colonoscopy demonstrated graft material within the upper rectum (Figure 1). A laparotomy was performed and the right limb of the graft was palpable within the colon. The large bowel was divided with a surgical staple device proximally and distally (Figure 2) and removed *en bloc* with the dacron graft (Figure 3). Vascular continuity was restored using a bifurcated graft comprising both superficial femoral veins from the infrarenal aorta to the common origins of the external and internal iliac arteries bilaterally (Figure 4). Postoperative recovery was uneventful and the patient remains well 9 months later.

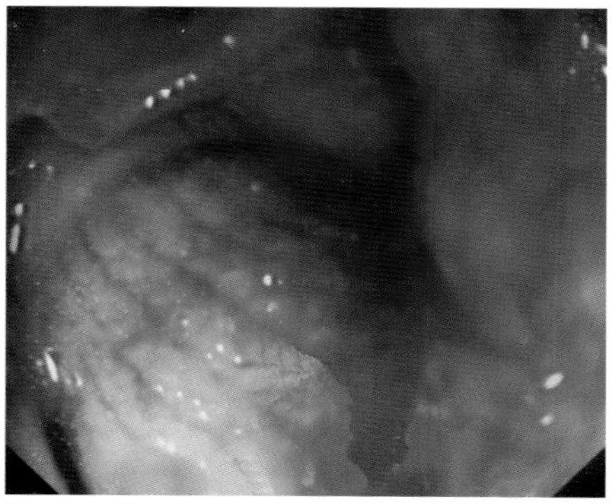

Figure 1.

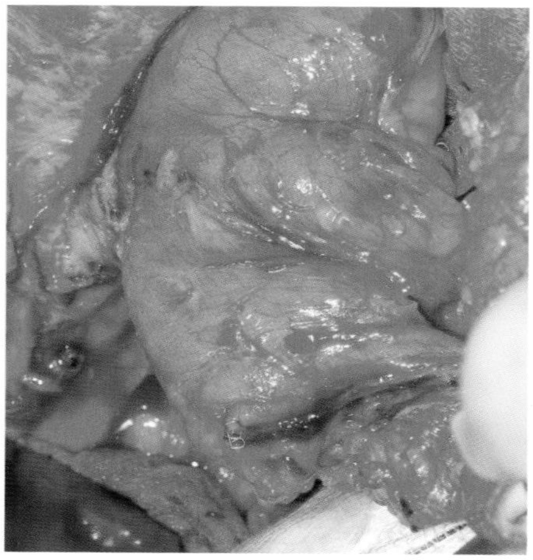

Figure 2.

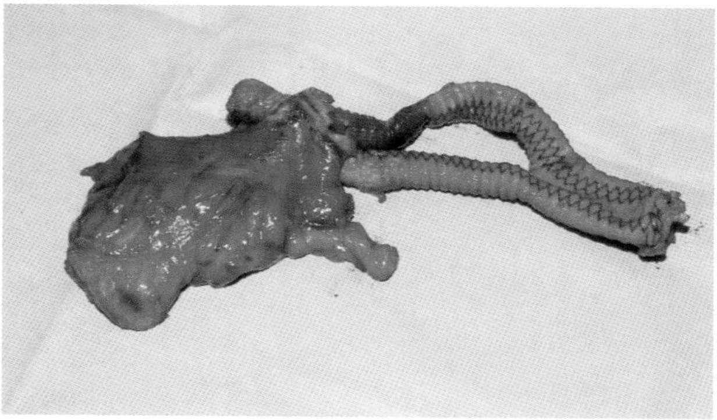

Figure 3.

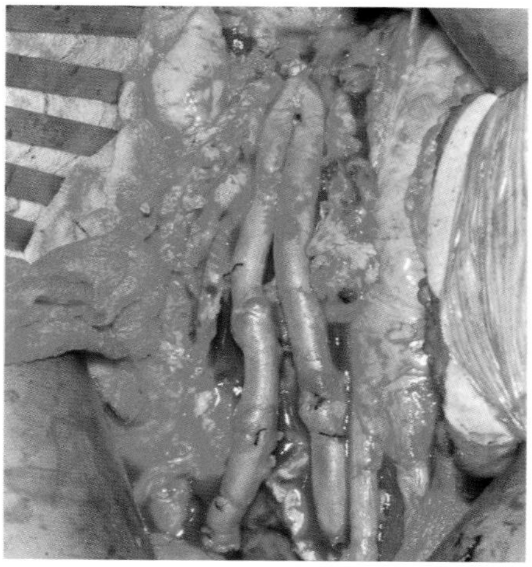

Figure 4.

Chapter 27

Aortic aneurysm associated with HIV

Matt Thompson MD FRCS, Professor of Vascular Surgery
Rob Morgan FRCR, Consultant Vascular Radiologist
Graham Munneke FRCR, Specialist Registrar, Vascular Radiology
Tom Loosemore MS FRCS, Consultant Vascular Surgeon
St. George's Hospital, London, UK

Introduction

The treatment of vascular disease in patients with HIV infection presents significant clinical, logistical and ethical challenges, which are likely to become more common [1]. The incidence of HIV infection continues to increase worldwide and recent advances in pharmacotherapy have improved patient survival. As survival increases, patients become more likely to present with vascular complications of HIV infection.

There is a high prevalence of cardiovascular disease in patients with HIV. A wide range of conditions have been described ranging from non-specific vasculitis to those associated with specific infective agents, e.g. cytomegalovirus (CMV) [2]. Patients with HIV have defined vascular cellular dysfunction that can lead to small vessel and large vessel pathology. In addition, accelerated atherosclerosis has been described in association with the protease inhibitors that are used in anti-retroviral therapy [3].

It is the large vessel disease that is likely to present to vascular surgeons. The spectrum of large vessel pathology has been described in several series to include occlusive disease, true and false aneurysms, mycotic aneurysms and arterial trauma [4,5]. Surprisingly, description of infective agents in pathological arterial tissue has not been particularly common and aetiologically many of the lesions may be due to a leococytoclastic vasculitis of the vasa vasorum or peri-adventitial vessels [2]. In a series of 16 patients with large vessel disease, Chetty *et al* described only one case of arterial infection with *S. aureus.* All vessels demonstrated characteristic pathological features with vasculitis of the peri-adventitial vessels, proliferation of vascular channels, chronic inflammation and fibrosis [6]. A similar low rate of documented infection has also been revealed in a larger study by Nair *et al* [5].

Patients with HIV-related aneurysms appear to form a discrete clinicopathological entity with distinct features [7]. They are usually younger, the aneurysms are commonly multiple and affect unusual vessels such as the carotid and upper limb vessels [5]. Patients may present with any features of aneurysm disease, but presentation with a pyrexia of unknown origin has also been described.

Series of aortic operations in patients with HIV are beginning to appear in the literature. Lin *et al* reported 48 patients with aorto-iliac occlusive disease (n=28), abdominal aneurysm (n=17) and mycotic aneurysms (n=3) [4]. All patients were treated with conventional

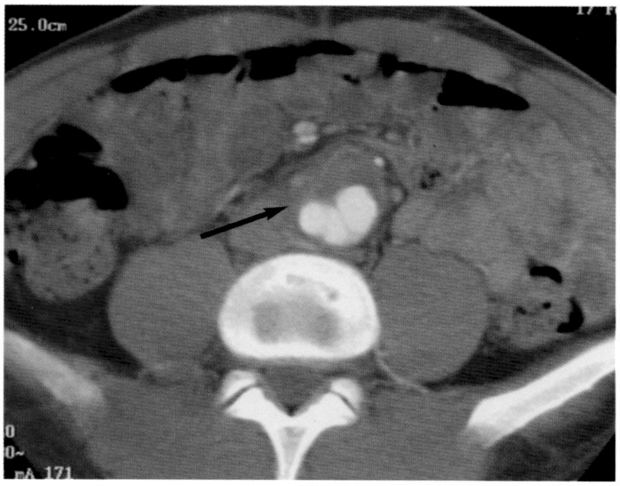

Figure 1. Pre-operative CT demonstrating a small aortic aneurysm affecting the aortic bifurcation.

surgical techniques with an in-hospital mortality of 15%. A multivariate analysis to determine factors associated with adverse morbidity implicated hypoalbuminaemia and a low CD4 count. Importantly, this series also reported that graft infection complicated 10% of the reconstructions, all in patients with a history of intravenous drug use. Other authors have also reported a high prevalence of late graft infection in patients with HIV-associated pathology. Both Curi *et al* [8] and Brock *et al* [9] have demonstrated a prosthetic graft infection rate exceeding 30% in patients with HIV. In both series, the infection rate was significantly higher in patients who had a history of intravenous drug use.

Case report

A 44-year-old Nigerian man had a one-month history of left groin and back pain. He had been resident in the UK for 10 years but travelled frequently to Uganda. His past history included tuberculosis and

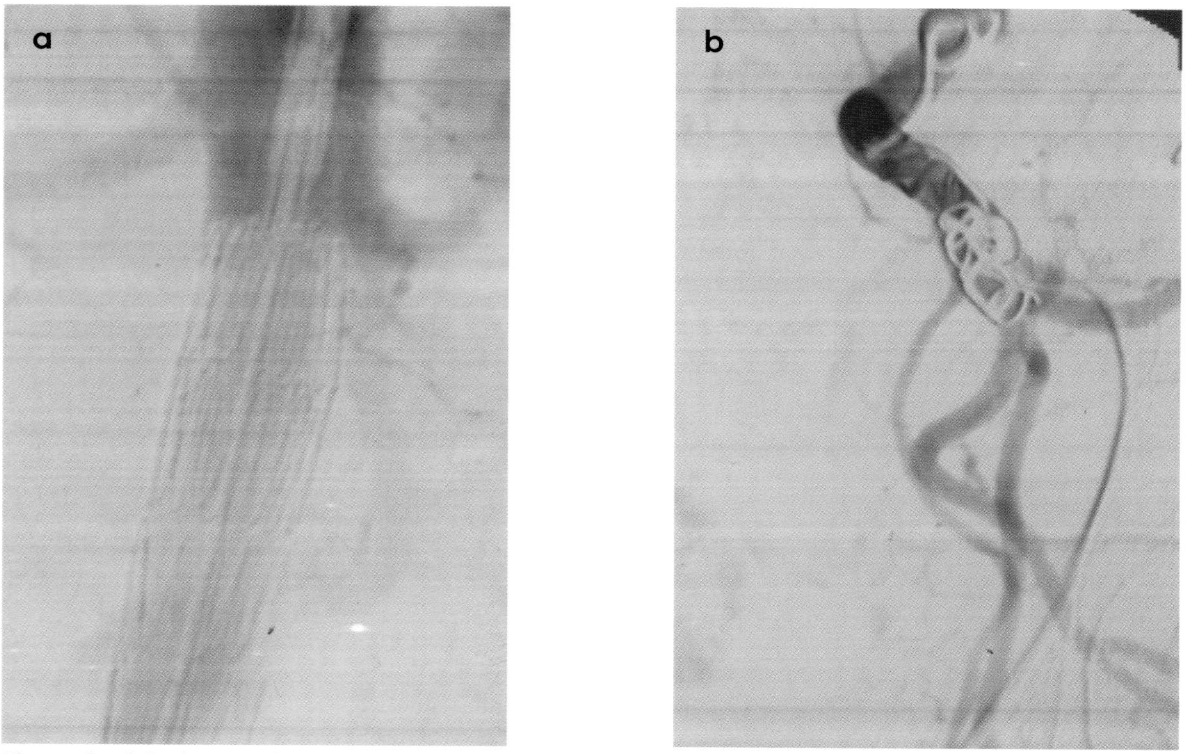

Figure 2. a) Endovascular repair of the HIV-associated abdominal aneurysm using an aorto-uni-iliac Zenith graft in association with b) embolisation of the left internal iliac artery.

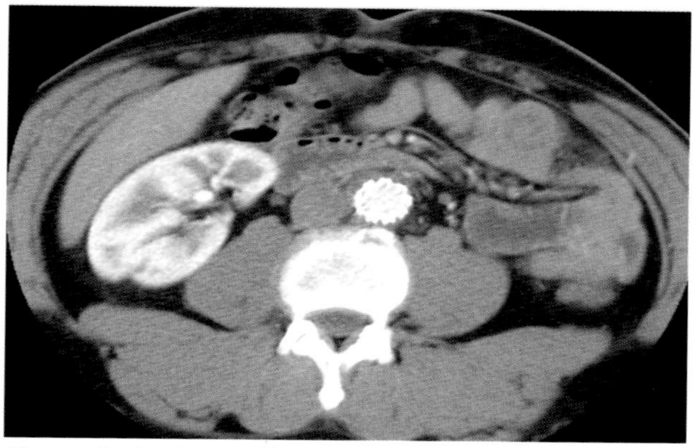

Figure 3. Postoperative CT demonstrating exclusion and regression of the aneurysm sac with a patent endovascular graft.

hypertension. He had a low-grade pyrexia with an elevated C-reactive protein level (90mg/l). Blood cultures were positive for *S. pneumoniae* and he was treated with intravenous benzylpenicillin. Plain X-rays of the chest and abdomen were unremarkable, but an ultrasound demonstrated a 4cm left femoral artery aneurysm. There were no clinical or echocardiographic signs of endocarditis.

Diagnostic femoral angiography demonstrated aneurysms of the infrarenal aorta, right common iliac and left common femoral arteries. CT confirmed a 3.7cm abdominal aortic aneurysm and an occluded left femoral artery aneurysm (Figure 1). The aneurysm was considered likely to be mycotic in origin. His left leg showed no signs of ischaemia, and his symptoms settled within a few days.

In view of his ethnic origin and likely mycotic aneurysm he underwent HIV testing, which was positive with a CD4 count of $257x10^6$/l and a viral load of 7,899 genomic copies/ml. He was hepatitis B and CMV positive. He commenced antiretroviral therapy and was discharged on long-term oral penicillin. He had a good response to antiretroviral therapy. His CD4 count rose above $400x10^6$/l and his viral load became undetectable.

Three months after initial presentation he developed more back pain and a CT demonstrated that the aortic aneurysm had expanded to 4.7cm in diameter. It was decided to repair the aneurysm and a decision was made to opt for an endovascular procedure under general anaesthesia. The left internal iliac artery was embolised and an aorto-uni-iliac endograft inserted via the right femoral artery (Figure 2). The procedure was performed uneventfully and the patient made a rapid recovery. Peri-operative antibiotics were continued for 4 weeks. Subsequent review has revealed complete exclusion of the aneurysm sac with excellent sac regression and no sign of infection (Figure 3). The patient has no recurrent symptoms and his HIV management has been uncomplicated.

Discussion

The case reported above raises some questions regarding the management of patients with HIV-associated aneurysms:

Should the aneurysm have been repaired at first presentation? The patient presented with back pain and a small abdominal aneurysm, presumably mycotic. His symptoms settled quickly on antibiotics and it was uncertain whether they could be attributed solely to the abdominal aneurysm. Another factor was that on presentation the patient was undiagnosed with HIV. On diagnosis his CD4 count was very low and viral load high. Intuitively, it was considered appropriate to offer him retroviral therapy before aneurysm repair. The association between CD4 count ($<200x10^6$/l) and morbidity suggests that patients with HIV-associated aneurysms should undergo medical therapy before intervention if possible.

Are the indications for repair different? Most series have described relatively successful aortic surgery in patients with HIV-associated aneurysms. The immediate peri-operative complications are similar to other large series of aneurysm repairs. However, most patients with HIV-associated aneurysms appear to present with symptoms, and surgery is often expedited to prevent rupture. It seems reasonable to suggest that patients with symptomatic aneurysms should be managed in a similar way to patients who are HIV-negative. The indication for repair of asymptomatic aneurysms is more difficult and requires more information regarding the long-term outcome of aortic reconstruction in patients with HIV. The high immediate infection rate must be a significant concern in this regard.

Is endovascular surgery appropriate? Endovascular surgery offers significant theoretical advantages for both the patient and the medical team. Endovascular aneurysm repair is less invasive, is associated with less blood loss, requires smaller incisions and does not require prolonged stay in critical care. All these factors help in controlling exposure to blood-borne viruses. In addition, endovascular repair has been associated with successful treatment of mycotic aneurysms and may be associated with less infection than standard surgical procedures. This obviously requires further study but may offer an advantage in patients prone to graft infection.

These advantages have to be weighed against the potential disadvantages of endovascular repair in a young patient, with the documented high incidence of graft failure and endoleak, and the need to occlude an internal iliac artery. It must be remembered, however, that patients with HIV have a reduced life expectancy, and the usual arguments about endovascular repair in the young may be less relevant.

HIV-associated aneurysms are likely to be seen more commonly in UK vascular units in the next few years. Our unit currently has four further HIV-associated aneurysms under surveillance. Endovascular techniques may play a significant role in the management of these patients and clearly close collaboration with physicians specialising in HIV is essential to minimise postoperative morbidity.

Key points

- **HIV-associated aneurysms are becoming more prevalent.**
- **HIV-associated aneurysms are often multiple.**
- **Infective agents are rarely cultured from the HIV-associated aneurysmal wall.**
- **Endovascular techniques are useful in dealing with these aneurysms.**

References

1. Dupont JR, Bonavita JA, DiGiovanni RJ, *et al.* Acquired immunodeficiency syndrome and mycotic abdominal aortic aneurysms: a new challenge? Report of a case. *J Vasc Surg* 1989; 10: 254-7.
2. Chetty R. Vasculitides associated with HIV infection. *J Clin Pathol* 2001; 54: 275-8.
3. Mirza H, Patel P, Suresh K, *et al.* HIV disease and an atherosclerotic ascending aortic aneurysm. *Rev Cardiovasc Med* 2004; 5: 176-81.
4. Lin PH, Bush RL, Yao Q, *et al.* Abdominal aortic surgery in patients with human immunodeficiency virus infection. *Am J Surg* 2004; 188: 690-7.
5. Nair R, Robbs JV, Naidoo NG, Woolgar J. Clinical profile of HIV-related aneurysms. *Eur J Vasc Endovasc Surg* 2000; 20: 235-40.
6. Chetty R, Batitang S, Nair R. Large artery vasculopathy in HIV-positive patients: another vasculitic enigma. *Hum Pathol* 2000; 31: 374-9.
7. Nair R, Abdool-Carrim A, Chetty R, Robbs J. Arterial aneurysms in patients infected with human immunodeficiency virus: a distinct clinicopathology entity? *J Vasc Surg* 1999; 29: 600-7.
8. Curi MA, Pappas PJ, Silva MB, Jr., *et al.* Hemodialysis access: influence of the human immunodeficiency virus on patency and infection rates. *J Vasc Surg* 1999; 29: 608-16.
9. Brock JS, Sussman M, Wamsley M, *et al.* The influence of human immunodeficiency virus infection and intravenous drug abuse on complications of hemodialysis access surgery. *J Vasc Surg* 1992; 16: 904-10.

Chapter 28

Mid-aortic syndrome

George Hamilton MD FRCS, Professor of Vascular Surgery
Royal Free & University College School of Medicine
Royal Free Hospital Hampstead NHS Trust, London, UK

Introduction

Mid-aortic syndrome, also known as middle aortic syndrome and abdominal coarctation, is a rare but well described condition which occurs primarily in children and younger adults. Severe hypertension is the usual presentation, but progression to renal failure is not uncommon. Although rare, this condition will typically be encountered on several occasions during the career of a vascular specialist.

Aetiology and pathology

The hallmark of this condition is narrowing of the visceral component of the abdominal aorta which can be variable in its severity, with stenosis of the renal and visceral branches. The condition was first described by Quain in 1847, but the first modern description of the condition was provided by Sen *et al* in 1963 [1, 2]. The exact aetiology of this condition remains unknown with the consensus being that it is primarily an aortic pathology since the stenotic disease is ostial, although the disease process with time extends out into the main renal and visceral arteries (Figure 1). The condition is thought to have a congenital component. One plausible theory is that aortic hypoplasia occurs during development of the abdominal aorta with failure of normal fusion of the two dorsal aortas [3]. Another hypothesis implicates intra-uterine injury or infection, particularly rubella as the factor that precipitates aortic hypoplasia.

Mid-aortic syndrome occurs in association with several other conditions that are broadly genetic in their aetiology. These include neurofibromatosis, a condition associated with other forms of renal artery stenosis. William's syndrome is an inherited disorder resulting from a microdeletion at the chromosome region 7q11 where the elastin gene is mapped. The condition results in children with elfin features, mental retardation, cardiovascular and renal abnormalities and renovascular hypertension. Hypertension is common in these children, as are stenotic abnormalities involving the visceral aorta and renal artery origins. Alagille syndrome, an autosomal dominantly inherited disorder involving chromosome 20, is characterised by triangular facies, abnormalities of the liver, eyes, heart and spine and is associated with the presence of abdominal coarctation. Other associations include mucopolycaccharidosis, foetal alcohol syndrome from excessive alcohol exposure in utero and neuroblastoma.

Mid-aortic syndrome may also be acquired as a result of inflammation, for example from rubella, but

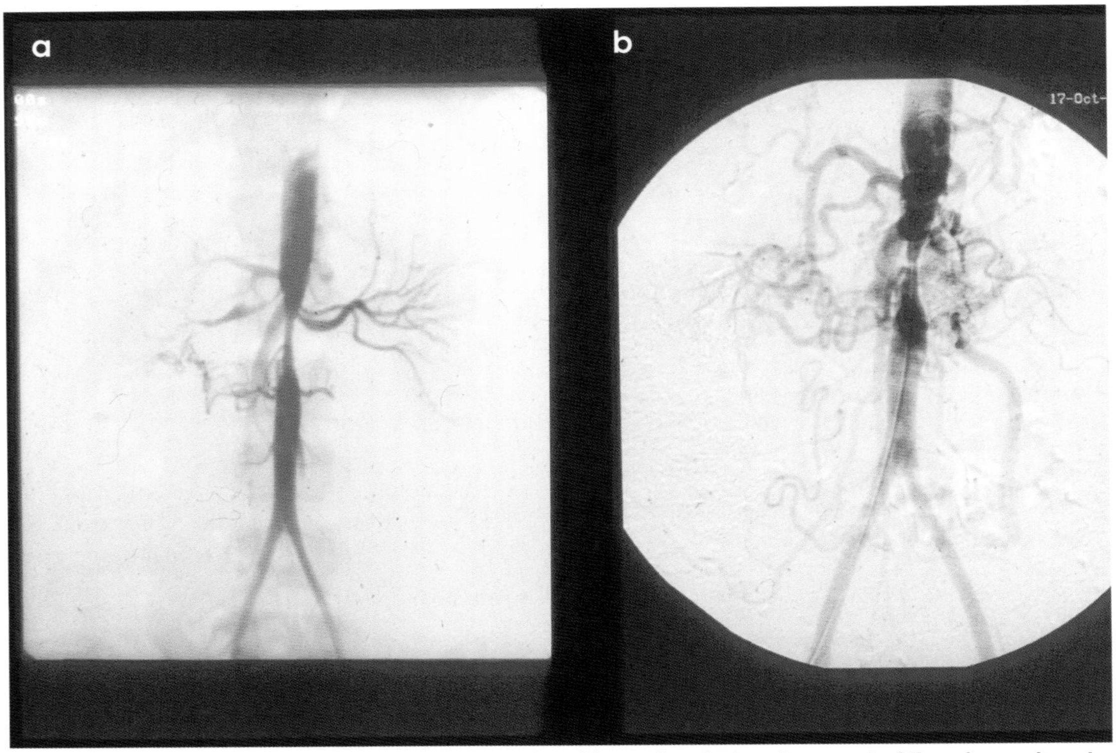

Figure 1. a) Mid-aortic stenosis in a 12-year-old with moderate involvement of the visceral aorta and renal arteries. b) Progression of the stenosis to occlusion of renal arteries after 5 years.

also from clinical variants of Takayasu's aortitis (see Chapter 5, Takayasu's arteritis). The relationship between mid-aortic syndrome and Takayasu's aortitis is controversial. Classically, Takayasu's disease presents with a combination of features including fever, myalgia, arthritis, rash and raised inflammatory markers. Particularly in the West, many patients present with the anatomical features of mid-aortic syndrome but with few of the clinical features suggesting an active aortitis. On this basis there is some support for the hypothesis that mid-aortic syndrome is the endpoint of a burnt-out vasculitis. In South Africa, Takayasu's aortitis presents frequently with mid-aortic syndrome and renovascular hypertension secondary to renal artery stenosis. This particular variant is associated with a high incidence of aneurysms, both fusiform and saccular, and a strong association with tuberculosis has been described [4] (Figure 2).

Histological analysis of aortic tissue from patients with mid-aortic syndrome (but without the clinical features of active vasculitis) shows intimal and subintimal fibrosis with fragmentation of the elastic lamina in the absence of inflammatory changes. The non-specific nature of these appearances, typical of a dysplastic process, is emphasised by many authors in support of the inherited hypothesis of aetiology [5]. Other histological analyses of mid-aortic syndrome, particularly from the East implicate segmental aortitis, suggesting that this syndrome is a variant of Takayasu's aortitis [6].

The aetiology remains obscure but probably varies in different parts of the world. In the West an inherited dysplastic process seems to be more prevalent while an acquired dysplasia secondary to an inflammatory process predominates in the East and South Africa.

Clinical features

Patients with mid-aortic syndrome typically present with severe hypertension, often with an abdominal

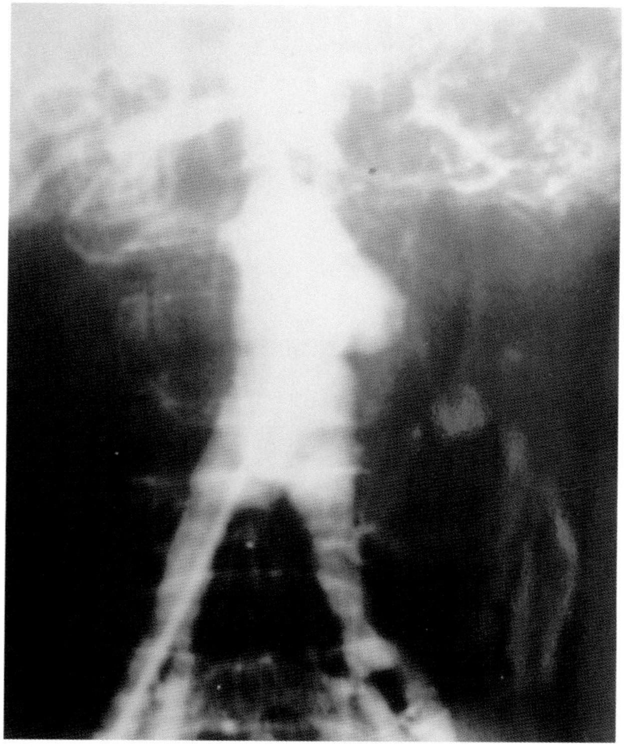

Figure 2. Takayasu's aortitis in a South African youth with mid-aortic stenosis and aneurysm formation; there is a strong clinical association with tuberculosis. Courtesy of Mr T. Abdool-Carim, University of Natal, South Africa.

Table 1. Clinical features of mid-aortic syndrome.
Severe hypertension Usually presents in children, adolescents or young adults Less common • renal failure • congestive cardiac failure • intermittent claudication • seizures Clinical examination • abdominal bruit • diminished leg pulses • reduced growth of the legs (rare finding)

bruit, diminished leg pulses and (less commonly) renal failure (Table 1). Usually the condition presents in children, adolescents or young adults, but it has been reported in a premature neonate, and also in a 58-year-old woman. Mid-aortic syndrome, if untreated, can result in severe hypertension, progressive renal failure, heart failure, cerebral aneurysm and death in young adulthood [7].

Anatomically, the condition is characterised by severe stenosis of the abdominal aorta in its visceral component. Review of the literature reveals progressive involvement of the renal arteries in over 90% of patients, with the coeliac axis and superior mesenteric artery involved in 20-40% and the inferior mesenteric artery almost never involved [8] (Figure 3). In children and young adults, renovascular disease is the cause of severe hypertension in up to 10% of patients referred for evaluation and 20% of these will have mid-aortic syndrome. An important association between mid-aortic syndrome and severe intracranial arterial disease has been reported by the Great Ormond Street group who recommend investigation of all such children before antihypertensive therapy is begun.

Diagnosis

Preliminary investigations include routine measurement of plasma urea and electrolytes, renal function and urinalysis, together with echocardiography to assess left ventricular function. Renal ultrasound and radio isotope scans will give functional and some structural information. Duplex ultrasonography is an important first-line investigation which, if performed by an accredited vascular ultrasonographer, can provide accurate anatomical information regarding the aorta and blood flow into the renal and visceral arteries. This is particularly so in children and young adults who are not obese.

Angiography remains the standard investigation of mid-aortic syndrome; this is supplemented by measuring systolic pressure gradients across the stenosis. The presence of renal artery stenosis is also assessed. With delayed imaging using digital subtraction angiography (DSA), collateral circulation to the kidneys can be assessed and a frequent finding

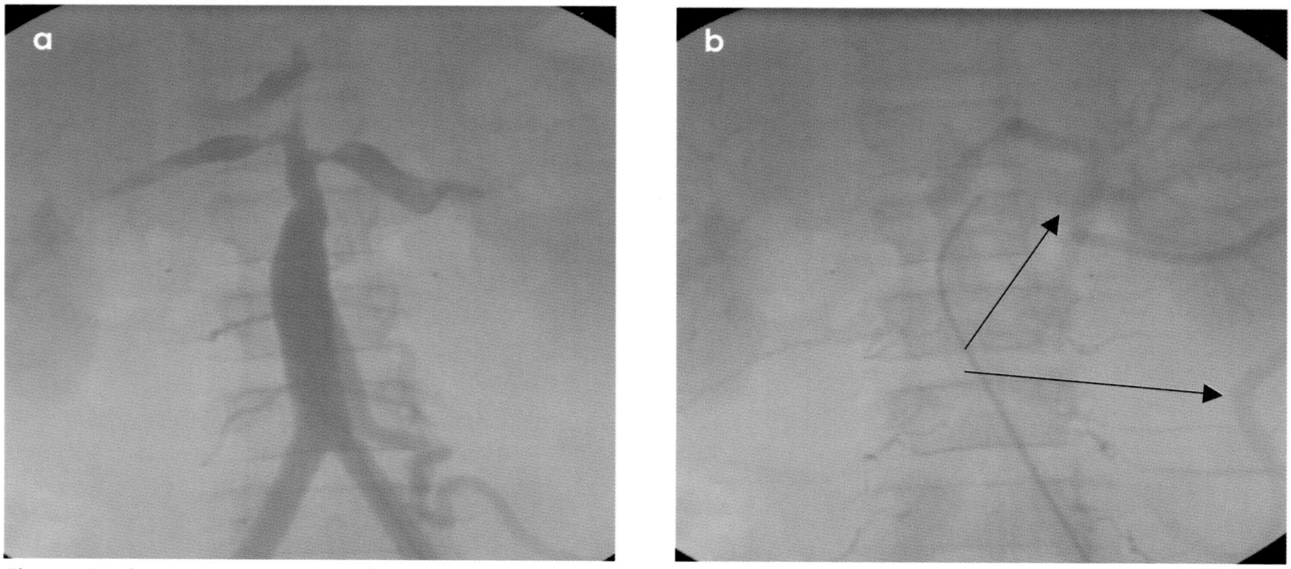

Figure 3. a) Angiogram of a 2-year-old with severe hypertension secondary to mid-aortic syndrome and with superior mesenteric artery occlusion; there was no clinical evidence of mesenteric ischaemia. b) Late phase images show collateral circulation including the marginal artery of Drummond (arrows).

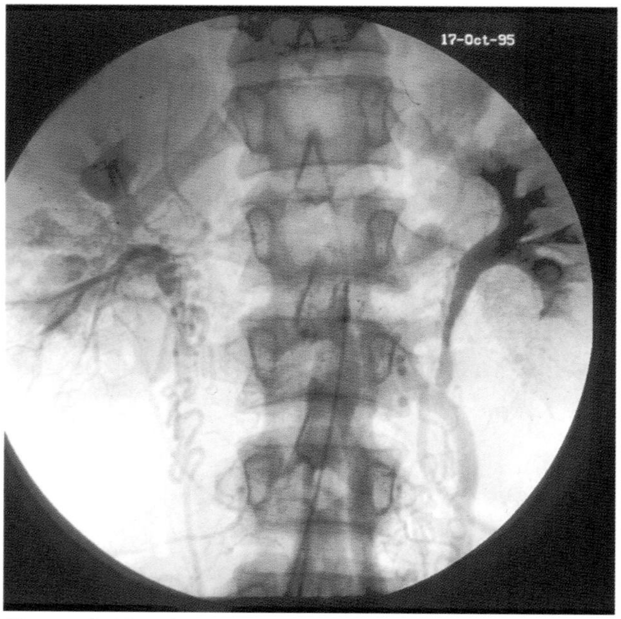

Figure 4. Massive renal collateral circulation in mid-aortic syndrome; these collaterals should be preserved during surgical intervention to maintain renal perfusion.

is of massive mesenteric collateral formation (Figure 4). Lateral views of the aorta should also be obtained in order to assess patency of the origins of the coeliac axis, the superior and inferior mesenteric arteries. Magnetic resonance angiography (MRA) with gadolinium enhancement is currently providing images that approach the specifity and sensitivity of DSA, but access to this investigation remains difficult in many centres. Excellent imaging of the aorta and its branches can also be obtained with spiral computed tomography angiography - a technique which is more readily available. This investigation has the disadvantage of needing intravenous contrast and delivers significant radiation dosage. However, the quality of images and the added insights provided by 3D reconstruction of the aorta and its branches are of value to the surgeon in pre-operative selection of a surgical procedure.

Lower limb ankle to brachial pressure index measurements (ABPI) following a treadmill exercise test are of value in assessing arterial blood supply to the legs. In children with mid-aortic syndrome, the possibility of disordered cerebral vasculature should be investigated, particularly where medical control of hypertension is being considered and where cerebral hypoperfusion may result. This can best be achieved by MRA of the cerebral circulation.

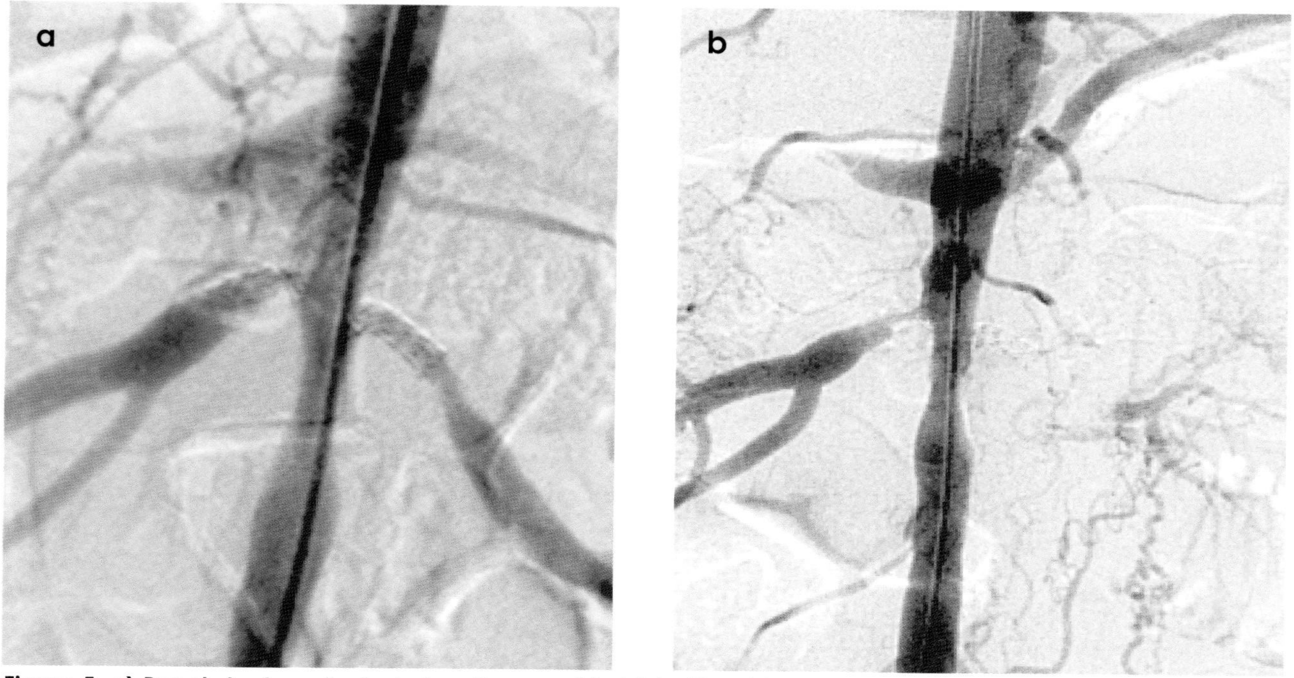

Figure 5. a) Renal stent angioplasty in a 3-year-old child with mid-aortic syndrome with good technical result and improvement in control of hypertension. b) In-stent restenosis of the right renal artery and occlusion of the left renal artery developed within 2 months. Surgical revascularisation was performed successfully by supracoeliac aortorenal bypass.

Treatment

Initial treatment is by control of hypertension which not infrequently in mid-aortic syndrome can be difficult. Typically, satisfactory control can be obtained only with multiple classes of antihypertensive agents. Medical treatment should also be directed towards any degree of cardiac failure. In children, medical treatment remains the mainstay of treatment providing hypertension can be controlled satisfactorily and renal function is maintained. However, the definitive treatment for mid-aortic syndrome and associated renal and visceral disease is surgical reconstruction. The ideal timing of this intervention in children is difficult and the goal is to reserve surgery until adolescence when a single-stage definitive reconstruction can take place.

In children where medical treatment of hypertension has failed or where renal failure is progressive, balloon dilatation of the aorta and of the renal arteries is a useful interim method of revascularisation. The overall success rate of angioplasty of renal artery stenosis in children lies between 30-50%. Angioplasty of mid-aortic stenosis has poor success rates with a not insignificant risk of aortic rupture. More recently, stent angioplasty of the renal arteries has been used as a result of the introduction of small diameter coronary stent angioplasty systems. The Paediatric Renovascular Group at Great Ormond St. Hospital for Sick Children recently reported a series of 22 renal artery stent angioplasties in children, with a technical success rate of 85%, with cure in 8% and improvement in 62%, but a high rate of in-stent restenosis of 56% over a median follow-up of 16 months [9] (Figure 5). Successful revascularisation by this method is short-lived but does not compromise subsequent surgery. Stent angioplasty of the abdominal aorta has also been used with partial success. The principle here is to use self-expanding stents with only moderate initial balloon angioplasty for deployment to minimise the risk of aortic rupture. The current role of stent angioplasty in the renal artery

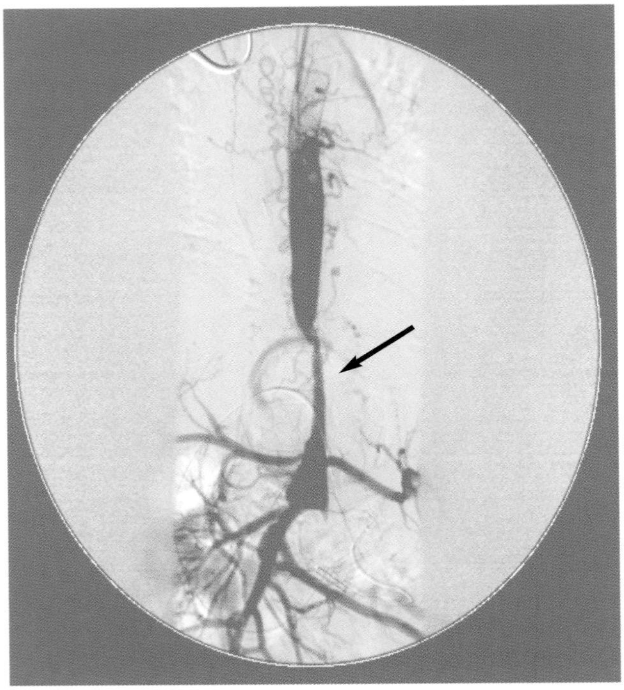

Figure 6. Aortogram of a 4-year-old child who previously had a thoraco-abdominal replacement of an acquired mid-aortic stenosis when 2 years old. This occluded as she grew bigger with a "hanging" segment of patent visceral aorta remaining (arrow). She underwent successful replacement of the mid thoracic to abdominal aorta with re-implantation of the visceral segment and aortofemoral bypass to treat incapacitating claudication, but faces the inevitability of a further aortic reconstruction when she nears puberty.

and aorta is in tiding over until the child has grown sufficiently to allow definitive one-stage surgical repair using a prosthetic graft.

Surgical intervention remains the treatment of choice for mid-aortic syndrome. Recent reviews of surgical series of paediatric patients document cure or improvement in over 90% [10]. Cure rates of 70-79% with improvement in a further 19-26% are reported in two recent large long-term series of surgically treated children with renal artery stenosis [11,12].

Surgical procedures

Careful pre-operative assessment by a multidisciplinary team comprising nephrologist, interventional radiologist and vascular surgeon must form the basis for choice of intervention. The primary indications for intervention are uncontrollable hypertension or, less commonly, progressive renal failure. Renal hypoperfusion may result from either the aortic stenosis or the renal artery stenosis or a combination of both. The degree of aortic stenosis can be assessed by angiography or by pull-through pressure measurement; a pressure drop across the stenosis of greater than 10-20mmHg is considered significant. In the presence of complete renal artery occlusion on angiography, delayed views of the main stem renal artery will almost always show patency of the distal renal artery via collateral perfusion. Careful assessment of the coeliac axis origin is of importance where either hepatorenal or splenorenal bypass is being considered. Because of the progressive nature of mid-aortic stenosis, such surgical approaches must only be considered if the coeliac axis is completely spared. Superior mesenteric artery revascularisation is very rarely required because of the extensive capacity for collateral formation in the mesenteric circulation. Superior mesenteric artery revascularisation is indicated only where there is good evidence that mesenteric angina and ischaemia is present - a condition that is extremely rare in mid-aortic syndrome.

The choice of vascular conduit is another factor that must be considered. The use of saphenous vein must be avoided since this becomes aneurysmal in over 20% of renal and mesenteric reconstructions in children and young adults. Dacron or PTFE grafts are suitable and have patency rates that are equivalent to those of the saphenous vein. The problem with prosthetics arises when used in young children where eventual growth will mandate secondary vascular reconstruction (Figure 6).

Extra-anatomic bypass by hepatorenal on the right, and splenorenal bypass on the left is an attractive option in that living arterial tissue can be used that will grow with the child. This approach can only be used as previously mentioned when the coeliac axis is not involved in the stenotic process and also where the aortic stenosis is not significant (Figure 7).

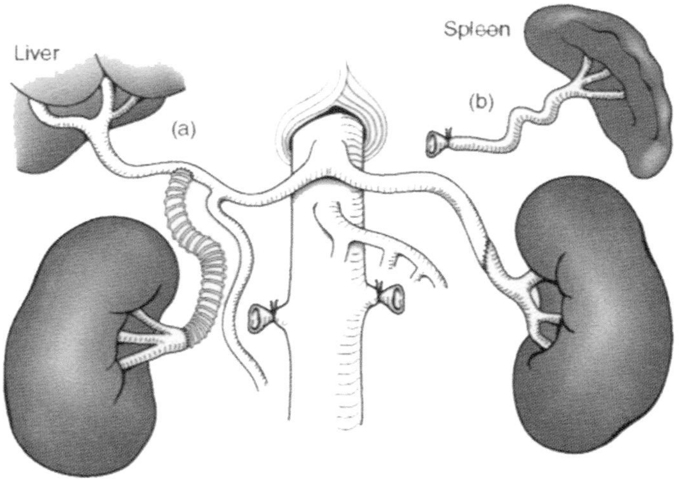

Figure 7. Extra-anatomic bypass for mid-aortic syndrome. This reconstruction has many advantages in a growing child but is only possible where the coeliac axis is widely patent. a) The gastroduodenal artery can be used for the hepatorenal bypass if it is of suitable calibre. b) In splenorenal bypass, splenectomy is not required because of adequate blood supply from the left gastro-epiploic and short gastric arteries.

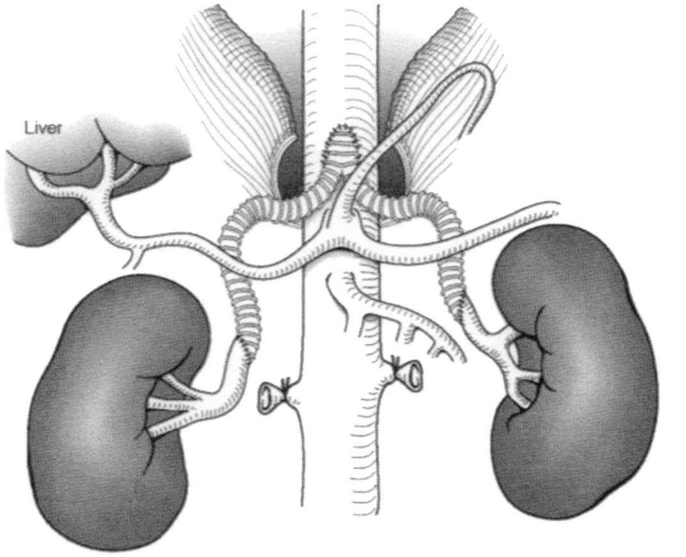

Figure 8. Aortorenal bypass using a bifurcated 12 x 8mm prosthetic graft. If indicated, a further limb can be taken for bypass onto the superior mesenteric artery.

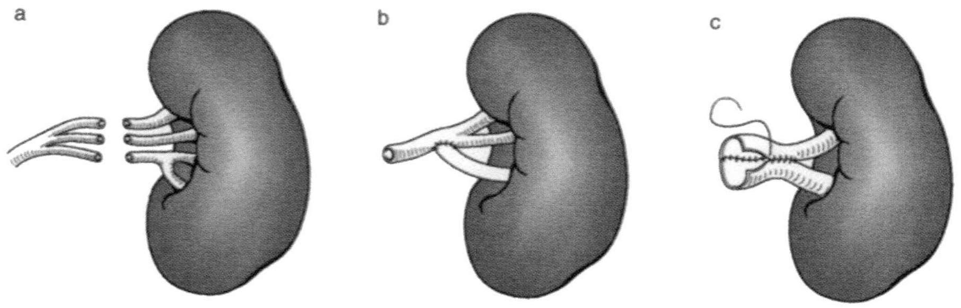

Figure 9. Bench surgery and autotransplantation is used where there is distal renal and/or segmental renal arterial involvement. a) The internal iliac artery is an ideal conduit (saphenous vein must not be used because of aneurysmal degeneration). b) & c) But a simpler reconstruction of the segmental arteries to form a common main renal artery is often possible.

An alternative approach where the coeliac axis is involved, is taking a prosthetic graft from the supracoeliac aorta with anastomosis end-to-end onto one, or both renal arteries. A 12 x 8mm dacron graft is suitable. Taking care to avoid kinking, a degree of redundancy in the length of the graft is maintained in the hope that some accommodation might take place as the child grows in order to delay or even avoid the need for graft replacement (Figure 8).

Where the aortic stenosis is significant, some form of aortic reconstruction will also be needed. In some cases, dacron patch angioplasty of the aorta may be possible, although this is technically difficult in most cases due to the fibrotic nature of the aorta. More frequently, a proximal to distal aortic bypass will be required. This can be performed using either a low thoraco-abdominal or a transperitoneal approach, taking the proximal aortic graft from the supracoeliac aorta exposed by division of the cura of the diaphragm. Pre-sewn 6 or 8mm dacron or PTFE jump grafts are taken sequentially from the main body of the aortic graft and anastomosed end-to-end onto the renal arteries, and, if needed, onto the mesenteric vessels. The distal end is then anastomosed onto the infrarenal abdominal aorta. Rarely, direct re-implantation of renal arteries or the superior mesenteric artery onto the aortic graft can be performed in situations where the disease is strictly ostial and where there is sufficient length of the main stem artery.

Where there is extensive involvement of the renal artery or involvement of the segmental renal arteries, removal of the kidney, bench reconstruction and autotransplantation into the iliac artery will be required. Obviously, adequate perfusion of the iliac arteries must be present and prior bypass of the middle aortic stenosis will be required in the presence of significant stenosis (Figure 9).

Key points

- Mid-aortic syndrome is a challenging condition presenting with hypertension in children or young adults.
- Stent angioplasty of renal artery stenosis and to a lesser extent of the aorta can buy time to allow a child to grow big enough for definitive repair.
- Stent angioplasty carries a high rate of restenosis and is not recommended as definitive treatment in the adolescent or young adult.
- Surgical reconstruction of the aorta and renal artery carries excellent long-term results.

References

1. Quain R. Partial Coarctation of the abdominal aorta. Transactions of the Pathological Society, London, 1847.
2. Sen PK, Kinare ST, Engineer SV, Parulkare GB. The middle aortic syndrome. *Br Heart J* 1963; 25: 610-8.
3. Arnot RS, Louw JH. The anatomy of the posterior wall of the abdominal aorta. Its significance with regard to hypoplasia of the distal aorta. *S Afr Med J* 1973; 47: 899-902.
4. McCullough M, Andronikou S, Goddard E, *et al.* Angiographic features of 26 children with Takayasu's aortitis. *Pediatr Radiol* 2003; 33: 230-5.
5. Poulias G E, Skoutas V, Diundoulakis N, *et al.* The mid-aortic dysplastic syndrome: surgical considerations with a 2-18 year follow-up and selective histopathological study. *Eur J Vasc Surg* 1990; 4: 75-82.
6. Pagni S, Denatale W, Boltax RS. Takayasu's aortitis: the middle aortic syndrome. *Am Surg* 1996; 62: 409-12.
7. Onart T, Zeran E. Coarctation of the abdominal aorta: review of 91 cases. *Cardiologia* 1969; 54: 140-57.
8. Panayiotopoulos YP, Tyrrell M R, Coffman G, *et al.* Mid-aortic syndrome presenting in childhood. *Br J Surg* 1996; 83: 235-40.
9. Hamilton G, Roebuck D, Lord RH, *et al.* Evaluation of outcomes of endovascular and surgical treatment of severe renovascular hypertension (SRT) in children. *Br J Surg* 2005; in press.
10. Stanley JC. Postoperative surgical intervention in pediatric renovascular hypertension. *Child Nephrol Urol* 1992; 12: 167-74.
11. Stanley JC, Zelenock JB, Messina LM, Wakefield TW. Pediatric renovascular hypertension: a thirty-year experience of operative treatment. *J Vasc Surg* 1995; 21: 212-27.
12. O'Neill J. Long-term outcome of surgical treatment of renovascular hypertension. *J Pediatr Surg* 1998; 33: 106-11.

Case vignette

Gastroduodenal artery aneurysm

Christopher P Gibbons MA DPhil MCh FRCS, Consultant Surgeon, Morriston Hospital, Swansea, UK

A 65-year-old man with a history of ischaemic heart disease and atrial fibrillation on warfarin was admitted with abdominal and back pain. Computed tomography showed an 8.5cm infrarenal aortic aneurysm and a 5cm visceral aneurysm, which was initially thought to arise from the hepatic artery (Figure 1). Whilst undergoing cardiac investigations the aortic aneurysm ruptured and was repaired as an emergency, leaving the visceral aneurysm intact. Angiography subsequently suggested that the aneurysm arose from the gastroduodenal artery with an abnormal origin of the right hepatic artery from the superior mesenteric artery (Figures 2 and 3), which was confirmed at laparotomy 10 weeks later. After control of the feeding vessels (Figure 4) the aneurysm was opened (Figure 5) and under-run from the inside without need for an arterial reconstruction.

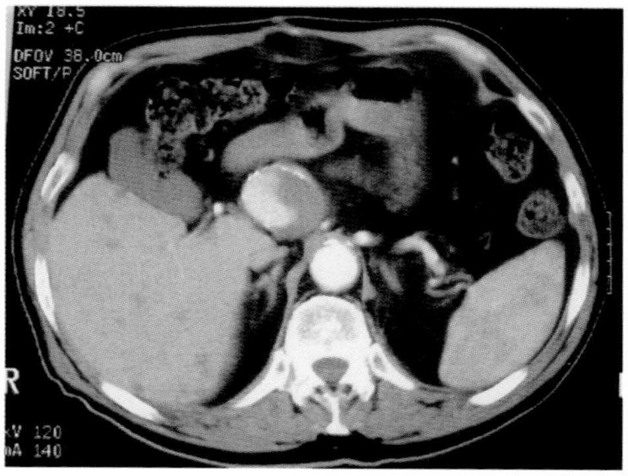

Figure 1.

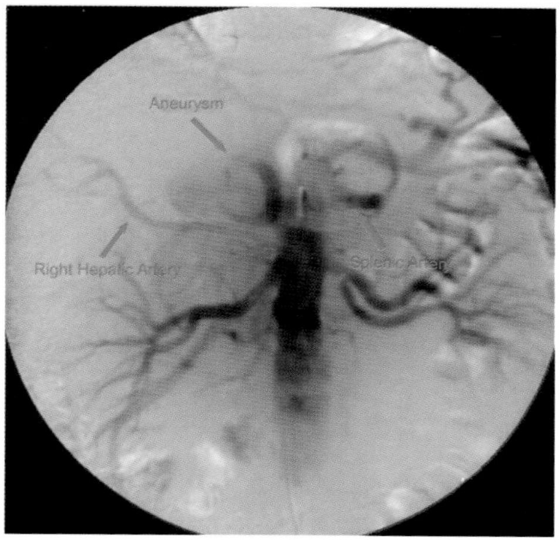

Figure 2.

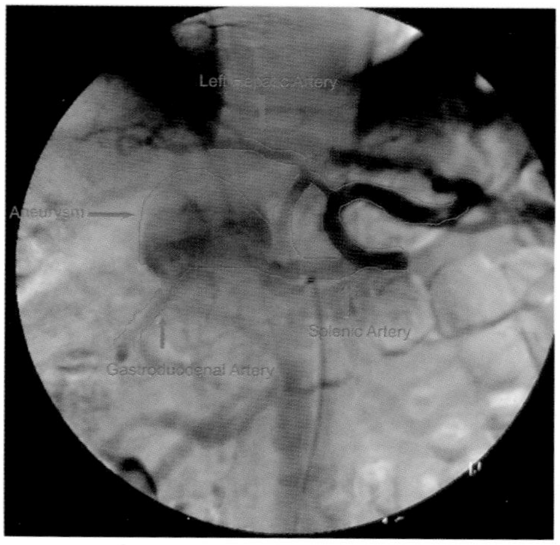

Figure 3.

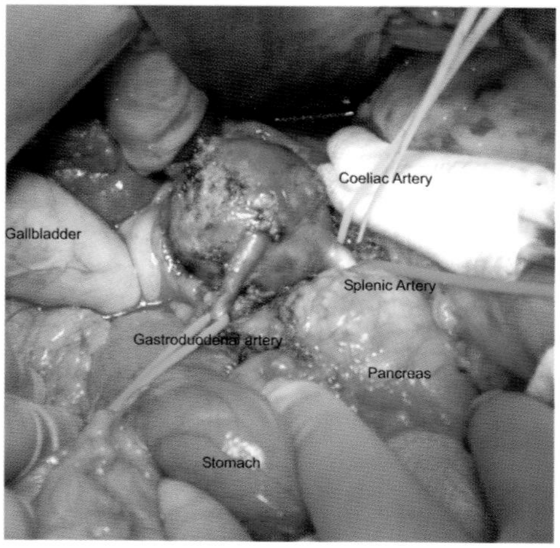

Figure 4.

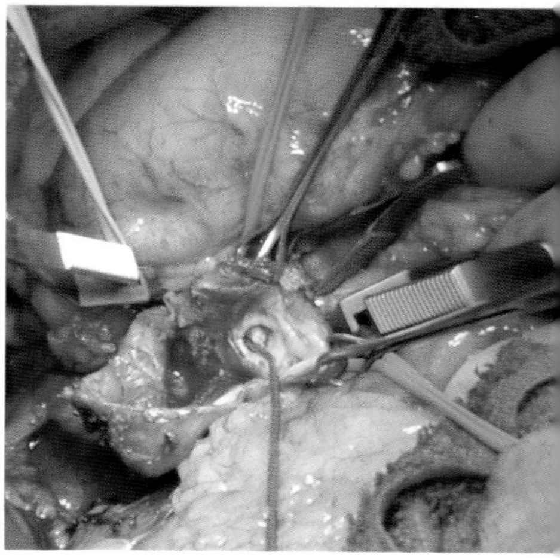

Figure 5.

Chapter 29

Visceral artery aneurysms

Frank CT Smith BSc MD FRCS FRCS (Ed) FRCS (Glas), Consultant Senior Lecturer
Bristol Royal Infirmary, UK

Introduction

Aneurysms may affect any of the arteries supplying the bowel, liver, pancreas and spleen, although, in comparison to aortic aneurysms and aneurysms of the major limb vessels, their incidence is small. They are particularly important as a potential cause of life-threatening retro- or intraperitoneal haemorrhage [1], and complicate a variety of degenerative, inflammatory and infective conditions. The incidence of individual visceral aneurysms is given in Table 1.

Each group of visceral aneurysms exhibits specific characteristic features. Aetiologies, although broadly similar, vary for aneurysms of different visceral arteries (Table 2).

Visceral artery aneurysms may be true or false. This classification is related to aetiology. Aneurysms arising because of fibromuscular dysplasia, segmental mediolytic arteriopathy and inherited vessel wall pathologies or vasculitis are usually true aneurysms. Pseudo-aneurysms occur secondarily to trauma, pancreatitis or surgery.

Treatment of visceral aneurysms and imaging modalities are evolving. During the last decade there has been a significant increase in the availability of minimally invasive and endovascular therapeutic techniques. Paradoxically, this has mirrored an increase in iatrogenic causes of visceral aneurysms such as surgery and percutaneous or transarterial catheterisation.

This chapter reviews individual visceral aneurysms with particular emphasis on the differences in aetiology, clinical presentation and current concepts in management.

Splenic artery aneurysms

Splenic artery aneurysms (SAA) comprise 60% of all visceral aneurysms. They may be multiple (Figure 1), are usually saccular in appearance (Figure 2), and arise most frequently in the distal third of the splenic artery. Reported incidences vary according to the population screened, occurring in approximately 0.1% of post mortem examinations, but in up to 10.4% of elderly patients when this condition is specifically sought at autopsy [2]. In 3600 patients undergoing abdominal arteriography (by definition a selected group with vascular pathology), SAAs were identified in 0.78% [3]. Women are four times more likely to develop a SAA than men. This reflects an increased propensity for aneurysms associated with

Table 1. The incidence of visceral artery aneurysms.

Visceral artery aneurysms	Incidence (% of total)
Splenic artery	60%
Hepatic artery	20%
Superior mesenteric artery	6%
Coeliac artery	4%
Jejunal, ileal, colic arteries	4%
Pancreaticoduodenal artery	2%
Gastroduodenal artery	2%
Inferior mesenteric artery	<1%

Table 2. Aetiology of visceral artery aneurysms.

- Degenerative
- Vasculitis
- Trauma
- Pancreatitis
- Pregnancy (splenic artery aneurysms)
- Fibromuscular dysplasia, segmental mediolytic arteriopathy
- Atherosclerosis
- Infection (SMA and hepatic artery aneurysms)
- Iatrogenic: surgery, percutaneous or transarterial catheterisation
- Liver disease, portal hypertension and splenomegaly (splenic artery aneurysms)
- Polyarteritis nodosa; systemic lupus erythematosus; Ehlers-Danlos syndrome; neurofibromatosis; Behcet's disease
- Post-stenotic (pancreaticoduodenal aneurysms due to coeliac axis or SMA stenosis)

SMA=superior mesenteric artery

physiological circulatory changes in pregnancy. There is an increased incidence in multiparous women.

Several important pathological conditions predispose to the development of splenic artery aneurysms. These include liver disease, particularly cirrhosis associated with portal hypertension [4]. SAA has been described in 7-17% of patients with cirrhosis and portal hypertension and also occurs more frequently in patients undergoing orthotopic liver transplantation [5]. Pancreatitis and blunt or penetrating trauma involving the pancreas may result in formation of a splenic artery pseudo-aneurysm [6]. Connective tissue disorders including polyarteritis nodosa, Ehlers-Danlos syndrome, medial fibrodysplasia, segmental mediolytic arteritis and systemic lupus erythematosus have also been implicated. Although atherosclerosis is associated with aneurysm development, it may be that the calcification, often seen in SAA, (with characteristic signet-ring appearances on plain

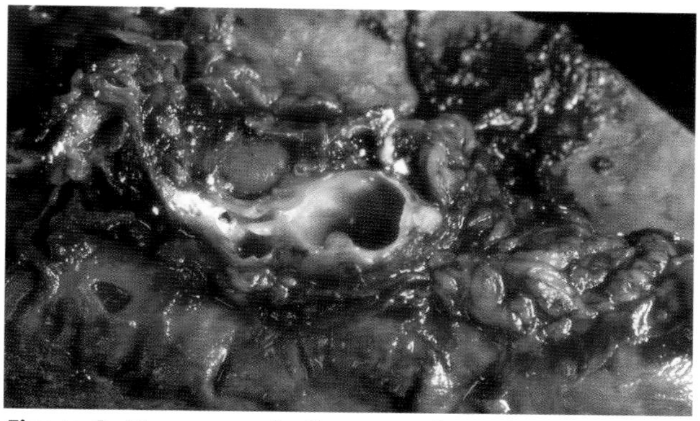

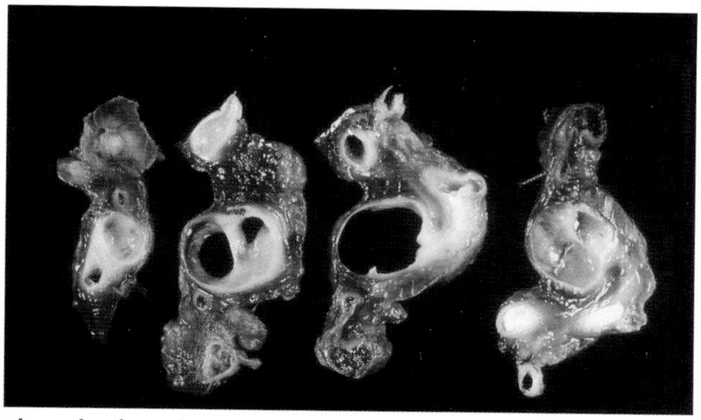

Figure 1. Macroscopic tissue sections demonstrating multiple splenic artery aneurysms. The patient was an 18-year-old girl with congenital hepatic fibrosis, portal hypertension and polycystic kidney disease. She presented with splenic artery rupture and retroperitoneal haemorrhage during pregnancy. Laparotomy, proximal splenic artery ligation and splenectomy were undertaken. The foetus did not survive.

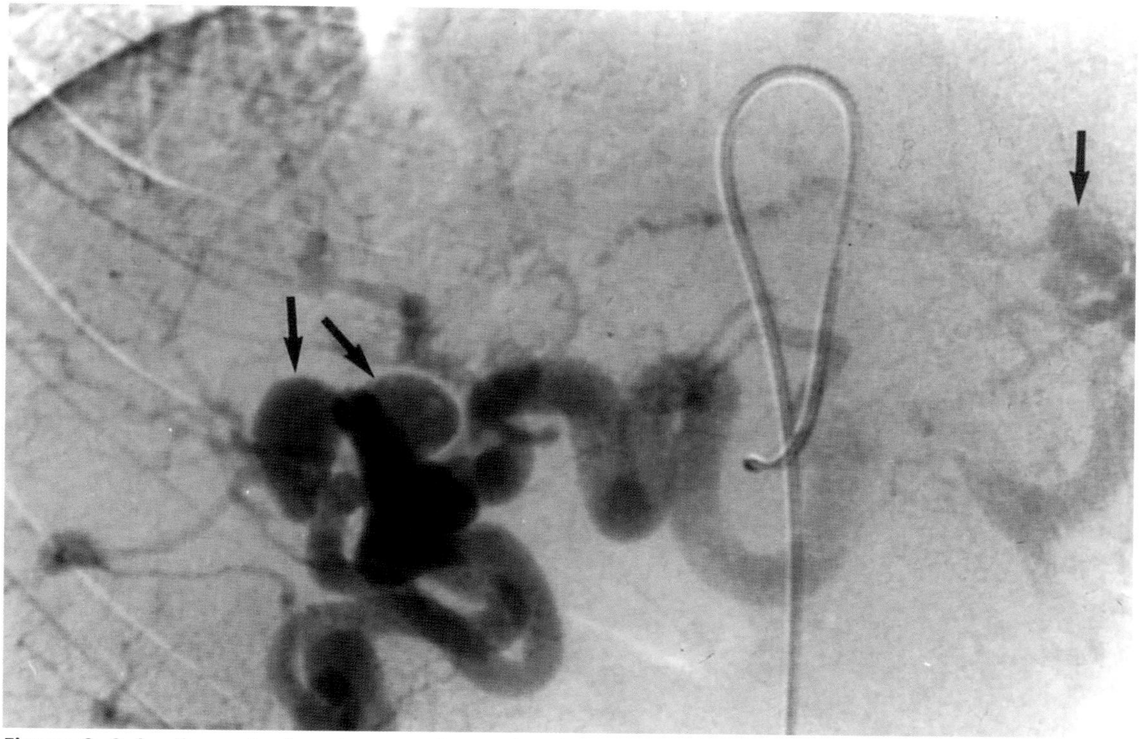

Figure 2. Selective splenic artery angiography demonstrating multiple small saccular aneurysms (arrows).

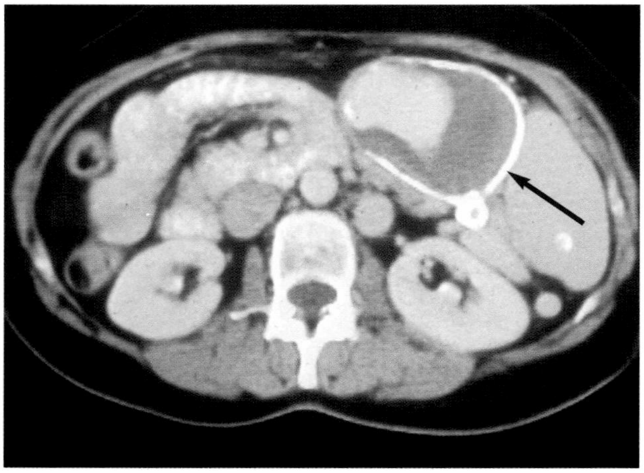

Figure 3. CT scan demonstrating a large saccular splenic artery aneurysm containing thrombus, arising from the afferent artery at the splenic hilum.

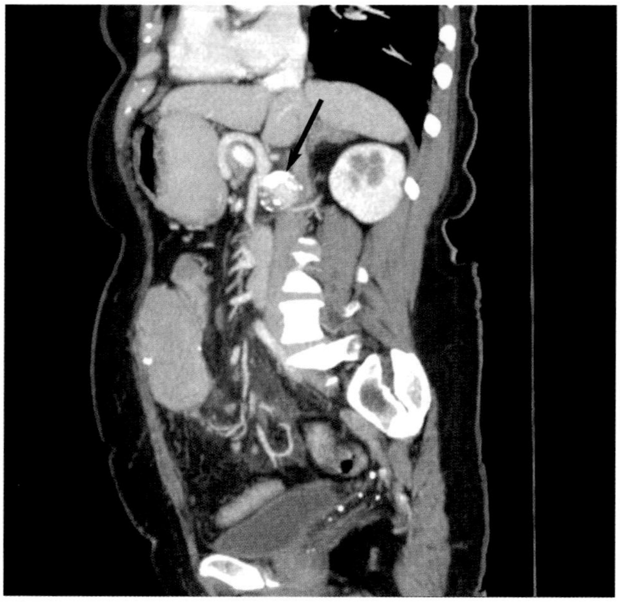

Figure 4. Sagittal contrast-enhanced CT scan of splenic artery aneurysm arising at the vessel origin (arrow). The arterial anatomy in this patient was anomalous with the hepatic artery arising from the aorta independently from the coeliac axis.

abdominal radiography), arises as a consequence of the aneurysm, rather than as part of an initiating atherosclerotic process.

Presentation of splenic artery aneurysms

The majority of SAAs are small (<2cm) and impalpable. Patients may occasionally suffer from left hypochondrial or epigastric discomfort, or back pain exacerbated by acute aneurysm expansion. Risk of rupture is highest in pregnant women when haemorrhage and collapse may mimic obstetric emergencies such as uterine rupture or placental abruption. Rupture of a true aneurysm occurs most commonly into the lesser sac. Initial tamponade affords a potential window of treatment which may be lost as blood tracks out through the foramen of Winslow with resulting intraperitoneal haemorrhage. Foetal and maternal mortality associated with SAA rupture in pregnancy have been reported to be as high as 75% and 70%, respectively.

Splenic artery pseudo-aneurysms secondary to pancreatitis may rupture into a pseudocyst, the stomach, adjacent bowel or the peritoneal cavity; bleeding through the pancreatic ducts may also occur.

The risk of SAA rupture increases after liver transplantation and in portal hypertension, resulting in significant morbidity and mortality. In one series, operative mortality after ruptured SAA was particularly high in patients with portal hypertension (56%) compared to patients who did not have portal hypertension (17%) [4]. Thrombocytopaenia due to hypersplenism and depleted coagulation proteins associated with liver disease may contribute to bleeding following aneurysm rupture. In the same series, mortality for elective repair of SAA was nil [4]. The majority of SAAs identified electively can safely be resected at the time of liver transplantation. Since the incidence of SAAs in patients with cirrhosis is high, CT or magnetic resonance angiography (MRA) has been recommended as an essential part of an evaluation protocol for liver transplantation.

Duplex ultrasound, selective mesenteric angiography, contrast CT and MRA all have potential roles to play in the diagnosis of SAAs (Figures 3 & 4).

Treatment of splenic artery aneurysms

Rupture occurs in fewer than 10% of SAAs overall and in approximately 2% of small aneurysms in low-risk groups. Treatment is indicated for symptomatic aneurysms, those that increase in size on surveillance, large aneurysms, and aneurysms in women of childbearing age or in patients undergoing liver transplantation. Small SAAs less than 2cm diameter in patients who are not in these high-risk groups may be managed conservatively with surveillance. A paucity of prospective data concerning treatment protocols, because of the small number of SAAs encountered by individual units, has led to proliferation of interventional techniques for treating SAAs. These can be grouped into endovascular and percutaneous interventions, laparoscopic procedures and open operative surgery.

Endovascular intervention

Transarterial catheter-directed embolisation via the femoral route has been employed successfully in a number of series to treat SAA. The collateral circulation usually preserves splenic function. Embolisation may be repeated if initially unsuccessful. Directed emboli have included steel coils, haemostatic sponge, N-butyl cyanoacrylate (glue) injection and detachable balloons. Embolisation techniques are less likely to be successful with large aneurysms. Embolisation may be particularly valuable in pseudo-aneurysms associated with pancreatitis, providing a temporary window for definitive surgery. More recently, successful exclusion of isolated SAAs with a covered stent has also been described.

Percutaneous and laparoscopic techniques

Percutaneous prothrombotic thrombin-collagen injection has recently been introduced to induce thrombosis in splenic artery pseudo-aneurysms.

The retrogastric and often intrapancreatic position of SAAs has discouraged many surgeons from laparoscopic treatment of this condition; however, a semi-lateral decubitus position allows laparoscopic access to the lesser sac. Intra-operative ultrasound may aid aneurysm location and successful laparoscopic interventions have involved clipping of the afferent and efferent splenic artery, aneurysmectomy and laparoscopic splenectomy when dictated by splenic hypoperfusion [6].

Open operative interventions

A variety of different open operative procedures have been used to treat SAAs. Interventions depend on the site and number of aneurysms and the nature of the underlying disease process. Splenic artery ligation alone has been described. Aneurysm resection with interposition vein grafting preserves splenic function but leaves scope for further aneurysm development. This seems unnecessarily complicated since restoration of arterial continuity is rarely necessary. Where a splenic artery pseudo-aneurysm arises as a result of trauma or pancreatitis, aneurysm resection may be necessary with, or without distal pancreatectomy, pseudocyst drainage and/or splenectomy. Resection in the presence of inflammation may be difficult and may require ligation or oversewing of the feeding vessel from within the sac [7]. When dealing with a ruptured aneurysm, early ligation or clamping of the proximal splenic artery, using an approach through the lesser sac after division of the gastrohepatic ligament, may facilitate control of haemorrhage. When splenectomy is necessary postoperative management should include appropriate antibiotic prophylaxis and immunisation against encapsulated bacteria and *Haemophilus influenzae*.

The appropriate intervention or combination of procedures to deal with an SAA should be tailored to the individual patient, the underlying pathology, the accessibility and size of the aneurysm(s). Elective treatment of simple SAAs should carry minimal mortality and low morbidity.

Hepatic artery aneurysms

True hepatic artery aneurysms (HAA) tend to occur after the fifth decade and are twice as common in men as in women. The majority of HAA affect the extrahepatic biliary tree with the common hepatic artery involved in approximately 60% of patients and the right hepatic artery in 30% (Figure 5). Intrahepatic pseudo-aneurysms are frequently associated with trauma. Most aneurysms are solitary, although multiple small aneurysms may occur in polyarteritis nodosa and other connective tissue disorders. Although some aetiologies are shared with SAA there is altered emphasis on predisposing conditions. Mycotic aneurysms, which in earlier eras were syphilitic in origin, now occur more commonly in intravenous drug users and immunocompromised patients, although intrahepatic pseudo-aneurysm has also been reported as a complication of amoebic liver abscess. As for SAA, atherosclerosis appears to be a secondary process rather than a primary cause of HAA. Acquired medial degenerative conditions predispose to aneurysm formation and increasing numbers of false aneurysms have arisen as a result of both blunt and penetrating trauma, iatrogenic instrumentation or damage incurred during laparoscopic cholecystectomy. Pseudo-aneurysms also arise as a significant complication of liver transplantation.

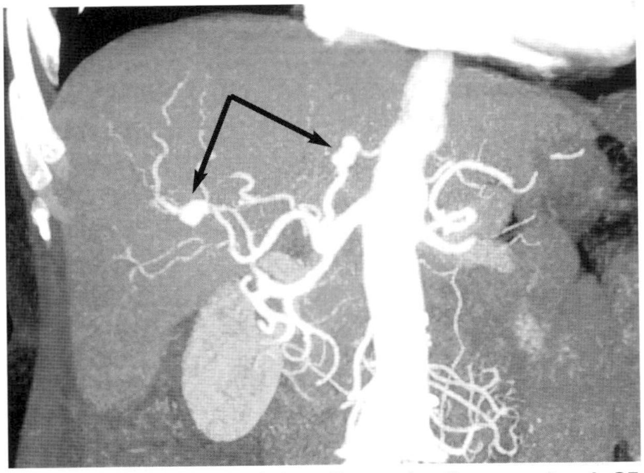

Figure 5. Maximum intensity projection contrast CT scan demonstrating two small hepatic branch artery aneurysms (arrows).

Most HAAs are asymptomatic although they may cause right hypochondrial or epigastric pain. Severe symptoms may mimic cholecystitis or pancreatitis. Up to 50% of HAAs are at risk of rupture and this mitigates intervention in an otherwise fit patient. Rupture is associated with mortality in excess of 30% [8]. HAAs may rupture into the peritoneum, the biliary tract or occasionally by erosion into surrounding structures. Rupture into the biliary tract (more common in traumatic intrahepatic pseudo-aneurysms) may cause frank haematobilia or haematemesis and, when protracted, is often associated with jaundice secondary to biliary obstruction by blood clots. Pyrexia may be a feature. Rupture can present more insidiously with chronic anaemia and melaena. Liver function tests are often deranged.

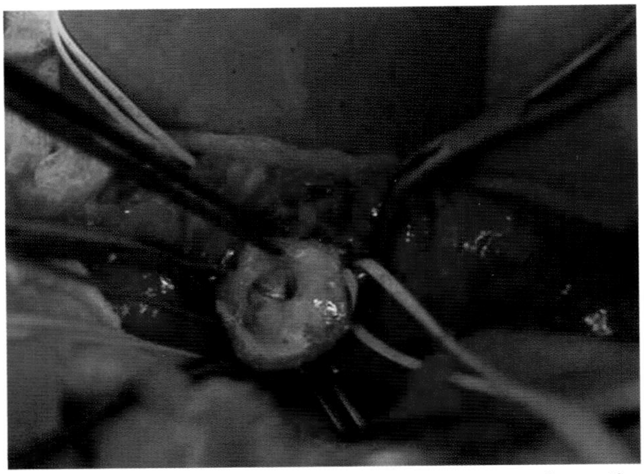

Figure 6. Operative illustration of a common hepatic artery aneurysm. The sac has been opened. Repair was undertaken with an inlaid interposition reversed vein graft.

Intervention for hepatic artery aneurysms

Intervention for HAA needs to take into account the location of the aneurysm, the blood supply of the liver and the potential need for liver resection in the event of open surgery for distal aneurysms.

In recent years, endovascular intervention by embolisation has achieved therapeutic prominence. In one contemporary series, open surgery for iatrogenic pseudo-aneurysms carried a 25% mortality, compared to 14% after embolisation [9]. Selective aneurysm embolisation was successful in 86% (12/14) of patients. Saccular pseudo-aneurysms may be easier to fill with coils than fusiform aneurysms [10]. In the former, flow may be maintained in the native vessel, whereas embolisation for fusiform aneurysms necessitates occlusion of the inflow and outflow tracts. Use of stent grafts to exclude a common hepatic artery aneurysm has been described, although the long-term durability of this procedure is unknown. Percutaneous thrombin injection is another technique reported in occasional cases.

Adequate exposure for open surgery can be achieved with either a "rooftop" or a midline incision. Patients should be adequately cross-matched and pre-operative coagulation deficits should be corrected, where possible. Vitamin K, fresh frozen plasma and platelets should be available. If the aneurysm involves the common hepatic artery then an adequate collateral blood supply via the right gastric and gastroduodenal arteries may allow simple ligation exclusion of the aneurysm sac. A period of trial clamping will demonstrate potential liver viability or compromise. Existing liver disease makes the need for arterial reconstruction more likely, as does the presence of a transplanted liver.

Surgical options include ligation exclusion, aneursymorrhaphy, or aneursymectomy with arterial reconstruction, employing reversed long saphenous vein or prosthetic graft as an interposition bypass (Figure 6). Use of autologous iliac artery or cadaveric iliac artery homograft for reconstruction, following aneurysm resection after liver transplantation, has also been described [11]. Intrahepatic or hepatic artery branch aneurysms may be treated by embolisation, or occasionally by ligation of the feeding branch artery. If these vessels are dissected, care must be taken to avoid damage to the bile ducts. Hepatic resection is rarely necessary, but when undertaken, the use of modern surgical adjuncts such as the cavitron ultrasonic surgical aspirator will reduce bleeding from the liver parenchyma. When it is not possible to site an interposition graft or to deal with an aneurysm by embolisation, ligation exclusion of the aneurysm sac with distal perfusion via an aorto-hepatic graft may be undertaken. Exposure of the right anterolateral border of the aorta can be achieved by right medial visceral rotation, employing an extended Kocher's manoeuvre. This allows anastomosis of a reversed vein graft in a retrograde fashion to the distal common or proper hepatic artery.

Superior mesenteric artery aneurysms

Since DeBakey and Cooley's description of resection of a mycotic aneurysm in 1953 [12], there have been numerous other reports of treatment of superior mesenteric artery (SMA) aneurysms. SMA aneurysms comprise approximately 6% of all visceral artery aneurysms. A major aetiological factor in this group, in contrast to other visceral aneurysms, is systemic infection. A significant proportion of SMA aneurysms are mycotic and they are often associated with subacute bacterial endocarditis. A variety of organisms have been implicated. Atherosclerosis, connective tissue disorders and trauma are other causes of SMA aneurysms. There is also a rare association with neurofibromatosis.

Patients presenting with a mycotic aneurysm are usually younger than 50, whilst aneurysms due to other pathologies are more common in older patients. There is an equal sex distribution.

The majority of aneurysms affect the proximal SMA. Unlike other visceral aneurysms, there is a predilection to dissection. When this occurs, occlusion of the SMA may result in thrombosis with distal thrombus propagation. The small intestine and proximal large bowel is dependent on its blood supply from the SMA, but receives a generous collateral blood supply from the coeliac axis via the pancreaticoduodenal artery, proximally, and from the middle colic artery via its marginal branch communication with the inferior mesenteric artery (IMA) distally. When this valuable collateral blood supply is lost due to extensive thrombus in the SMA, the risk of mesenteric ischaemia and bowel infarction is increased significantly.

SMA aneurysms appear prone to rupture and, when detected incidentally, should probably be dealt with electively. A variety of interventional methods have been described.

Treatment of SMA aneurysms

Originally, open operative procedures were undertaken. Selective mesenteric angiography helps plan surgery. A distal SMA aneurysm can be tackled via a mid-line incision and transperitoneal approach, but when the proximal vessel is involved, exposure may necessitate a retroperitoneal approach with medial visceral rotation of the left colon, kidney and spleen in order to obtain access to the aorta and proximal SMA. If the collateral circulation allows adequate bowel perfusion after a period of trial clamping, then simple ligation exclusion or aneursymorrhaphy may be sufficient. However, aneurysm resection and interposition grafting, ideally with autologous reversed vein, may be necessary. If intervention is undertaken for a mycotic aneurysm, then long-term adjunctive antimicrobial therapy should be considered.

Occasionally it may be possible to ligate a proximal aneurysm and to achieve distal SMA perfusion by undertaking aorto-SMA bypass, a procedure more commonly employed for mesenteric revascularisation in the presence of proximal SMA stenosis or occlusion. The graft is usually taken from the front of the aorta to the distal SMA, employing end-to-side anastomoses (see Chapter 30, Mesenteric ischaemia). If the aneurysm has not arisen due to infection, a short segment ring-reinforced ePTFE graft is ideal in this situation since it will tend to resist kinking and potential occlusion (to which vein grafts are prone) when the bowel mesentery is replaced in its normal position.

Endovascular procedures have also been described for treatment of SMA aneurysms. It has been suggested that transcatheter arterial embolisation with coils or with N-butyl cyanoacrylate may carry lower morbidity and mortality than open surgery, although prospective data to support this are lacking. Small (coronary) covered stents have been deployed to exclude SMA aneurysms and percutaneous injection with thrombin has also been undertaken with success.

Coeliac artery aneurysms

Coeliac artery aneurysms constitute approximately 4-6% of visceral artery aneurysms [13]. Atherosclerosis, medial degenerative conditions, trauma and infection have been implicated as causative factors and a proportion arise in conjunction with aortic aneurysms. Post-stenotic dilatation associated with proximal occlusive disease, in common with the SMA, may progress to true aneurysm development. Coeliac aneurysms often occur synchronously with other visceral aneurysms.

Epigastric pain radiating to the back is the most common clinical symptom, although mesenteric angina (abdominal pain after meals) is a rare presenting feature, particularly if there is also occlusive disease of the SMA and IMA. Contrast CT and gadolinium-enhanced MRA are useful imaging methods.

The mainstay of open surgical interventions to date has involved operative exposure via a thoraco-abdominal incision with medial visceral rotation of the left colon, kidney, spleen and pancreas. The left crus of the diaphragm is divided to enable control of the aorta, in a manner similar to that employed for Type IV thoraco-abdominal aortic aneurysm repair. Resection of the aneurysm with arterial reconstruction by interposition graft or aortocoeliac bypass with a graft originating from the supracoeliac aorta is the most commonly employed technique. Coeliac axis ligation, however, has also been described. If this is undertaken, liver perfusion must be monitored carefully and revascularisation may be necessary.

Endovascular procedures to control coeliac aneurysms have included transcatheter embolisation and placement of stent grafts. Endovascular exclusion with visceral revascularisation may have some potential for treatment of these aneurysms and the development of side-branched modular endografts holds promise.

Other visceral vessel aneurysms

These include aneurysms of the gastric and gastro-epiploic vessels, the gastroduodenal, pancreatic and pancreaticoduodenal arteries and jejunal, ileal and colic artery aneurysms. They occur predominantly in men. Medial degeneration, often in association with local inflammatory processes or vasculitis, is likely to be the cause of the majority of these aneurysms. Pancreaticoduodenal aneurysms may arise in association with coeliac axis stenosis or compression

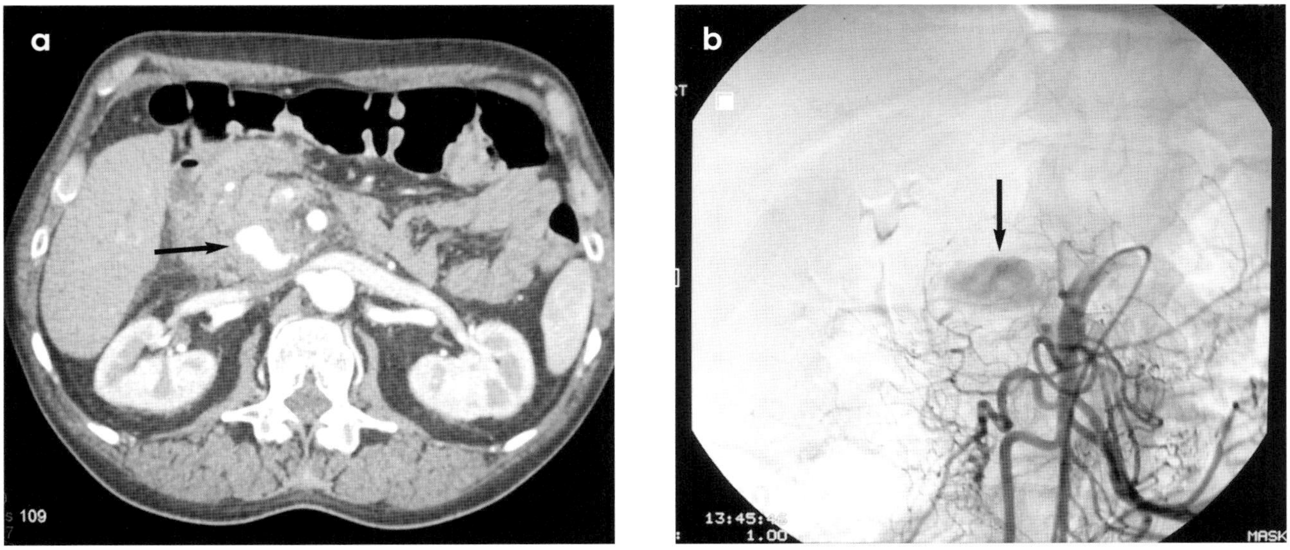

Figure 7. a) CT scan demonstrating a pancreaticoduodenal artery aneurysm (arrow). b) A contrast blush can be seen in the aneurysm sac on selective SMA angiography (arrow). The patient was a 55-year-old man with pancreatitis. The aneurysm was treated by percutaneous transhepatic thrombin injection through the right lobe of the liver. Follow-up at 9 months revealed persistent thrombosis of the aneurysm sac.

by the median arcuate ligament. Pancreatitis, however, is a more common aetiological factor. False aneurysms of the pancreaticoduodenal artery are more common than true aneurysms.

Most aneurysms present with symptoms of rupture, or as a coincidental finding on abdominal imaging or angiography. When ruptured, these visceral aneurysms result in high mortality and surgery is directed at controlling life-threatening haemorrhage. Open operative procedures involving aneurysm ligation and oversew of feeding vessels, often from within the sac, provide the mainstay of emergency surgical treatment. Surgery may be made difficult by local inflammation and, particularly where gastroduodenal or pancreaticoduodenal aneurysms arise as a complication of pancreatitis, pancreatic pseudocyst drainage and pancreatic resection or necrosectomy may be necessary. The emerging role of transcatheter arterial embolisation, particularly in an initial phase prior to definitive surgery, is important and intra-operative thrombin injection of visceral branch aneurysms has been reported as a useful adjunctive procedure (Figure 7).

Acknowledgements

Thanks are due to Dr. Mark Callaway and Dr. Hugh Roach, Consultant Radiologists at Bristol Royal Infirmary, UK, for providing the illustrations used in Figures 4, 6 & 7.

Key points

- **Visceral artery aneurysms are uncommon, but may be a life-threatening cause of intra-abdominal haemorrhage.**
- **Aetiologies and clinical presentations vary. Different groups of visceral aneurysms should be regarded as individual clinical entities.**
- **Intervention demands careful assessment of the collateral circulation and the effects of ischaemia on end-organs.**
- **Elective surgical treatment should carry low morbidity and mortality.**
- **Interventional radiological procedures including embolisation and stent graft placement hold therapeutic promise.**

References

1. Carr SC, Mahvi DM, Hoch JR, *et al.* Visceral artery aneurysm rupture. *J Vasc Surg* 2001; 33: 806-11.
2. Bedford PD, Lodge B. Aneurysm of the splenic artery. *Gut* 1960; 1: 312-20.
3. Stanley JC, Fry WJ. Pathogenesis and clinical significance of splenic artery aneurysms. *Surgery* 1974; 76: 898-909.
4. Lee PC, Rhee RY, Gordon RY, *et al.* Management of splenic artery aneurysms: the significance of portal and essential hypertension. *J Am Coll Surg* 1999; 189: 483-90.
5. Kobori L, van der Kolk MJ, de Jong KP, *et al.* Splenic artery aneurysms in liver transplant patients. Liver Transplant Group. *J Hepatol* 1997; 27: 890-3.
6. Arca MJ, Gagner M, Heniford BT, *et al.* Splenic artery aneurysms: methods of laparoscopic repair. *J Vasc Surg* 1999; 30: 184-8.
7. Tessier DJ, Stone WM, Fowl RJ, *et al.* Clinical features and management of splenic artery pseudoaneurysm: case series and cumulative review of literature. *J Vasc Surg* 2003; 38: 969-74.
8. Abbas MA, Fowl RJ, Stone WM, *et al.* Hepatic artery aneurysm: factors that predict complications. *J Vasc Surg* 2003; 38: 41-5.
9. Tessier DJ, Fowl RJ, Stone WM, *et al.* Iatrogenic hepatic artery pseudoaneurysms: an uncommon complication after hepatic, biliary, and pancreatic procedures. *Ann Vasc Surg* 2003; 17: 663-9.
10. Kasirajan K, Greenberg RK, Clair D, Ouriel K. Endovascular management of visceral artery aneurysm. *J Endovasc Ther* 2001; 8: 150-5.
11. Muralidharan V, Imber C, Leelaudomlipi S, *et al.* Arterial conduits for hepatic artery revascularisation in adult liver transplantation. *Transpl Int* 2004; 17: 163-8.
12. DeBakey ME, Cooley DA. Successful resection of mycotic aneurysm of superior mesenteric artery; case report and review of the literature. *Am Surg* 1953; 19: 202-12.
13. Stone WM, Abbas MA, Gloviczki P, *et al.* Celiac arterial aneurysms: a critical reappraisal of a rare entity. *Arch Surg* 2002; 137: 670-4.

Chapter 30

Mesenteric ischaemia

Christopher P Gibbons MA DPhil MCh FRCS, Consultant Surgeon
Morriston Hospital, Swansea, UK

Introduction

Intestinal ischaemia usually presents as a surgical emergency which has a high mortality. In a Swedish population-based study with an 87% autopsy rate, mesenteric ischaemia had an incidence of 8.6/100,000 and accounted for 6/1000 deaths [1]. By contrast with lower limb ischaemia, few patients present with chronic symptoms that would otherwise enable surgical or endovascular treatment to prevent catastrophic intestinal necrosis.

Anatomy

Three aortic branches supply the intestine: the coeliac axis supplies the foregut region (stomach, duodenum, liver and pancreas), the superior mesenteric artery (SMA) supplies the midgut (the small intestine, right and transverse colon) and the inferior mesenteric artery (IMA) the hindgut (left colon and rectum). Variations in anatomy are common, particularly of the coeliac axis, where the right hepatic artery frequently originates from the superior mesenteric artery [2]. There is an extensive collateral circulation so that ischaemia is rare despite the frequent (29%) finding of stenoses or occlusion of at least one mesenteric vessel in unselected autopsies [3]. In patients with superior mesenteric artery occlusion, the middle colic and marginal arteries often hypertrophy to form the "wandering artery of Drummond" to supply the small bowel from the inferior mesenteric artery (Figure 1).

The venous drainage is via the superior and inferior mesenteric veins into the portal vein to the liver. Acute portal venous occlusion results in the pooling of blood in the intestine, hypotension and intestinal necrosis, whereas the gradual onset of chronic portal vein obstruction or portal hypertension due to cirrhosis allows the development of portosystemic collaterals in the form of oesophageal, gastric or rectal varices, or distended veins around the umbilicus (caput medusae). Localised intestinal necrosis can also result from venous occlusion due to strangulating intestinal obstruction.

Acute mesenteric ischaemia

Embolic arterial occlusion is the commonest cause of acute mesenteric ischaemia (45%), with smaller numbers of arterial (12%) and venous thomboses (5-17%). In approximately 20% of cases, ischaemia occurs in the absence of either arterial or venous occlusion (non-occlusive mesenteric ischaemia) [4,5].

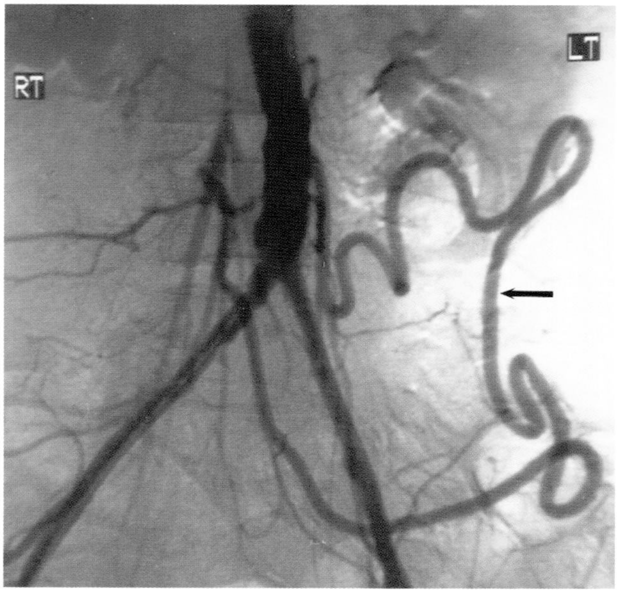

Figure 1. Mesenteric angiogram showing hypertrophied marginal artery (arrow) supplying the superior mesenteric artery territory from the inferior mesenteric artery: the wandering artery of Drummond. Courtesy of Mr. SD Parvin.

Diagnosis

The diagnosis of acute mesenteric ischaemia is notoriously difficult and, in the Swedish study, was delayed until autopsy in 67% [1]. Patients usually present with severe acute abdominal pain, which is initially central, colicky and accompanied by few physical signs. Later, the pain becomes constant and generalised with guarding and rigidity as intestinal necrosis occurs. There may be diarrhoea, which can be bloodstained and usually has a characteristic smell of dead tissue. Nausea and vomiting may occur but are not invariable. Atrial fibrillation or a recent myocardial infarction may point to an embolic cause; a few patients give a history of chronic abdominal pain and weight loss suggesting acute on chronic mesenteric thrombosis.

With further deterioration, patients become shocked, acidotic and anuric. Leucocytosis (>20,000) is typical but not always present. Other possible markers of intestinal necrosis are D-dimer [6], fatty acid binding protein [7] and lactate but none of these is specific. Serum amylase may be raised, leading to a misdiagnosis of pancreatitis. A small amount of intraperitoneal fluid may be present which may be bloodstained on aspiration and have a characteristic odour.

Plain abdominal X-ray films are often unhelpful but may show moderately dilated small bowel loops or mucosal oedema and, in the later stages, gas in the bowel wall or portal vein. CT with contrast or CT angiography is often more helpful and may show an absence of contrast in the SMA, thickening and lack of contrast enhancement of the small intestine or gas within the portal vein or bowel wall. This can be confirmed by conventional angiography.

Treatment

Acute mesenteric arterial occlusion

If the diagnosis of acute mesenteric ischaemia has been made pre-operatively, the patient should be given 5000u heparin intravenously to limit further propagation of thrombus. Most patients will require careful pre-operative resuscitation with fluid replacement and some may require urgent control of fast atrial fibrillation.

Whilst there have been reports of successful thrombolysis ± percutaneous SMA angioplasty and laparoscopy to determine bowel viability [8, 9], laparotomy is strongly advisable because the extent of bowel necrosis is often more extensive than clinical signs would suggest and difficult to assess by laparoscopy. Moreover, in most cases, the diagnosis of intestinal ischaemia is only secured at emergency laparotomy performed on clinical grounds for a presumed intra-abdominal catastrophe of uncertain cause.

Laparotomy usually reveals extensive small bowel infarction. The absence of arterial pulsation in the mesentery points to an arterial occlusion and the pattern of intestinal ischaemia may suggest the cause. In patients with superior mesenteric embolus, the first 30cm of jejunum is usually spared as emboli tend to lodge in the SMA at the origin of the first major branch (usually the middle colic artery) leaving the first few jejunal arteries perfused. Lesser degrees of infarction may also occur, particularly with small emboli (Figure

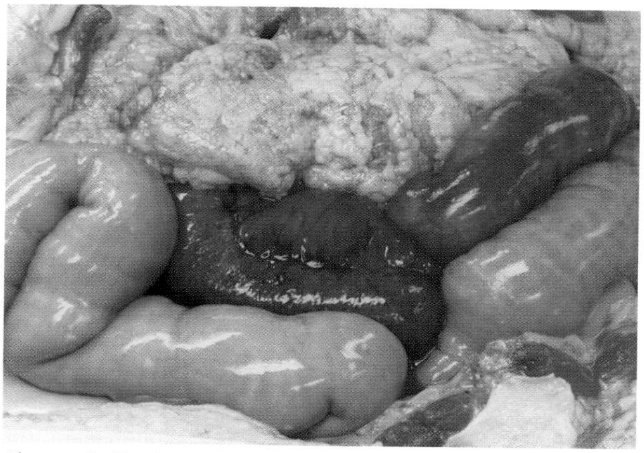

Figure 2. Post mortem photograph of localised small bowel gangrene resulting from superior mesenteric embolus.

2). By contrast, superior mesenteric artery thrombosis usually occurs as a result of atheroma at, or near its origin, leading to infarction of the whole midgut territory from the duodenojejunal flexure to the transverse colon.

In rare cases where the bowel is found to be viable at laparotomy, superior mesenteric embolectomy or bypass may be worth attempting. The superior mesenteric artery is best exposed as it passes in front of the third part of the duodenum to enter the mesentery. After isolating a suitable length of the SMA and controlling the branches, embolectomy can be performed through a longitudinal arteriotomy using a 3 Fr Fogarty catheter. If good inflow and outflow are obtained, the arteriotomy is closed using a vein patch. If an adequate inflow cannot be achieved, a bypass can be taken from the infrarenal aorta or the iliac artery and anastomosed to the arteriotomy. Under these circumstances, a reversed vein bypass using long saphenous or femoral vein is preferable to a prosthetic bypass because of the possible need for bowel resection, and the potential risk of graft infection. Re-implantation of the SMA into the aorta is an alternative but more difficult approach.

Marston[10] advocated embolectomy through a longitudinal arteriotomy in the ileocolic artery and, if an adequate inflow was not achieved, anastomosing it side-to-side to the iliac artery. Because the ileocolic artery is smaller than the SMA, upstream clot is more difficult to extract. Moreover, the anastomosis of the arteriotomy to an often-calcified iliac artery can be difficult. This approach would therefore appear to have little, if any advantage.

Unfortunately, distal propagated clot is usually present after embolectomy and cannot be extracted from the jejunal and ileal arcades. On-table thrombolysis is unlikely to be successful and bowel resection is usually required. In most cases there is already extensive irreversible intestinal ischaemia, so that revascularisation would be futile. The choice then lies between massive bowel resection and palliative treatment, which may be preferred in elderly patients with less than 30cm viable small intestine.

The necessary extent of resection is not always easy to judge, but after a suitable period of observation (at least 20-30 minutes if revascularisation was necessary) the presence of mesenteric pulsations, the colour of the bowel, the persistence of peristalsis and bleeding of the cut end are indicators of viability. Mucosal necrosis is usually greater than suggested by the serosal appearance but there may be considerable capacity for mucosal regeneration. Seeking Doppler signals in the mesentery has also been advocated for the determination of viability, but adds little to the accuracy of clinical judgement. The demonstration of luminescence on ultraviolet illumination after intravenous injection of fluorescein is said to determine viability accurately but the equipment is rarely available [11].

After bowel resection, the author's preference is to re-anastomose the ends so as not to waste intestinal length in the production of a stoma and to avoid a high-output jejunostomy. Others advocate terminal jejunostomy and mucous fistula or stapling the distal end. In very unstable patients "damage limitation surgery" involves stapling the bowel ends, with later re-anastomosis. In any case a second-look laparotomy should be performed in survivors after 24-36 hours to assess the need for further resection, and can be repeated if necessary 24-48 hours later.

Patients with emboli should be anticoagulated postoperatively with heparin, followed by warfarin. Those with atheromatous disease should have maximal medical therapy (antiplatelet agents, statins, smoking cessation and rigorous blood pressure and diabetic control, where appropriate).

Most patients endure a complicated postoperative course requiring intensive care, prolonged parenteral and later enteral nutritional support. Whilst the regenerative capacity of the intestine is often surprising, up to a third of patients with very extensive bowel resections require long-term intravenous feeding and for some younger patients small bowel transplantation may be a late option.

Despite advances in intensive care, the mortality of acute mesenteric ischaemia remains high in population-based studies (93%)[1], although there have been a number of published individual series with lower mortality [7].

Mesenteric venous thrombosis

Mesenteric venous occlusion is less common than arterial thrombosis but has a better prognosis [12]. The extent of thrombosis is more variable than in arterial occlusion. It is associated with thrombotic states such as factor V Leiden, antithrombin III deficiency, protein C and S deficiency or anticardiolipin antibodies, and septic hypercoagulable states such as portal vein thrombosis following intra-abdominal sepsis such as appendicitis or diverticulitis.

The presentation is similar, but CT with contrast may reveal thrombus within the mesenteric or portal veins. At laparotomy, the bowel is usually oedematous, haemorrhagic and purple in colour with areas of necrosis. Arterial pulsations are usually present in the mesentery, but dark thrombus is visible in the mesenteric veins. Histological examination of resected bowel confirms the diagnosis.

Successful thrombolysis has been reported [13] but is rarely a viable option, as emergency laparotomy is essential to determine the extent of bowel infarction and there is a considerable risk of haemorrhage. The treatment is primarily resection and anastomosis with second-look laparotomy after 24-48 hours. Superior mesenteric venous thrombectomy has also been reported and is worth considering to limit the extent of thrombosis [12]. Any underlying cause, such as an intra-abdominal septic focus, should be dealt with at the same time. Subsequent anticoagulation with heparin and warfarin has been shown to reduce mortality and should be continued long-term unless there is a remediable cause for the thrombotic episode. Recurrent thromboses may occur in a third of patients [12].

Non-occlusive mesenteric ischaemia

The fact that up to 20% of patients presenting with acute mesenteric ischaemia have no demonstrable arterial or venous thrombosis [5] was first documented in 1943 by Thorek. Non-occlusive mesenteric ischaemia may be associated with low-flow states or splanchnic vasoconstriction, as may occur in ergot or cocaine poisoning, congestive cardiac failure, prolonged hypotension, digitalis overdose or intra-abdominal sepsis. It is also seen in 4% of patients undergoing operative repair of aortic coarctation. Arteriography is said to show diagnostic attenuation of the intestinal arcades and direct injection of papaverine to alleviate spasm has been advocated. In most cases the diagnosis is made at laparotomy and confirmed by histological examination of the resected bowel.

Chronic intestinal ischaemia

Chronic mesenteric ischaemia is surprisingly rare in view of the known high incidence of significant atheromatous disease of the mesenteric vessels from post mortem studies [3]. It affects women more commonly than men, despite the greater male predisposition to atherosclerosis elsewhere.

Diagnosis

The typical presentation is a female smoker in her 50s or 60s with a history of colicky central abdominal pain after eating, often leading to "food phobia" and severe weight loss (usually over 20lb). Whilst most patients are cachectic at presentation, the occasional patient may appear well nourished despite significant weight loss. There is often some bowel disturbance (either constipation or diarrhoea) or nausea and vomiting. The weight loss often gives rise to a

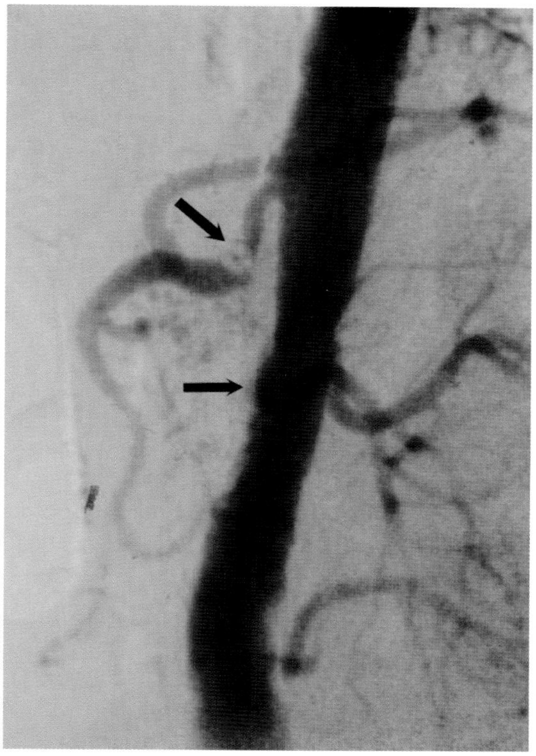

Figure 3. Lateral view of aortic angiogram in a patient with severe mesenteric ischaemia showing a severe stenosis of the coeliac axis (upper arrow) and an occlusion of the superior mesenteric artery (lower arrow).

mistaken diagnosis of gastric or pancreatic carcinoma, and multiple investigations of the gastro-intestinal tract such as gastroscopy, barium studies, CT and abdominal ultrasound may be undertaken before the diagnosis is considered. Other manifestations of generalised atheroma may be present such as claudication, ischaemic heart disease or cerebrovascular disease.

Mesenteric duplex imaging, if available, will usually demonstrate significant mesenteric occlusive disease; this is best confirmed by intra-arterial digital subtraction angiography with lateral views to display the origins of the mesenteric vessels (Figure 3). CT angiography and magnetic resonance angiography are increasingly useful. Typically, two mesenteric vessels are occluded or severely stenosed but mesenteric angina does occur occasionally with single vessel disease. However, the mere presence of mesenteric vessel disease does not necessarily confirm the diagnosis of mesenteric ischaemia because large collaterals may be sufficient to prevent postprandial ischaemic pain (Figure 1). Unfortunately, there is no specific diagnostic test, so the clinician must rely on a classical clinical presentation together with duplex or arteriographic evidence of SMA occlusion or severe stenosis (>70%), preferably with an occluded or severely stenosed coeliac axis. In patients with single vessel disease but a good history, the diagnosis is difficult and the only conclusive way of confirming the diagnosis is by assessing the result of revascularisation. This is usually best achieved by percutaneous angioplasty of the superior mesenteric artery. A good angiographic result combined with symptomatic improvement points to mesenteric ischaemia as the primary diagnosis.

Treatment

Once the diagnosis of chronic mesenteric ischaemia has been made, treatment should take place as soon as possible to prevent further nutritional deterioration. However, most patients who need surgery will benefit from a period of pre-operative intravenous feeding, especially if they have a low serum albumin.

Percutaneous transluminal angioplasty may be possible for non-ostial stenoses or short occlusions and a good therapeutic response may be helpful in securing the diagnosis in doubtful cases. Success rates of 80-90% have been reported [14]. Although less durable than surgery, angioplasty may be preferable in elderly or unfit patients. Stenting may be useful in patients in whom the stenosis reforms after dilatation, or for short occlusions, but the patency is probably no better than angioplasty alone [14]. If restenosis occurs, further angioplasty or stenting can be performed, but surgery offers a more durable option.

Open surgery offers the best hope of long-term symptom relief in patients able to withstand anaesthesia and may be the only option for ostial lesions and long occlusions. Transaortic endarterectomy through a thoracoabdominal incision or via laparotomy and medial visceral rotation is advocated by some [15]. The major disadvantages are

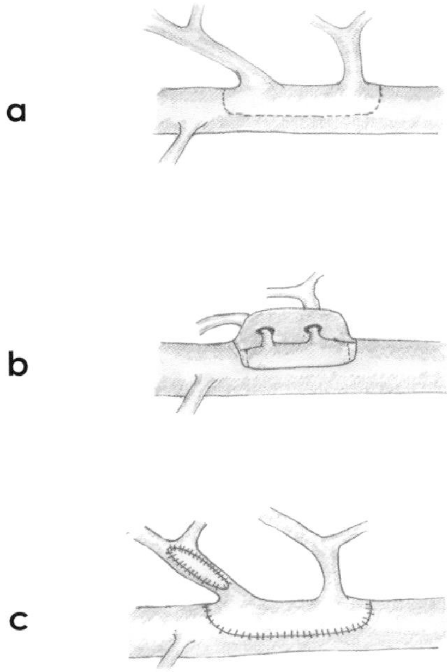

Figure 4. Transaortic endarterectomy. a) Trapdoor incision. b) Endarterectomy. c) Closed endarterectomy incision with a vein patch at the endpoint on the superior mesenteric artery.

that supracoeliac clamping is required and that the eversion endarterectomies of the coeliac axis and SMA do not allow easy inspection of the endpoint and there remains the potential to leave a distal intimal flap. For this reason the first few centimetres of the SMA and coeliac arteries may require exposure in case a patch angioplasty of their origins is required (Figure 4).

Bypass surgery is certainly the most popular and probably the best option. The standard approach is to perform a short bypass to the SMA from the infrarenal aorta. However, the feasibility depends on the degree of aortic calcification. If the aorta is severely diseased an aortic endarterectomy may be required and the mesenteric graft can be anastomosed to a dacron aortic patch. Where the aorta is too calcified to clamp, a common or external iliac artery may be used as the inflow. In other cases an aortobifemoral graft may be used to provide inflow (Figures 5 and 6). Under most circumstances a ringed prosthetic graft (e.g. an 8mm externally supported PTFE) is probably best (Figure 7) as vein grafts tend to kink as they pass over the duodenojejunal flexure from the infrarenal aorta to the SMA. If sepsis or intestinal perforation is present, an autologous graft is essential. Superficial femoral vein

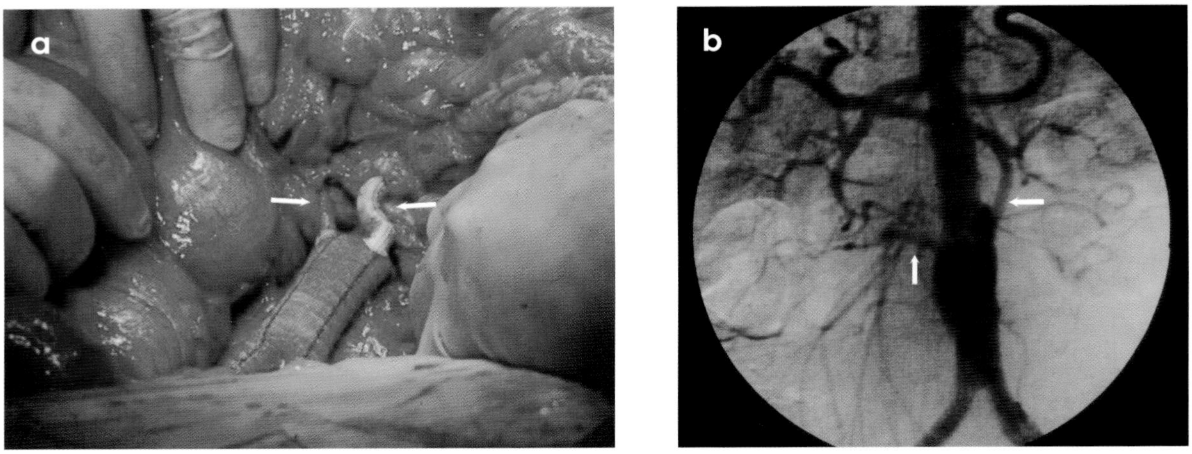

Figure 5. Aorto-superior mesenteric artery vein graft (left arrow) and aortohepatic PTFE graft (right arrow) originating from the hood of an aortobifemoral dacron graft: a) intra-operative photograph; b) postoperative angiogram.

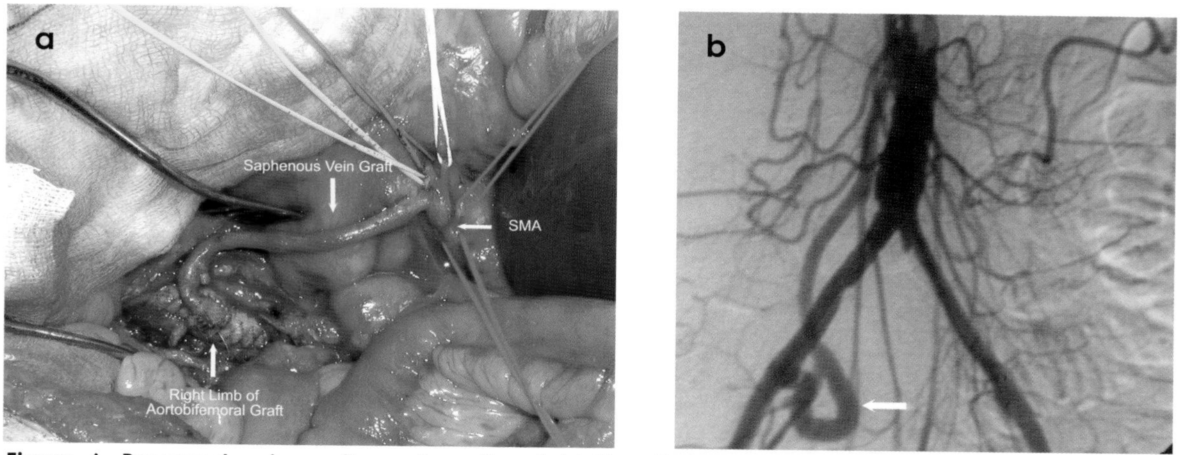

Figure 6. Reversed vein graft run from the right iliac limb of an aorto-iliac graft to the superior mesenteric artery (SMA): a) intra-operative photograph; b) postoperative angiogram (arrow shows a patent graft). Courtesy of Mr. SD Parvin.

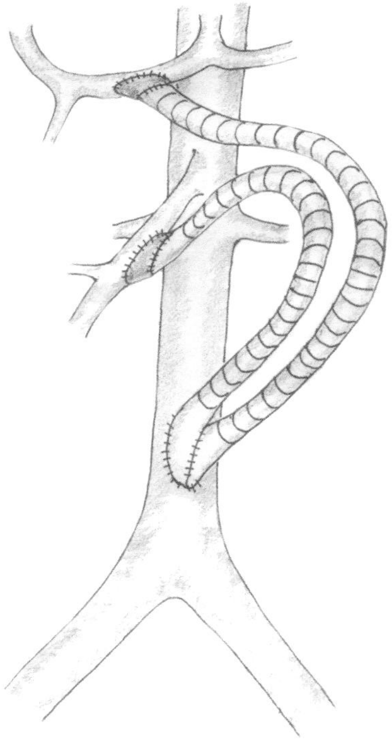

Figure 7. Diagram of infrarenal PTFE aorto-superior mesenteric artery and aortohepatic grafts.

is probably better than long saphenous vein under these circumstances as it is wider and its patency may be superior [16]. If kinking occurs, the graft may be kept under stretch by interposing the greater omentum between it and the duodenum. The need for a second bypass to the coeliac axis is contentious but in most cases is strictly unnecessary provided the SMA is well revascularised. Excellent 4 to 5-year patency rates of about 90% and survival rates of 80% have been recorded for single grafts [14] and the frequency of recurrent symptoms is similar for single and double grafts [17]. However, if a bypass to the coeliac territory is deemed necessary it is most easily accomplished end-to-side to the common hepatic artery (Figures 6 & 7), run either behind the pancreas or anteriorly with interposed omentum to prevent erosion of the posterior wall of the stomach. It is the author's preference to use a vein cuff at the mesenteric anastomosis.

If the infrarenal aorta and iliac arteries are unusable, a bifurcated graft may be run from the supracoeliac aorta at the level of the diaphragmatic crura [18] or from the descending thoracic aorta to the coeliac axis and SMA (passed behind the pancreas). Here, an end-to-end anastomosis can easily be fashioned without any tendency to kink (Figure 8). The need for supracoeliac clamping undoubtedly increases morbidity and is often associated with thrombocytopenia and clotting problems towards the end of the operation. For this

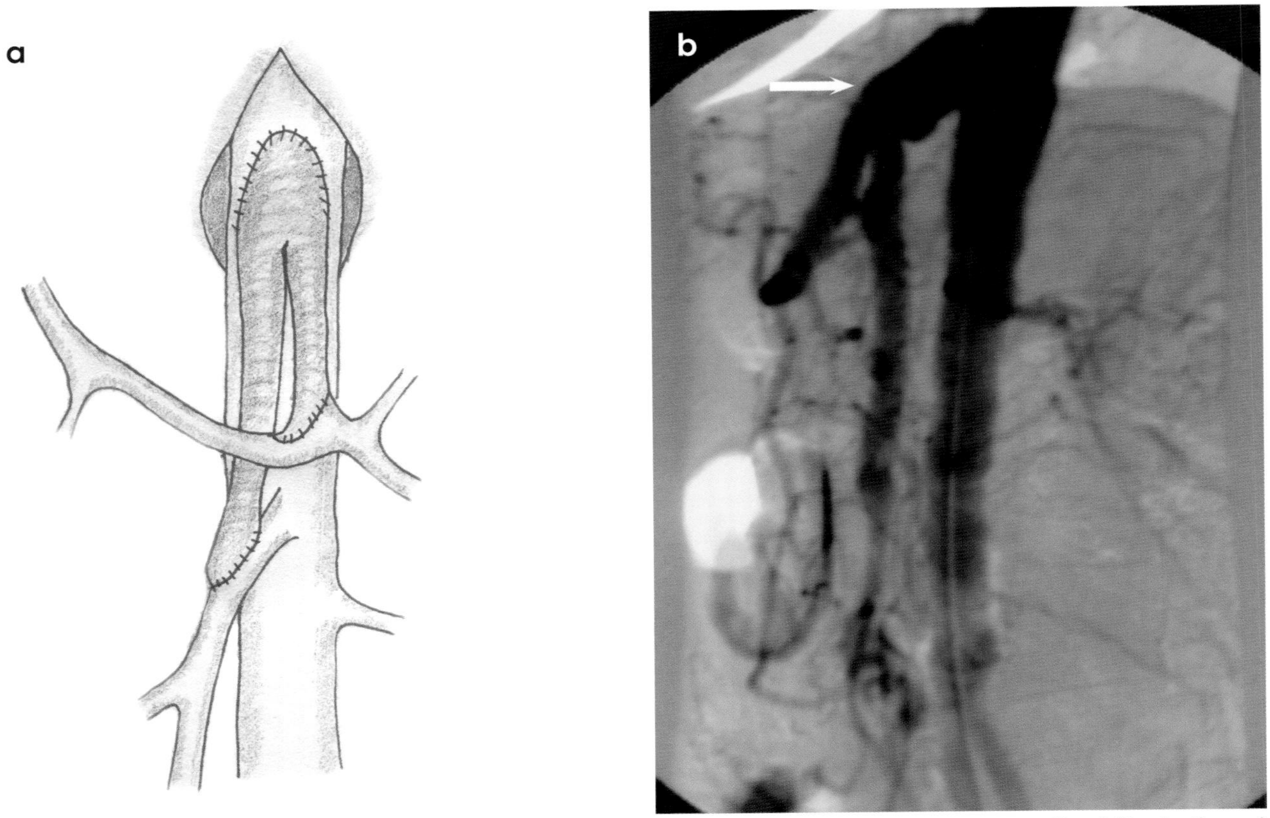

Figure 8. Antegrade aorto-superior mesenteric artery and aortocoeliac dacron trouser graft: a) illustration of graft; b) postoperative angiogram.

reason an infrarenal aortomesenteric bypass is preferable in most cases.

Postoperative complications such as chest infection, persistent diarrhoea and steatorrhoea are common and mortality is relatively high (10% in most series). Postoperative ascites (which may be chylous) may result from hypoproteinaemia and division of lymphatic channels in the mesentery on exposure of the mesenteric vessels. These problems are usually self-limiting.

The results of successful revascularisation are gratifying, with improvements in appetite, and weight gain. Patency rates for surgery are in the order of 85% at a mean of 30 months and are better than those reported for angioplasty (70%) or stenting (63% at a mean of 9 months) [14].

Coeliac artery compression syndrome (Dunbar's syndrome)

The coeliac artery compression syndrome was first described by Harjola in 1963 in a patient with coeliac artery stenosis and postprandial abdominal pain which was relieved by surgical release of a fibrous coeliac ganglion. It is rare but more common in women and has since been described in patients from 13 to 84 years. The coeliac stenosis is now usually attributed to external compression by the median arcuate ligament of the diaphragm.

The syndrome presents with vague postprandial abdominal pain and variable weight loss. An epigastric bruit may be audible. Mesenteric artery duplex, CT angiography or conventional arteriography demonstrates a significant coeliac artery stenosis with post-stenotic dilatation. The stenosis is worse during deep expiration and in the standing position [19].

Division of the median arcuate ligament at laparotomy [20] or laparoscopy [21] improves coeliac artery blood flow and relieves the symptoms in most reported cases. In some series, intra-operative Doppler measurements showed improved coeliac blood flow in a proportion of patients after division of the median arcuate ligament and the remaining patients underwent aortocoeliac bypass, patch angioplasty or coeliac re-implantation [22].

Recurrent symptoms are frequent and usually associated with restenosis or occlusion of the coeliac axis [20]. Angioplasty is probably ineffective but the results of stenting are uncertain.

Most reports consider the coeliac artery compression syndrome to be a true entity but it has been questioned by several authors on the basis of the known excellent collateral circulation to the coeliac axis branches, the vague and variable symptomatology and the frequent angiographic demonstration of coeliac artery compression in normal asymptomatic individuals [23].

Ischaemic colitis

The excellent collateral blood supply of the colon from the SMA via the marginal artery and from the internal iliac arteries via the middle and inferior rectal vessels protects it from the potential effects of inferior mesenteric artery (IMA) occlusion. Such collaterals are adequate in the vast majority of patients, allowing safe routine high ligation of the IMA in most anterior rectal resections and aortic aneurysm repairs.

IMA occlusion in the absence of adequate collaterals causes colonic ischaemia of varying severity. In the worst cases, left colonic necrosis occurs with a high mortality. Lesser degrees of ischaemia cause isolated mucosal damage, resulting in acute left-sided abdominal pain and bloodstained diarrhoea. In some cases, an ischaemic stricture develops over the ensuing weeks leading to large bowel obstruction. The cause of IMA occlusion is usually atheroma but embolisation has also been reported [24].

IMA ligation during aortic surgery may result in colonic ischaemia when the collateral supply is inadequate. In the Swedvasc Registry, postoperative ischaemic colitis occurred in 2.8% after elective aortic surgery and 7.3% after surgery for ruptured aortic aneurysms [25]. Lesser degrees of ischaemia can be detected by colonoscopy in up to 36% of ruptured aneurysms [26]. Systemic hypotension and blood loss are major causative factors. Attempts to identify patients at risk of ischaemic colitis intra-operatively using IMA stump pressures have been disappointing [27]. Nevertheless, some surgeons advise clamping the IMA until the pelvic circulation is re-established and colonic perfusion is adequate before ligating it. This allows IMA re-implantation if the distal colon appears ischaemic. Bilateral internal iliac artery occlusion increases the risk of colonic ischaemia and should be avoided if possible. However, if bilateral internal iliac occlusion is required for endovascular repair of aorto-iliac aneurysms, embolisation is best performed as a two-stage procedure before insertion of the endograft [28].

Right colonic ischaemia is rare and often associated with cardiac disease or chronic renal failure. It is frequently non-occlusive and can be drug-related. Spontaneous rectal ischaemia can occur but is more often a part of generalised pelvic ischaemia, resulting from bilateral internal iliac artery thrombosis or ligation during aorto-iliac surgery.

Diagnosis

The clinical presentation is very variable. *De novo* colonic ischaemia usually presents with bloodstained diarrhoea with variable degrees of left-sided abdominal tenderness, which may progress to generalised rigidity if full-thickness colonic necrosis occurs. With colonic infarction, tachycardia, hypotension, renal failure and eventually multi-organ failure are seen. Sigmoidoscopy or colonoscopy is useful to exclude ulcerative colitis and stool cultures may exclude infective causes. There is usually leucocytosis (often >20,000) and acidosis. Plain abdominal X-ray may show colonic dilatation, thumb printing or intramural gas. If perforation occurs, there may be free intraperitoneal gas. CT with contrast may demonstrate colonic oedema or lack of contrast enhancement of the bowel wall. Angiography and duplex imaging are generally unhelpful. In less acute cases, a barium enema may show thumb printing.

Colonoscopy or flexible sigmoidoscopy may show mucosal necrosis or lesser degrees of inflammation, in which case biopsy may confirm the diagnosis. In the experimental setting, sigmoid pH monitoring detects minor degrees of ischaemia but is not generally useful in clinical practice [29]. Intra-operative Doppler, photoplethysmography or laser Doppler have also been used to assess colonic perfusion [24].

Treatment

In mild cases resolution may be awaited with careful observation, but increasing abdominal tenderness and tachycardia indicate the need for urgent laparotomy. If, on the other hand, the patient improves, a barium enema at 6-8 weeks is wise to detect any developing colonic stricture. More acute cases demand immediate laparotomy and colonic resection (usually left hemicolectomy). Re-anastomosis is unwise and the procedure should be completed with an end colostomy and closure of the rectal stump (Hartmann's procedure). Mortality depends on the stage of the disease but reaches about 50% in patients with colonic infarction.

Key points

- **Acute mesenteric ischaemia has a high mortality and the mainstay of treatment remains bowel resection, although in occasional cases continuing bowel viability allows superior mesenteric embolectomy or bypass. Second-look laparotomy is essential following resection or revascularisation for acute mesenteric ischaemia.**
- **There are no reliable tests for chronic intestinal ischaemia. The diagnosis is based on clinical presentation and the presence of a severe stenosis or occlusion of the superior mesenteric artery, usually in combination with a severe stenosis or occlusion of the coeliac axis.**
- **Percutaneous angioplasty with stenting, if necessary, is effective in non-ostial lesions of the SMA and may help confirm the diagnosis of chronic mesenteric ischaemia, but mesenteric bypass is more durable. Bypass from the infrarenal aorta or iliac arteries is probably the procedure of choice in most fit patients.**
- **The coeliac artery compression syndrome is a controversial entity, but division of the median arcuate ligament or coeliac reconstruction may relieve symptoms of postprandial pain in some patients.**
- **Ischaemic colitis presents with self-limiting bloody diarrhoea or colonic necrosis. It may arise *de novo* or following aortic surgery. The diagnosis is best made by colonoscopy and the treatment of colonic infarction is Hartmann's resection.**

References

1. Acosta S, Ogren M, Sternby NH, *et al.* Incidence of acute thrombo-embolic occlusion of the superior mesenteric artery- - a population-based study. *Eur J Vasc Endovasc Surg* 2004; 27: 145-50.
2. Shukla CJ, Ellis H. Normal and variant anatomy and collateral mesenteric circulation. In: *Diseases of the Visceral Circulation.* Geroulakos G, Cherry KJ, Eds. Arnold, London, 2002. Ch 1: 1-23.
3. Jarvinen O, Laurikka J, Sisto T, *et al.* Atherosclerosis of the visceral arteries. *Vasa* 1996; 24: 9-14.
4. Rius X, Escalante JF, Llaurado MJ, *et al.* Mesenteric infarction. *World J Surg* 1979; 3: 489-93.
5. Rivers S. Acute nonocclusive mesenteric ischaemia. *Semin Vasc Surg* 1990; 3: 172
6. Acosta S, Nilsson TK, Bjorck M. D-dimer testing in patients with suspected acute thromboembolic occlusion of the superior mesenteric artery. *Br J Surg* 2004; 91: 991-4.
7. Krijgsman B, Hamilton G. Acute intestinal ischaemia. In: *Vascular Emergencies.* Branchereau A, Jacobs M, Eds. Blackwell/Futura, New York, 2003. Ch 14: 137-48.
8. Leduc FJ, Pestieau SR, Detry O, *et al.* Acute mesenteric ischaemia: minimally invasive management by combined laparoscopy and percutaneous transluminal angioplasty. *Eur J Surg* 2000; 166: 345-7.
9. Simo G, Echengusia AJ, Camunez F, *et al.* Superior mesenteric arterial embolism: local fibrinolytic treatment with urokinase. *Radiology* 1997; 204: 775-9.
10. Marston A. Acute intestinal failure. In: *Intestinal Ischaemia.* Marston A. Edward Arnold, London, 1977. Ch 5: 70-104.
11. Bulkley GB, Zuidema GD, Hamilton SR, *et al.* Intraoperative determination of small intestinal viability following ischaemic injury: a prospective controlled trial of two adjuvant methods (Doppler and fluorescein) compared with standard clinical judgement. *Ann Surg* 1981; 193: 628-37.
12. Kazmers A. Intestinal ischemia caused by venous thrombosis. In: *Vascular Surgery.* Rutherford RB, Ed. 5th Edition, 2000. Ch 111: 1524-31.
13. Robin P, Gruel Y, Lang M, *et al.* Complete thrombolysis of mesenteric vein occlusion with recombinant tissue-type plasminogen activator. *Lancet* 1988; 1: 1391.
14. Robless P, Belli A, Geroulakos G. Endovascular versus surgical reconstruction for the management of chronic visceral ischaemia: a comparative analysis. In: *Diseases of the Visceral Circulation.* Geroulakos G, Cherry KJ, Eds. Arnold, London, 2002. Ch 10: 108-18.
15. Cherry KJ. Visceral revascularisation for chronic visceral ischemia: transabdominal approach. In: *Diseases of the Visceral Circulation.* Geroulakos G, Cherry KJ, Eds. Arnold, London, 2002. Ch 8: 94-100.
16. Modrall JG, Sadjadi J, Joiner DR, *et al.* Comparison of superficial femoral vein and saphenous vein as conduits for mesenteric arterial bypass. *J Vasc Surg* 2003; 37: 362-6.
17. Park WM, Cherry KJ, Chua HK, *et al.* Current results of open revascularization for chronic mesenteric ischemia: a standard for comparison. *J Vasc Surg* 2002; 35: 853-9.
18. Kazmers A. Operative management of chronic mesenteric ischaemia. *Ann Vasc Surg* 1998; 12: 299-308.
19. Erden A, Yurdakul M, Cumhur T. Marked increase in flow velocities during deep expiration: a duplex Doppler sign of celiac artery compression syndrome. *Cardiovasc Intervent Radiol* 1999; 22: 331-2.
20. Reilly L, Ammar A, Stoney R, *et al.* Late results following operative repair for celiac artery compression syndrome. *J Vasc Surg* 1985; 2: 79-91.
21. Roayaie S, Jossart G, Gitlitz D, *et al.* Laparoscopic release of celiac artery compression syndrome facilitated by laparoscopic ultrasound scanning to confirm restoration of flow. *J Vasc Surg* 2000; 32: 814-7.
22. Takach TJ, Livesay JJ, Reul GJ Jr, *et al.* Celiac compression syndrome: tailored therapy based on intraoperative findings. *J Am Coll Surg* 1996; 183: 606-10.
23. Szilagyi D, Rian R, Elliot J, *et al.* The celiac artery compression syndrome. Does it exist? *Surgery* 1972; 72: 849-63.
24. Stansby G, Thomas HW, Goldin RD. Ischemic colitis. In: *Diseases of the Visceral Circulation.* Geroulakos G, Cherry KJ, Eds. Arnold, London, 2002. Ch 15: 193-296.
25. Bjorck M, Bergqvist D, Troeng T. Incidence and clinical presentation of bowel ischaemia after aortoiliac surgery - 2930 operations from a population-based registry in Sweden. *Eur J Vasc Endovasc Surg* 1996; 12: 139-44.
26. Champagne BJ, Darling RC 3rd, Daneshmand M, *et al.* Outcome of aggressive surveillance colonoscopy in ruptured abdominal aortic aneurysm. *J Vasc Surg* 2004; 39: 792-6.
27. Killen DA, Reed WA, Gorton ME, *et al.* Is routine postaneurysmectomy hemodynamic assessment of the inferior mesenteric artery circulation helpful? *Ann Vasc Surg* 1999; 13: 533-8.
28. Mehta M, Veith FJ, Darling RC, *et al.* Effects of bilateral hypogastric artery interruption during endovascular and open aortoiliac aneurysm repair. *J Vasc Surg* 2004; 40: 698-702.
29. Bjorck M, Lindberg F, Broman G, *et al.* pH monitoring of the sigmoid colon after aortoiliac surgery. A five-year prospective study. *Eur J Vasc Endovasc Surg* 2000; 20: 273-80

Chapter 31

Retroperitoneal lymph node dissection for metastatic germ cell tumours

Jonathan D Beard MB BS BSc ChM FRCS, Consultant Vascular Surgeon
Nandan Haldipur MB BS AFRCSI MRCS Ed., Specialist Registrar, General Surgery
Sheffield Vascular Institute, The Northern General Hospital, Sheffield, UK

Introduction

Testicular carcinoma is one of the most common solid malignancies in men between 15 and 35 years of age. Testicular tumours transform into one of two main histological groups: seminomas and non-seminomatous tumours [1]. These tumours frequently metastasise to the retroperitoneal lymph nodes and lungs. Seminomas are very radiosensitive and therefore radiotherapy is administered to the retroperitoneum in the early stages of the disease. Retroperitoneal lymphadenectomy plays a key role in the management of metastatic testicular teratoma, which is not so radiosensitive.

Traditionally, retroperitoneal lymphadenectomy is an operation performed by a urologist. However, in Sheffield, patients who need retroperitoneal lymphadenectomy for metastatic testicular cancer have been referred to a single vascular surgeon, via the germ cell tumour multidisciplinary team. This chapter reviews an experience and argues that vascular surgeons should take a greater role in the management of this condition.

Patients

A total of 861 patients in South Yorkshire were diagnosed with a germ cell tumour between 1990 and 2004 and were entered into the National Teratoma Database. Fifty of these were referred for retroperitoneal lymph node dissection. The indications for retroperitoneal surgery were: patients with teratoma who had a residual mass of >1cm after chemotherapy or patients with either teratoma or seminoma who relapsed with enlarging masses and rising serum tumour markers after treatment.

Surgical technique

An experienced anaesthetist was involved, since the bleomycin used in the chemotherapy regime can damage the lungs [2]. A low inspired oxygen concentration was used to avoid pneumonitis. During the operation a cell-saver was used routinely, but the salvaged blood was not reinfused unless absolutely necessary because of the theoretical risk of dissemination of tumour cells.

Surgical access was usually via a curved transverse upper abdominal incision, as this can be extended laterally to facilitate nephrectomy, if required, and is covered by a thoracic epidural. The commonest site for metastatic tumour is the left side of the aorta, below the left renal vein, usually involving the origin of the inferior mesenteric artery. Not uncommonly, the tumour extends behind or around

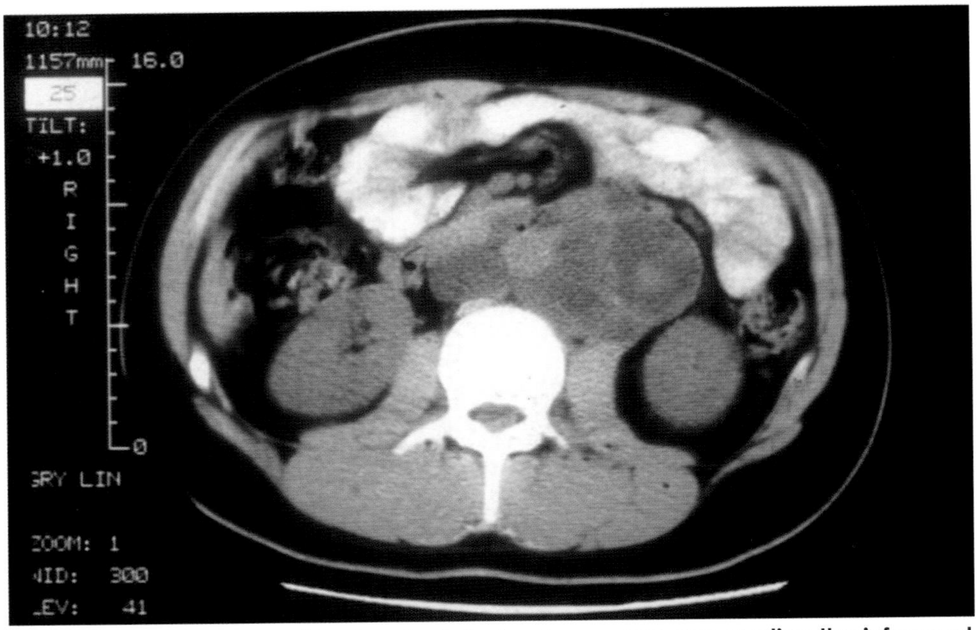

Figure 1. CT of a large residual metastatic teratoma mass surrounding the infrarenal aorta and displacing the IVC forwards. The mass is typically partially cystic and is invading the left psoas muscle.

the aorta and inferior vena cava (IVC), laterally into the renal pelvis and posteriorly into the psoas muscle, often causing back pain (Figure 1).

The inferior mesenteric artery is usually ligated and divided flush with the aorta. There is not a problem with colonic ischaemia in these young patients but retrograde ejaculation, due to damage to the postganglionic sympathetic fibres, is common and patients must be warned about this pre-operatively. The aorta can be mobilised to improve access to a posterior tumour by ligating and dividing the lumbar arteries. The lumbar veins can be ligated and divided in the same way to mobilise the infrarenal IVC (Figure 2). The amount of mobilisation of the great vessels achieved by this manoeuvre is surprising. In the present series, spinal cord ischaemia has never been a problem. The tumour can usually be excised from the great vessels by sharp dissection in the adventitial plane but occasionally, the vena cava and/or aorta may need to be resected *en bloc*, because of tumour involvement; this may contribute to a prolonged tumour-free interval [3]. A small defect in the aorta can be repaired with a piece of the abdominal wall fascia. Resection of the IVC causes some postoperative leg swelling but this can be controlled with compression hosiery. Use of prosthetic material to replace the aorta is best avoided to prevent the risk of infection in these immunocompromised patients. If necessary, the aorta can be reconstructed using a spiral vein graft. The long saphenous vein is harvested, opened longitudinally and sutured in a spiral fashion around a syringe of the same diameter as the aorta (Figure 3). This procedure can take a long time and one patient in the series subsequently required fasciotomies for compartment syndrome.

To prevent the formation of chylous ascites, lymphatics are either ligated with sutures or clips. The ureter can usually be dissected off the tumour mass, but involvement of the renal pelvis usually requires nephrectomy. Posterior invasion into the psoas requires partial resection of the muscle, then oversewing of lumbar arteries and veins once the tumour mass has been removed (Figure 4). Table 1 indicates the number of patients that required additional intra-operative procedures in the authors' series.

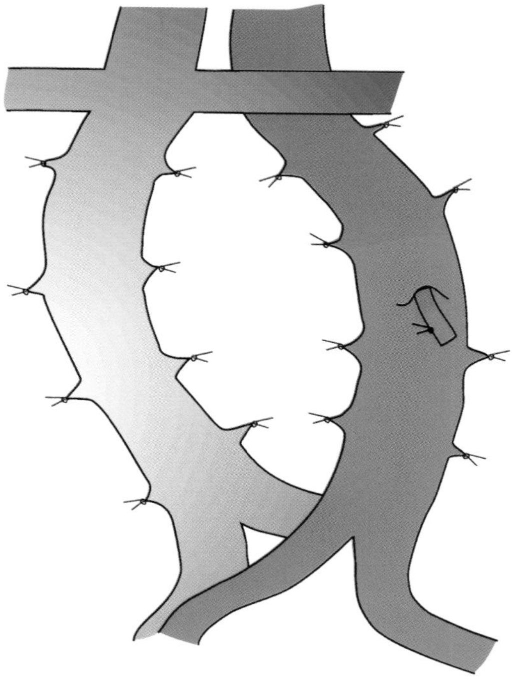

Figure 2. The lumbar arteries and lumbar veins can be ligated and divided to increase the mobility of the infrarenal aorta and IVC, thereby facilitating the dissection of posterior tumours.

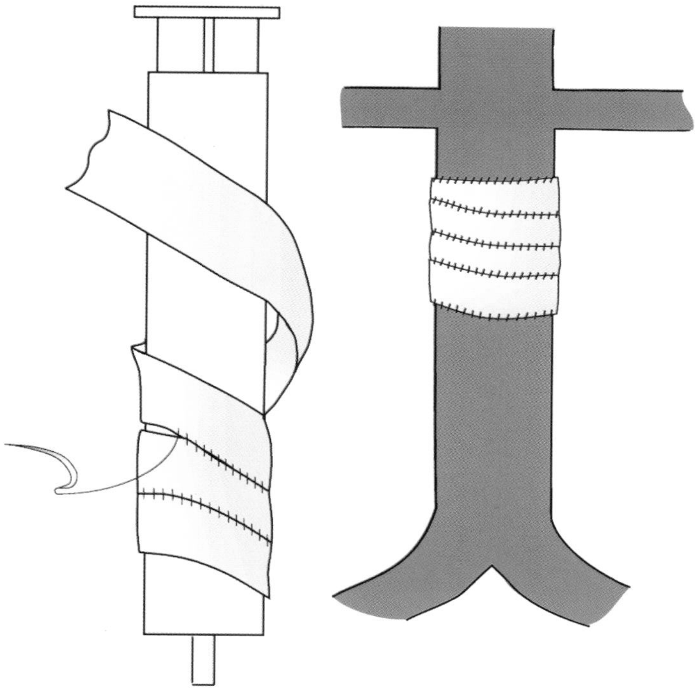

Figure 3. a) The long spahenous vein is opened longitudinally and sutured in a spiral fashion over a syringe of the same diameter as the aorta to form a tube. b) This can then be used to replace the infrarenal aorta.

Outcome

All 50 patients were male with an age range at diagnosis of 16-47 years (median 29 years). All but one patient originally had a teratoma; one had a seminoma. The cancer originated in the testes in 49 men while one germ cell tumour was extragonadal. Histology of the resected specimens showed viable tumour in 32 patients (64%), necrosis/fibrosis only in nine patients (18%), and data were not available in nine patients (18%).

Blood loss ranged from 0-10,500ml (mean 934ml). In this series, 13 patients (27%) had one or more postoperative complications (Table 2). One patient, a Jehovah's Witness, died in the early postoperative period from haemorrhage from the renal bed.

Table 1. Intra-operative procedures.

Procedure	Total (%)
Aortic repair (fascia)	4 (8%)
Aortic replacement (spiral graft)	3 (6%)
IVC resection	3 (6%)
Iliac artery replacement	2 (4%)
Iliac vein resection	2 (4%)
Nephrectomy	7 (14%)
Ureter divided and repaired (over stent)	10 (20%)

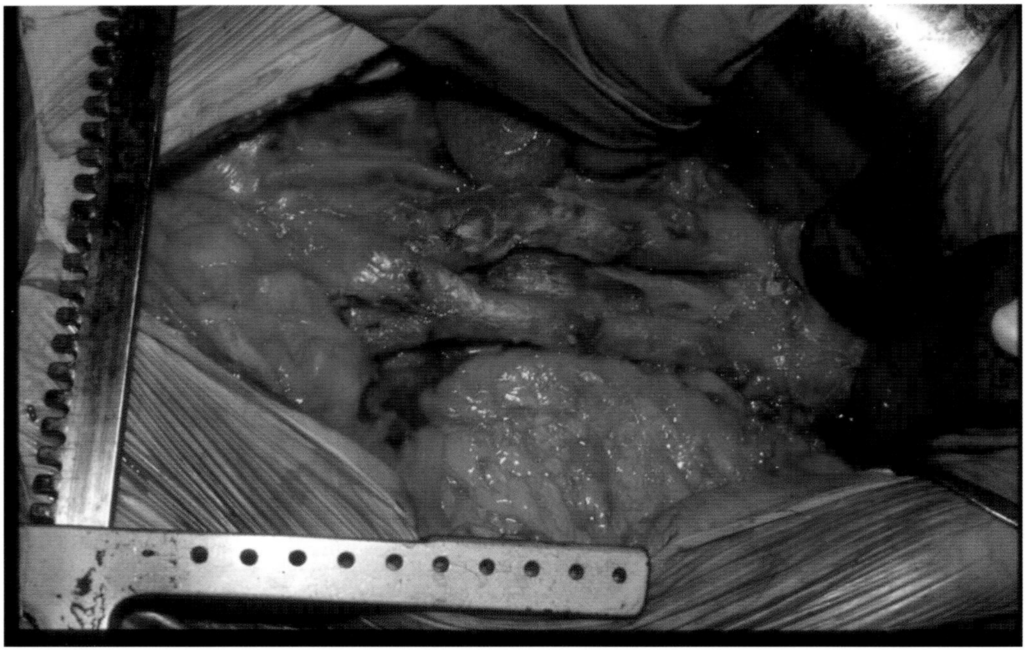

Figure 4. Completed dissection after tumour removal showing skeletonisation of the aorta and IVC. Head end is to the right.

Table 2. Postoperative complications after retroperitoneal tumour resection.

Complication	Total (%)
Postoperative bleeding	2 (4%)
Chest infection	5 (10%)
Pancreatitis	1 (2%)
Prolonged ileus	6 (12%)
Chyloperitoneum	2 (4%)
Pulmonary embolus	1 (2%)
Wound infection	2 (4%)
Compartment syndrome	1 (2%)

Follow-up

At the time of review, the length of follow-up ranged from 3 months to 12 years, median 4 years 11 months. Ten patients died, eight from tumour recurrence and one from septicaemia during chemotherapy; one committed suicide. Of the 40 survivors, seven were well with a residual retroperitoneal mass and the remainder were disease-free at last follow-up.

The role of lymphadenectomy

The role of lymphadenectomy in the management of testicular cancer has changed over the last decade and continues to evolve. There is no consensus on the treatment of early stage teratomas. CT may stage these tumours inadequately. Up to 30% of patients with early stage disease on radiology have involved retroperitoneal lymph nodes at surgery [4]. Therefore, in North America and in some centres in Europe, patients with early testicular teratomas are offered prophylactic retroperitoneal lymph node dissection. Alternatively, these patients may be monitored closely with regular tumour markers and CT. In patients with involved retroperitoneal nodes, studies have shown a clear benefit from retroperitoneal lymphadenectomy. It has been established that this stage disease can be cured by adjuvant retroperitoneal lymphadenectomy [5].

In other reports, a multicentre study of 327 patients undergoing retroperitoneal lymph node dissection revealed a postoperative complication rate of 17% and a mortality rate of 2% [6]. The commonest complications were wound infection and prolonged ileus; major complications included chylous ascites, pulmonary embolism, small bowel obstruction and pancreatitis. The overall complication rate reported in the literature varies between 25-30% [7]. Late recurrence (after 2 years) occurs in 2-5% of patients treated with testicular cancer and the prognosis in these patients is poor [8,9].

Advances in chemotherapy, radiological staging and a multidisciplinary approach have dramatically improved the prognosis for patients with testicular tumours. Surgery in experienced hands carries a low mortality and a good prognosis. Complete tumour clearance can usually be achieved but often involves mobilisation and/or resection and replacement of major vessels. This surgery may best be undertaken by a vascular surgeon, who should be a member of the multidisciplinary team [10].

Key points

- **The successful management of metastatic germ cell tumours requires an experienced surgeon working with a multidisciplinary team.**
- **Metastatic disease is commonly located to the left of the infrarenal aorta and extends around the aorta and IVC.**
- **Division of the inferior mesenteric artery, lumbar arteries and veins permits extensive mobilisation of the aorta and IVC.**
- **Sharp dissection in the adventitial plane is required.**
- **If necessary, the IVC can be resected but the aorta requires replacement with a spiral vein graft.**

References

1. Diekmann KP, Skakkebaek NE. Carcinoma *in situ* of the testis, review of biological and clinical features. *Int J Cancer* 1999; 83: 815-22.
2. Goldiner PL, Schweizer O. The hazards of anesthesia and surgery in bleomycin-treated patients. *Semin Oncol* 1979; 6: 121-4.
3. Spitz A, Wilson TG, Kawachi MH, *et al.* Vena caval resection for bulky metastatic germ cell tumors: an 18-year experience. *J Urol* 1997; 158: 1813-18.
4. Donohue JP, Thornhill JA, Foster RS. Primary retroperitoneal lymph node dissection in clinical stage A nonseminomatous germ cell testes cancer: a review of the Indiana University experience (1965-1989). *Br J Urol* 1993; 71: 326-35.
5. Foster RS, Donohue JP. Retroperitoneal lymph node dissection for the management of clinical stage I nonseminoma. *J Urol* 2000; 163: 1788-92.
6. Heidenreich A, Albers P, Hartmann M, *et al.* Complications of primary nerve-sparing retroperitoneal lymph node dissection for clinical stage I nonseminomatous germ cell tumors of the testis: experience of the German Testicular Cancer Study Group. *J Urol* 2003; 169: 1710-14.
7. Baniel J, Sella A. Complications of retroperitoneal lymph node dissection in testicular cancer: primary and post-chemotherapy. *Semin Surg Oncol* 1999; 17: 263-7.
8. Gerl A, Clemm C, Schmeller N, *et al.* Late relapse of germ cell tumors after cisplatin-based chemotherapy. *Ann Oncol* 1997; 8: 41-7.
9. Baniel J, Foster RS, Einhorn LH, *et al.* Late relapse of clinical stage I testicular cancer. *J Urol* 1995; 154: 1370-2.
10. Christmas TJ, Smith GL, Kooner R. Vascular interventions during post-chemotherapy retroperitoneal lymph-node dissection for metastatic testis cancer. *Eur J Surg Oncol* 1998; 24: 292-7.

Case vignette

Carotid patch infection treated with resection and vein graft replacement

Jonothan J Earnshaw DM FRCS, Consultant Vascular Surgeon, Gloucestershire Royal Hospital, Gloucester, UK

A 56-year-old man underwent block dissection of the left side of his neck followed by radiotherapy for a squamous carcinoma of the tonsil. Six months later he had a palpable lump in the neck which was biopsied by an ENT surgeon under local anaesthetic. The catastrophic haemorrhage that resulted was repaired using a dacron patch to the damaged common carotid artery.

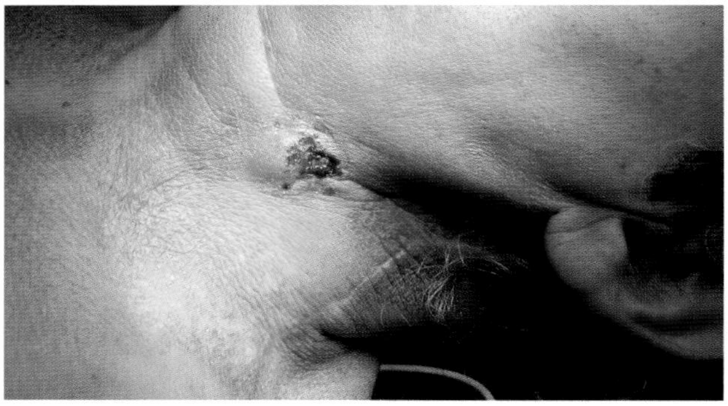

Figure 1.

The wound in irradiated skin failed to heal and two months later he presented with a sinus oozing pus and altered blood with the patch visible at its base (Figure 1). At re-operation under general anaesthetic, it was possible to expose normal common carotid below and internal carotid artery above the patch (Figure 2). After heparinisation and clamping, the carotid was resected and the external carotid artery oversewn. Long saphenous vein previously harvested from the groin was reversed and threaded over a Javid shunt (Figure 3). It was sutured end-to-end to internal and then common carotid arteries with 6/0 Prolene (Figure 4). The defect in the irradiated skin was then repaired with a vascularised flap of pectoralis major muscle and skin (Figure 5). The patient made an uncomplicated early recovery.

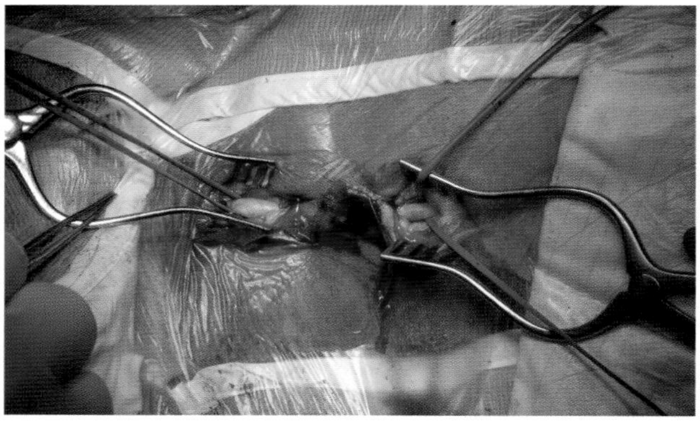

Figure 2.

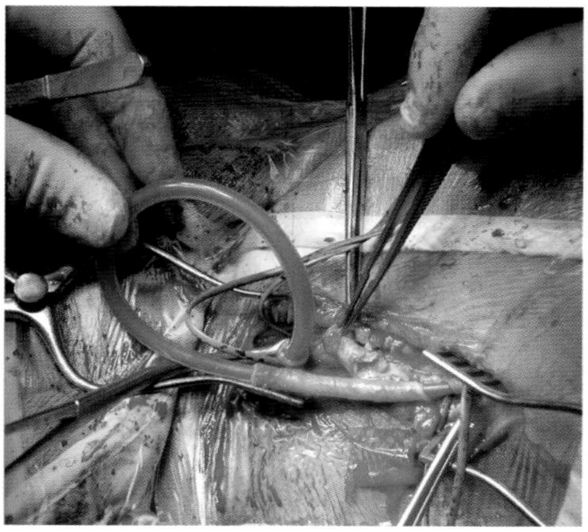

Figure 3.

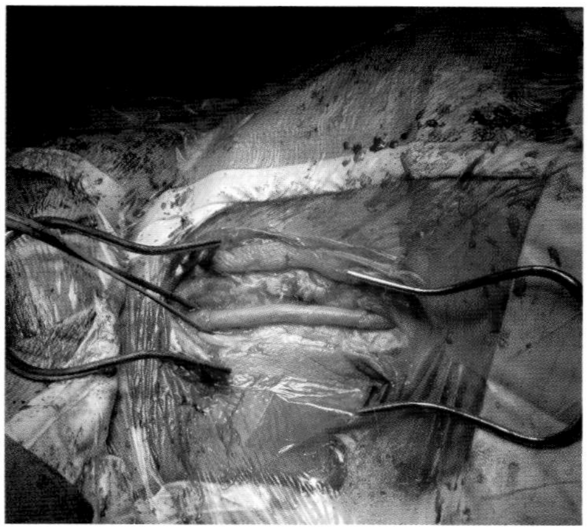

Figure 4.

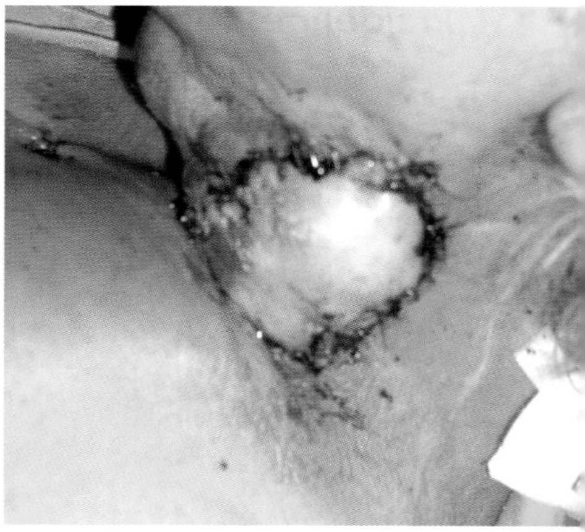

Figure 5.

Chapter 32

Infection following aortic and carotid surgery

A. Ross Naylor MD FRCS, Professor of Vascular Surgery
Leicester Royal Infirmary, Leicester, UK

Introduction

Infection is, justifiably, one of the most feared complications following vascular reconstruction and is associated with considerable morbidity and mortality. Although the principles of management (regardless of the anatomical site) are relatively straightforward: (i) control of haemorrhage, (ii) eradication of infection, (iii) minimise morbidity and mortality and (iv) optimise distal perfusion, these goals can be difficult to meet and largely depend on patient fitness and mode of presentation.

Carotid patch infection

Incidence

Many surgeons employ prosthetic material (PTFE or dacron) as a patch angioplasty to repair the arteriotomy after carotid endarterectomy. There is therefore a potential for patch infection, though only 53 cases have been reported in the world literature. This equates to an overall prevalence of 0.5-1.0%. Accordingly, most surgeons have relatively limited experience of dealing with this type of problem [1-3].

Aetiology

Table 1 summarises the timing of patch infection relative to the original procedure. As with infections elsewhere, there appears to be a biphasic onset. Approximately 40% of infections become evident within 2 months of carotid endarterectomy (CEA) and tend to be associated with virulent micro-organisms (*Staphylococcus aureus*, *Streptococcus*). Many follow a documented early wound complication (infection, haematoma), stressing the importance of prevention[1-3]. The majority of patch infections (almost 60%) present after 6 months and follow infection with less virulent bacteria such as *Staphylococcus epidermidis*. Interestingly, and presumably reflecting the relatively superficial location of the patch to skin and airway, 90% of micro-organisms responsible for carotid patch infection are either *Staphylococci* or *Streptococci*. [1].

Clinical

Table 1 summarises the various modes of presentation for patch infection. Early infections (within 2 months) tend to present with overt sepsis (deep infection, cellulitis, abscess), false aneurysm formation and, rarely, patch rupture. Thereafter,

Table 1. Mode of presentation in 53 patients with prosthetic carotid patch infection.

	Timing of prosthetic patch infection after carotid endarterectomy		
	<2 months	**2-6 months**	**>6 months**
Presentation			
Wound infection/abscess	14	-	4
Patch rupture	2	-	2
False aneurysm	5	3	7
Chronic sinus discharge	-	1	17

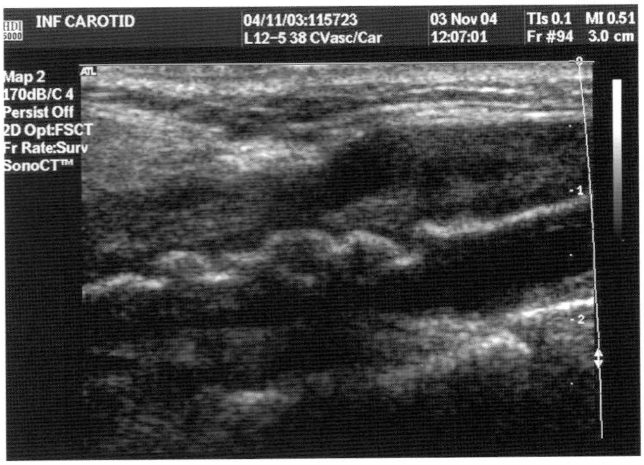

Figure 1. Corrugation of a prosthetic patch on duplex ultrasound. Recognition of this phenomenon may precede diagnosis of patch infection by 6-12 months.

varying combinations of false aneurysm formation and chronic sinus discharge predominate. Late infections (>12 months) almost exclusively present with chronic sinus discharge. Only four patients in the world literature have presented with rupture of a prosthetic patch, (usually in association with methicillin-resistant *Staphylococcus aureus* [MRSA]). This low reported incidence (inevitably an underestimate) is extremely fortunate as the management of catastrophic haemorrhage can be extremely difficult, due mostly to the difficulty in gaining distal control in the emergency situation. Stroke or transient ischaemic attack (TIA) is, however, a surprisingly rare mode of presentation, but does tend to be more prevalent in patients presenting with a false aneurysm[1-3].

The key to management and optimising outcome is early diagnosis. Sometimes this can be quite difficult, but the surgeon should start to be suspicious when the patient complains of persisting deep wound discomfort, particularly if a duplex scan suggests corrugation of the patch (Figure 1). In the Leicester series, patch corrugation (without false aneurysm formation) preceded overt infection by up to 12 months in several patients [4].

Investigation

For patients with acute patch rupture and major haemorrhage, there is no time for investigation and the patient should get to theatre as soon as possible.

For patients (the majority) with a less dramatic presentation, there is scope for work-up and this will have to be tailored individually. There is, currently, no consensus on what constitutes appropriate investigation. Some surgeons advocate varying combinations of CT, angiography and labelled white cell scans but these, in our experience, rarely alter management. Differentiation should be made between investigations undertaken to confirm the diagnosis of patch infection and those that contribute towards planning an operative procedure. In Leicester, greater reliance is placed on duplex imaging to diagnose false aneurysm formation, determine the extent of peri-arterial induration/inflammation and demonstrate the presence/absence of patch corrugation (Figure 1). Duplex can usually inform the surgeon as to distal

Table 2. Management strategies and outcomes in 52 patients with prosthetic carotid patch infection.

	First 30 postoperative days			Post 30-day survivors follow-up	
	no problems	died	stroke	no re-infection	re-infected
Debridement, patch left in situ					
Postoperative antibiotic irrigation (n=1)	1	-	-	1	0
Sternomastoid flap (n=2)	2	-	-	2	0
Abscess drainage alone (n=1)	1	-	-	0	1 (8wks)
Oversew bleeding point (n=1)	1	-	-	1	0
Excision of granulation track (n=1)	1	-	-	0	1 (9wks)
Debridement, patch removal					
Ligation ECA/ICA/CCA (n=4)	3	1	-	3	0
Ligation ECA + CCA (n=2)	2	-	-	2	0
Vein patch insertion (n=19)	19	-	-	18	0
Reversed vein bypass (n=12)	10	-	2	12	0
Dacron patch insertion (n=6)	5	1	-	2	3 (12,12,17mths)
Dacron graft bypass (n=2)	2	-	-	0	2 (2,24mths)
Primary closure (n=1)	1	-	-	1	0

ECA= external carotid artery
ICA=internal carotid artery
CCA=common carotid artery

patency (occlusion is not uncommon with infection). However, if there is any doubt as to the integrity of the distal internal carotid artery, an angiogram or magnetic resonance (MR) study should be performed. It is also immensely helpful to have information regarding the likely organism. The management of an MRSA-infected patch is totally different from one caused by *Staph. epidermidis*.

Before undertaking any operative intervention, it is extremely helpful to review the original operation notes. Key factors to observe include: (i) were any problems encountered with distal access? (ii) if the operation was done under loco-regional anaesthesia, did the patient suffer a focal neurological deficit following test clamping? If yes, this patient will clearly not tolerate carotid ligation and (iii) how high up the carotid artery did the patch extend? A 2cm patch will obviously be easier to treat than a 4cm one and the approach to the distal internal carotid artery will be different. Finally, re-operation is associated with a higher incidence of cranial nerve injury; bilateral recurrent laryngeal nerve palsies can be fatal. If there is any doubt, the vocal cords should be checked pre-operatively.

Management

Table 2 summarises the treatment strategies adopted in 52 patients from the world literature. As can be seen, there is a wide spectrum of therapeutic options ranging from debridement and some form of adjunctive procedure or, more commonly,

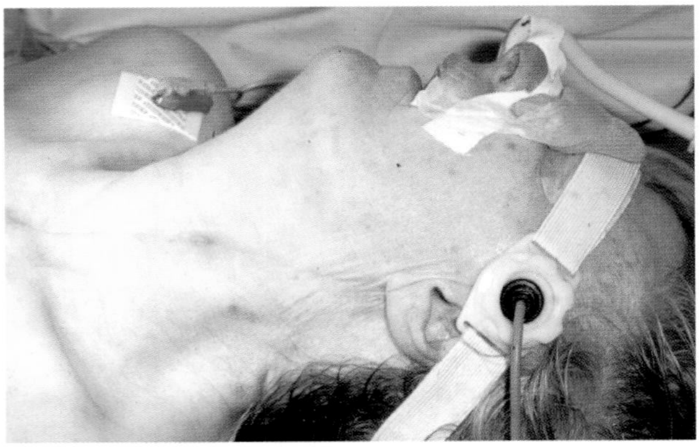

Figure 2. Patient with a discharging abscess in the mid-point of the wound. The clinical appearance looks innocuous but ultrasound (Figure 1) showed extensive inflammatory change extending high into the neck.

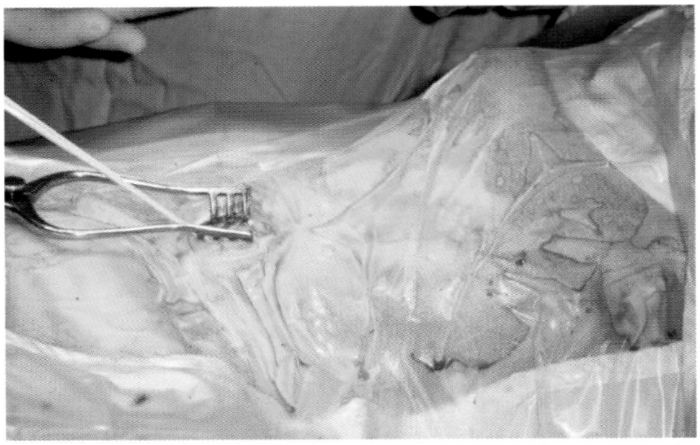

Figure 3. The proximal common carotid artery is controlled well below the original wound.

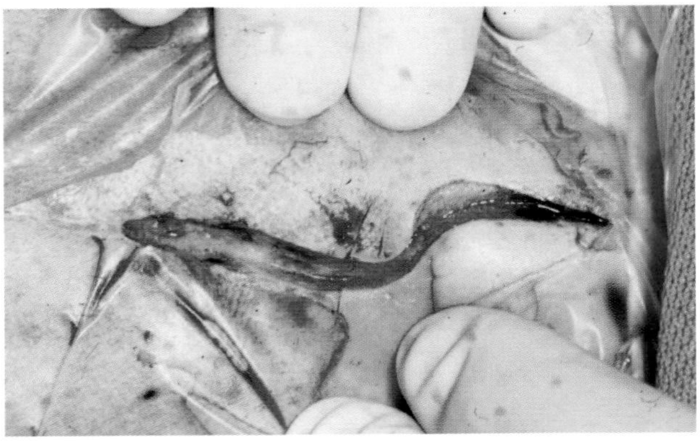

Figure 4. Distal control is secured using an incision that extends anterior to the ear and then swings postero-inferiorly.

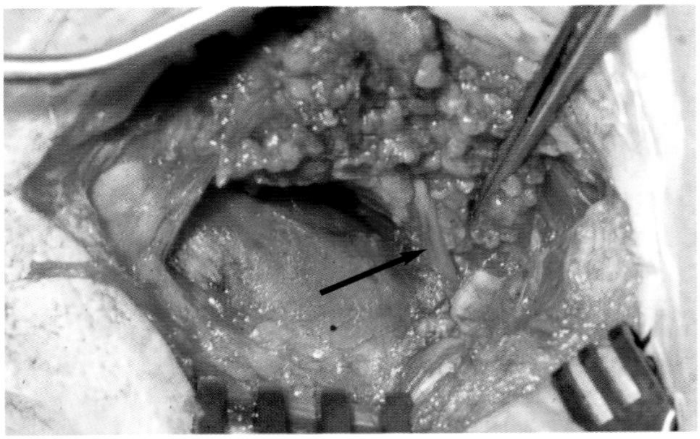

Figure 5. Securing distal control. The parotid gland is mobilised supero-medially and the facial nerve preserved (arrow). No attempt is made to divide the posterior belly of digastric as this can precipitate anastomotic disruption.

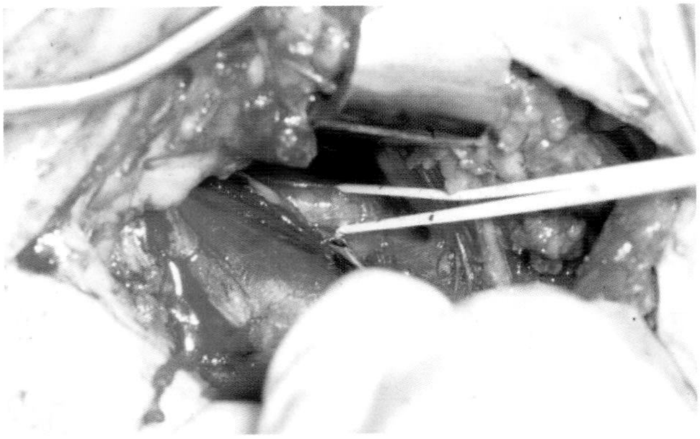

Figure 6. Dissection continues above digastric until the distal internal carotid artery is mobilised and slung.

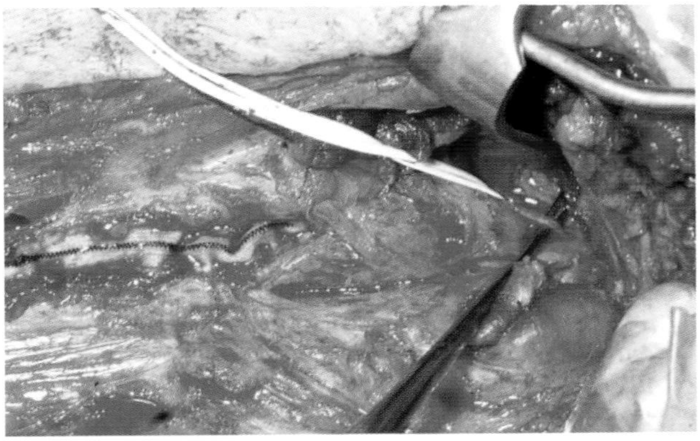

Figure 7. The main wound can now be reopened. The patch usually emerges with little need for dissection. Note the corrugations in the patch (identical to that predicted on ultrasound in Figure 1). The white sling encircles the distal internal carotid artery. The Watson-Cheyne dissector identifies the glossopharyngeal nerve.

debridement followed by patch removal and revascularisation. Table 2 also summarises rates of re-infection.

The actual choice of management will obviously depend on the overall status of the patient. Frail, elderly patients with a "relatively" limited infection can be treated initially with antibiotics or debridement with a muscle flap. Occasionally, it can be difficult to determine the extent of infection. Figure 2 shows a discharging sinus (following spontaneous abscess drainage) four months after CEA. Microbiological cultures from the sinus yielded no growth. However, the duplex scan (Figure 1) showed corrugation and an extensive area of induration and inflammation surrounding the patch, which was directly continuous with the cutaneous sinus. A trial of antibiotic therapy was considered until the ultrasound scan revealed the true extent of the inflammatory/infective process. Microbiological culture was negative, but at surgery a deep-seated collection of pus was encountered yielding MRSA. If a more conservative approach had been adopted in this situation, it is highly likely that the anastomosis would have disrupted.

Once the decision has been taken to operate, the surgeon essentially has a choice between carotid ligation and revascularisation following debridement and patch excision. Carotid ligation should only be considered a "last resort" in the face of uncontrolled haemorrhage, because 50% of patients will suffer a stroke as a consequence. This difficult decision can be made easier if the surgeon knows whether cerebral perfusion was adequate during carotid clamping under locoregional anaesthesia at the original operation. For those surgeons who operate under general anaesthesia, transcranial Doppler can be a useful adjunct and a mean middle cerebral artery velocity >20cm/sec usually means that the patient will tolerate carotid ligation.

The available evidence (Table 2) suggests that revascularisation with autologous vein is the treatment of choice[1-3]. To date, no patient who had autologous revascularisation has developed re-infection and cumulative freedom from operative stroke/death and/or late re-infection is about 92% at 2 years. Revascularisation using prosthetic material should be avoided. Table 2 indicates that 5/6 patients who had prosthetic reconstruction developed re-infection within 24 months.

A few general points may be useful to anyone contemplating re-operation for carotid patch infection. First, this is not the type of operation to be doing unassisted for the first time. If the diagnosis is suspected, seek the input of more experienced colleagues, either locally or regionally. Second, if faced with major haemorrhage in the emergency situation, it is often possible to control this with local pressure whilst seeking assistance or even transfer to a more specialised unit. It is impossible to transfer a bleeding patient once the operation has commenced. Third, ensure that it is a "golden rule" that no one incises an abscess over a carotid wound (no matter how old or innocuous) without a vascular surgeon being present. Fourth, parenteral antibiotics should be started as soon as the diagnosis is suspected. The author's first-line preference is for cefuroxime and metronidazole. If the infection has occurred early, there is a high risk that this may be due to MRSA and it is, therefore, advisable to add vancomycin to the antibiotic regimen. Obviously the antibiotic policy can be revised following microbiological review.

Re-operation

The worst possible problem during re-operation is uncontrolled haemorrhage. Occasionally this cannot be avoided, but steps should be taken to minimise the risks. In Leicester, re-operation for patch infection is a joint procedure between a vascular surgeon and ENT surgeon. The familiarity of the ENT surgeon in dealing with high neck dissections can be invaluable.

The patient is positioned on the operating table as for primary CEA. This operation should not be performed under locoregional anaesthesia. Nasolaryngeal intubation opens up the space between the mandible and mastoid process and so facilitates distal access. The first step is to achieve proximal control through a small incision placed well below the original wound (Figure 3). Second (and more difficult) is distal control. This is best done by an ENT surgeon. The distal incision is made anterior to the ear, which then curves posteriorly below the pinna but not onto the area of induration (Figure 4). The parotid gland is

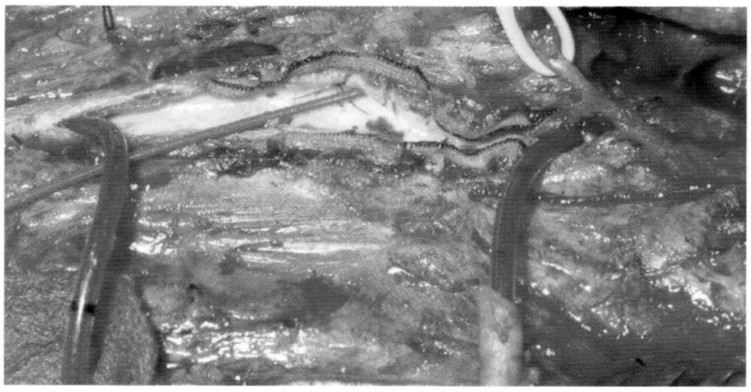

Figure 8. Intra-operative view with the carotid opened and a Pruitt-Inahara shunt inserted. The distal limb of the shunt already has a segment of reversed saphenous vein on it.

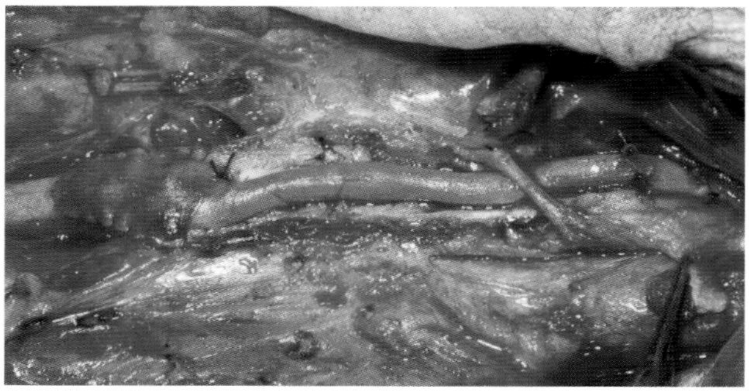

Figure 9. Completed saphenous vein bypass graft. In this case the external carotid artery origin has been oversewn. The distal anastomosis is under the styloid musculature and distal to the glossopharyngeal nerve.

mobilised supero-medially and the facial nerve identified (Figure 5). No attempt is made to divide digastric at this stage as this may cause disruption of the friable anastomosis. Having protected the facial nerve, dissection is then continued above to digastric and the distal internal carotid artery is controlled with a sling (Figure 6).

The main wound can now be reopened in the knowledge that proximal and distal control has been achieved. From this point onwards, any unexpected bleeding can be controlled immediately by clamping followed by insertion of a Pruitt-Inahara shunt or Fogarty balloon catheter. Once the main wound has been reopened, the patch usually exposes itself without much dissection (depending on the extent of infection) and digastric can now be divided to reveal the full extent of the operative field (Figure 7), including the styloid apparatus and glossopharyngeal nerve.

At this point the patient should be systemically heparinised and the vessels cross-clamped. The patch is opened longitudinally (the external carotid artery can be controlled with a Fogarty balloon catheter and three-way tap) and a Pruitt-Inahara shunt is inserted into the upper reaches of the internal carotid artery, having first placed a segment of reversed saphenous vein over the distal limb of the shunt (Figure 8). The advantage of inserting a shunt at this stage is that it prevents bleeding from a disrupted anastomosis during distal mobilisation. These tissues are incredibly friable and, with the shunt in place, distal dissection can continue safely.

The external carotid artery can either be ligated or included in any subsequent vein bypass (Figure 9). The distal venous anastomosis is undertaken first, using a spatulated anastomosis and interrupted 6:0 Prolene sutures. Once the distal anastomosis is completed, the distal shunt balloon can be deflated and the Pruitt shunt retracted to just below the distal anastomosis. If there is any bleeding from the anastomosis it should be dealt with early. Once the proximal anastomosis is completed, it may be impossible to deal with bleeding from the posterior aspect of the distal anastomosis.

Gentamicin-impregnated collagen sponge may be placed around both anastomoses and in those areas subjected to extensive debridement. The wound is then closed in the usual manner. There is no consensus as to whether postoperative antibiotic irrigation is advisable, but it is not usually necessary. If there is any question about the integrity of overlying skin and subcutaneous tissues, then a rotated sternomastoid muscle flap and secondary skin graft should be considered.

Postoperative care

There is no consensus regarding how long antibiotics should be continued. The author's practice is to keep the patient on appropriate systemic and then oral antibiotics for at least 6 weeks postoperatively.

In the early postoperative period, caution must be exercised regarding starting feeding, as these patients are very prone to swallowing difficulties due to a higher incidence of cranial nerve injury than following primary CEA. If there is any question about the integrity of the swallowing reflex, then a formal assessment should be performed. Problems with swallowing are usually transient, but may require a variable period of enteral feeding.

Long term, the prognosis is extremely good provided autologous vein has been used. Patients should be reviewed regularly for up to 5 years. Carotid vein bypass patients should be entered into a graft surveillance programme, as they have a 20% 2-year risk of severe restenosis.

Aortic graft infection

Incidence

Major aortic graft infection complicates about 1-2% of reconstructions for occlusive disease and 2-3% of aortic aneurysm repairs. The incidence increases if there are any groin anastomoses, re-explorations (e.g. for graft thrombosis), a history of seroma formation and in patients undergoing emergency aortic surgery (e.g. for ruptured aneurysm).

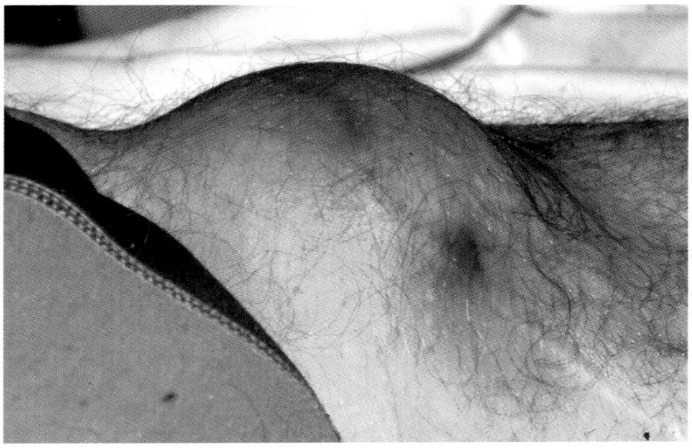

Figure 10. False aneurysm of the anastomosis between the common femoral artery and graft limb of an aortofemoral bypass. This aneurysm appeared within 5 days of discomfort being reported by the patient, 5 years after graft insertion. Note the general redness of the swelling with focal areas of blue-black discolouration. The latter is a warning of impending rupture.

Aetiology

In the 1980s, the principal infecting organisms were *Staphylococcus epidermidis*, *Staphylococcus aureus* and *Streptococcus faecalis* (Enterococcus). By the late 1990s, however, MRSA emerged as the major pathogen in graft infection in the UK and has, undoubtedly, changed the way in which many surgeons approach treatment.

As with carotid patch infection, aortic graft infection has a biphasic mode of presentation. Early infections are almost always seeded at the time of primary surgery and the organisms are usually more virulent. Late infections tend to involve *Staphylococcus epidermidis* or follow the development of graft-enteric or aorto-enteric fistulae. Whilst there is no debate that graft-enteric fistula is a form of aortic graft infection, some feel that aorto-enteric fistulae may be due to mechanical trauma as opposed to true infection. However, in practical terms, this is usually irrelevant. Late infections can also follow haematogenous or lymphatic seeding. This is an important point to remember as relatively few vascular units specifically advise their aortic graft patients to ask for antibiotic prophylaxis should they undergo any invasive procedure (e.g. dental extraction).

Clinical features

Aortic graft infection can present with a wide spectrum of septic or, otherwise, non-specific clinical features, so that the most important factor (for the patient) is the surgeon being suspicious. Early aortic infection tends to present with overt signs of sepsis, including any combination of pyrexia, septicaemia, abscess formation, anaemia, purulent wound discharge or haemorrhage. Late infections tend to have a more insidious presentation, although haemorrhage and false aneurysm formation can still be a major problem (Figure 10). Typical clinical features of late infection include: discomfort, malaise, weight loss, anorexia, anaemia wound sinus formation, pulsatile swellings (Figure 10), septic

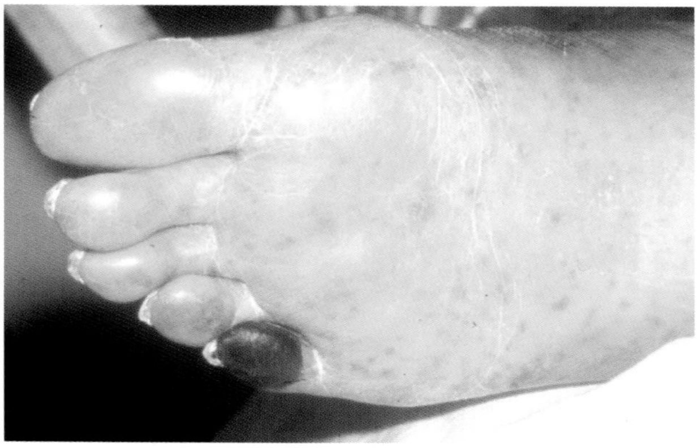

Figure 11. Septic emboli in the skin of the right foot of a patient who had undergone repair of a symptomatic aortic aneurysm 2 years earlier.

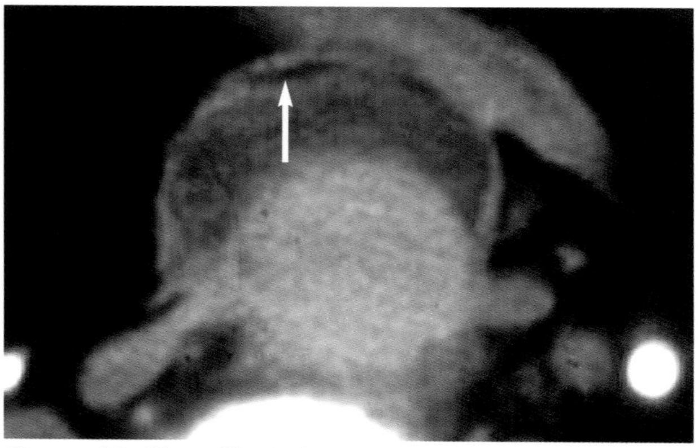

Figure 12. Magnified view of a CT scan in a patient who had undergone elective aortic aneurysm repair 15 months before. He presented with acute upper gastro-intestinal haemorrhage. The bright white structure is the anterior aspect of a lumbar vertebra. The sac surrounds the body of the graft. There is a gas/fluid interface within the sac with close proximity to the overlying bowel (arrow). At operation an aorto-enteric fistula was confirmed.

emboli (Figure 11) and graft thrombosis. The presence of gastro-intestinal haemorrhage in the presence of a known aortic graft should alert the clinician to the likelihood of aorto-enteric fistula until proven otherwise.

Investigation

As with carotid patch infection, the key to investigation and management is awareness. Investigations are, otherwise, dictated by the mode of presentation and severity of onset. Massive gastro-intestinal blood loss is the only reason for not undertaking some form of pre-operative assessment.

Depending upon urgency, the most important investigation remains the CT. CT can identify peri-graft fluid collections, air/fluid interfaces (Figure 12), graft patency and proximity to vital structures (e.g. renal arteries). CT also enables the clinician to obtain guided needle aspirates under aseptic conditions, so that organisms can be cultured and antibiotic sensitivities established early. Supplementary investigations include angiography and labelled white cell scans. Angiography can be invaluable in planning complex reconstructions, especially in the current era of endovascular interventions. Duplex ultrasound imaging is of less importance in this condition. Labelled white cell scanning may be of value in patients in whom a diagnosis of aortic graft infection is suspected, but not certain. A positive scan is strongly supportive of the diagnosis, but a negative scan does not mean that infection is not present.

Management

There are few more challenging problems in vascular surgery than the operative treatment of aortic graft infection. Because the overall incidence is low, most surgeons do not gain significant experience in its management and most published series are immediately historical because they usually span at least a decade of experience.

Previously, total graft excision (TGE) with oversewing of the aortic stump and extra-anatomic bypass was considered the gold-standard treatment, but many now question this assumption. In reality, the gold standard will always be the most appropriate treatment for the individual patient that enshrines the guiding principles of infection eradication, minimising morbidity and mortality, and ensuring distal perfusion. Clearly, the management of a frail, unstable patient with an aorto-enteric fistula will be quite different from

Table 3. Strategies for treating major aortic graft infection.

Antibiotic therapy		
Catheter-guided/open irrigation		
Endovascular "lining" of existing grafts with covered stents		
Placement of coils to occlude bleeding fistulae		
Partial or total graft excision plus:		
	closure of arteriotomies with autologous vein	
	oversew aortic stump with:	
		delayed revascularisation as necessary
		primary amputation
		extra-anatomic bypass
	in situ replacement with:	
		unbonded prosthesis
		rifampicin-bonded prosthesis
		silver coated prosthesis
		cryopreserved allograft
		superficial femoral vein

treating a younger patient with a large intra-abdominal collection.

The principal management strategies available to the surgeon are summarised in Table 3 and their rationales and outcomes are summarised below.

Antibiotic therapy

Antibiotic therapy should be considered standard; however, for some patients it may be decided (after due assessment) that they are too unfit for any other intervention and long-term antibiotic treatment may be recommended. This choice of treatment is clearly palliative, but it may be the most appropriate strategy in highly selected individuals.

Catheter-guided/open irrigation

Irrigation catheters can be inserted into retroperitoneal collections, either under ultrasound/CT guidance or at open surgery. The advantage of the latter is that it also enables debridement of the abscess cavity. For the most part, this treatment strategy is palliative, but may be ideal in an unfit patient in whom the only alternative is major surgery with little prospect of survival. As a rule, microbiologists are not keen on irrigation! Potential irrigants include aqueous iodine and/or appropriate antibiotics. On a practical point, the irrigant should be kept within the cavity for at least 30 minutes before drainage for it to be effective. This is achieved by having an inflow catheter and an outflow drain that can be clamped temporarily.

Endovascular delivery of covered stents

Aortic graft infection is an excellent example of how modern innovations can alter the management of a very difficult problem. As a consequence, some patients with acutely bleeding aorto-enteric fistulae can be stabilised by the insertion of a covered stent across the defect in the aortic anastomosis (usually proximal). This should not be considered a curative strategy, but it can serve as a valuable bridge before performing a more definitive procedure when the patient is more stable. Alternatively, it can function as a palliative intervention in patients considered unfit for major surgery. Covered stents can also be used to treat difficult or inaccessible false aneurysms.

Placement of coils in bleeding fistulae

Having completed major surgery some time previously for aortic graft infection, it is extremely disappointing to find that a small number return with a recurrent aorto-enteric fistula. Most are usually related to fistulation between the oversewn aortic stump and the bowel, despite omentoplasty. This problem is extremely difficult to treat surgically, because there is usually very little residual aorta below the renal arteries. Operative strategies include further attempts at exclusion of the fistula, but for many, it may be necessary to perform an aortorenal bypass so as to achieve safe oversewing of the aortic stump. This is a formidable undertaking in an unstable patient with acute haemorrhage. However, we have recently treated one patient who refused redo open surgery by inserting coils into the fistula via an arterial catheter in the brachial artery. Although this was only a palliative strategy, it did enable him to have 2-3 months of further life.

Partial or total graft excision, *plus*:

This strategy remains the cornerstone for managing aortic graft infection. Partial graft excision (PGE) is generally indicated when investigations or surgical exploration either reveal evidence of only limited infection (e.g. one graft limb), or that the patient is totally unfit to undergo total graft excision (TGE). In the latter situation, PGE is a compromise that promotes survival (initially), but which is accepted to render the patient at greater risk of re-infection in the long term. Following partial excision, revascularisation has traditionally been performed via the extra-anatomic route (e.g. obturator bypass, femoro-femoro crossover, axillofemoral), although an increasing number of surgeons might now consider *in situ* reconstruction using the superficial femoral vein or saphenous vein.

Total aortic graft excison can be a formidable undertaking and is associated with significant morbidity and mortality. It is usually undertaken as a semi-elective procedure unless the patient presents with massive gastro-intestinal blood loss secondary to an aorto-enteric fistula. In the past, the latter type of patient had a limited chance of survival. However, the evolution of endovascular interventions can be of immense help in this difficult situation, for example by positioning an aortic balloon catheter within the aorta at the beginning of the procedure, via the common femoral artery. This can be immediately inflated in the event of severe haemorrhage and is an additional safeguard should the anastomosis fall apart during mobilisation. Surgeons with no access to emergency endovascular interventions can achieve much the same effect by inserting a Foley catheter up the common femoral artery via a cut-down in the groin. The balloon can then be inflated if the patient becomes unstable. It is not as good as a carefully placed aortic balloon catheter, but it may prevent uncontrolled haemorrhage in an otherwise very difficult clinical situation.

The first step is to gain control of the aorta at the level of the diaphragm. Thereafter, TGE can be performed through the traditional transperitoneal approach with mobilisation of the small bowel to the patient's right hand side; this requires the surgeon to dissect through the root of the small bowel mesentery and the inevitable inflammatory mass to gain vascular control. At any point, the anastomosis can disrupt. An alternative strategy is to perform a right medial visceral rotation, as used by transplant surgeons to harvest the right kidney. The rationale is that the surgeon is now operating through virgin tissue planes and the juxtarenal aorta can be exposed relatively easily.

The right colon peritoneal reflection is incised throughout its length and the right colon mobilised medially as for a colectomy. Dissection continues posterior to the duodenum, but superficial to the right kidney. The duodenum and head of pancreas are mobilised superomedially whereupon the common bile duct becomes the principle tethering tissue. The result is full exposure of the IVC, left renal vein and aorta above the inflammatory mass. Despite what is often documented in the operation notes, it is still usually possible to mobilise sufficient infrarenal aorta for either oversewing or *in situ* revascularisation (Figure 13). Once the aorta has been controlled in this way, it is then possible to enter the inflammatory mass directly via the standard approach (if needed), without the fear of uncontrolled haemorrhage.

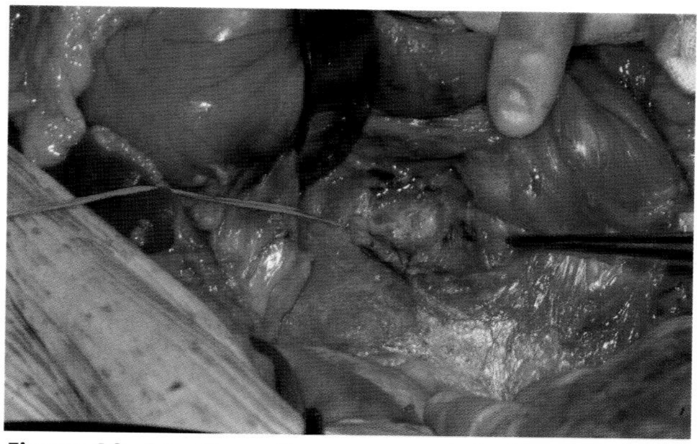

Figure 13. An alternative approach to the juxtarenal aorta in a patient with an infected aortic graft. The surgeon incises the peritoneum overlying the right paracolic gutter and mobilises the right colon, small bowel, duodenum and pancreas to the patient's left. The left renal vein is identified at its junction with the IVC and mobilised superiorly (blue sling). The juxtarenal aorta is then mobilised and can be clamped.

Aortic stump closure and delayed revascularisation as necessary

The standard method for oversewing the aortic stump is to close it in two layers with non-absorbable monofilament sutures, possibly buttressed with pledgets made from the rectus sheath. The aortic stump should then be covered with a vascularised pedicle of omentum (omentoplasty) wherever possible. The remainder of the aortic graft can then be removed in its entirety, followed by debridement of the retroperitoneal tissues.

Occasionally, surgeons prefer to stop at this point on the basis that the patient has already undergone a physiologically stressful procedure and that, sometimes, immediate revascularisation is unnecessary. This may be true if the original procedure was for occlusive disease, but it is less likely to be successful if the original pathology was an aneurysm. The main risk is that the patient can rapidly deteriorate in the early postoperative period due to the sequellae of severe acute limb ischaemia. For the most part, this strategy is not to be recommended unless: (i) the patient's overall condition mandates haemodynamic stabilisation before continuing any further and (ii) the legs are viable at the end of the operation.

Closure of arteriotomies with autologous vein

This strategy is only possible in aortic graft infection patients who have undergone aortobifemoral/iliac bypass for occlusive disease in whom the proximal anastomosis was end-to-side. Selected patients can undergo TGE with closure of the proximal aortic and femoral/iliac anastomoses using autologous vein, provided limb viability is established. In reality this is rarely possible, but it does remain an option.

Oversew aortic stump and primary amputation

For some patients, the only reasonable prospect of survival may be to perform TGE, aortic stump closure and primary amputation with no attempt being made at revascularisation. This is usually done after extensive discussion with the patient pre-operatively, particularly if there is any question of him/her being unable to withstand prolonged surgery. This strategy may also be necessary if the patient presents from the outset with severe limb-threatening ischaemia. The other situation that may merit adopting this approach is where the patient suffers an acute coronary event in the operating theatre and the priority then becomes survival rather than limb salvage.

Oversew aortic stump and extra-anatomic bypass

This, for a long time, has been considered the gold standard. Following aortic closure, the blood supply to the lower limbs is maintained by extra-anatomic bypass (either biaxillo-femoral/popliteal or axillo-bifemoral/popliteal bypass). There has been much debate as to the timing of the graft excision and revascularisation procedures. This ranges from doing the extra-anatomic bypass: (i) 2-3 days before TGE, (ii) immediately before TGE or (iii) immediately after TGE. Surgeons rarely adopt the first strategy nowadays (because of the increased risk of cross-infection of the new graft), but there is no systematic evidence that either of the other two strategies is preferable. However, the theoretical advantage of performing the bypass immediately before TGE is that there is no period of leg ischaemia during the operation. This is the preferred option in Leicester.

The literature contains much conflicting data. However, a review of 688 cases treated by TGE, aortic closure and extra-anatomic bypass and published in the literature between 1990-2004 was undertaken for purposes of this chapter. Overall, the 30-day mortality rate was 20%, the 30-day amputation rate was 10% and the prevalence of aortic stump "blowout" in the early postoperative period was about 5%. Although considerable, these early risks represent a significant reduction on parallel data for 442 patients treated during the period 1965-1989, when the respective figures were 31%, 24% and 15%. One-year survival in the group reported between 1990-2004 was 63%, but 27% of patients suffered graft occlusion at some point in their follow-up and 15% of extra-anatomic bypasses became re-infected. These late risks have not changed at all compared with outcomes published between 1965-1989.

In situ replacement with an unbonded prosthesis

There was a period in the late 1980s and early 1990s when this strategy was common. The reason for its introduction was that it was becoming increasingly recognised that long-term patency rates were much better if the aortic inflow could be reinstated. This approach was, not surprisingly, associated with a higher rate of re-infection and has now been superceded by other *in situ* techniques.

In situ replacement with a rifampicin-bonded prosthesis

In the early 1990s it became apparent that rifampicin bonded well with the gelatin sealant used to coat polyester grafts. From a practical point of view, 600mg of rifampicin is mixed with 10ml of solute, applied to the graft and then left for 15-20 minutes. A number of centres have reported outcomes in patients treated with TGE followed by *in situ* replacement with a rifampicin-bonded graft. The aim was to achieve maximum inflow and better long-term patency and hope that antibiotic bonding of the graft reduced the risks of late re-infection. To date only 45 patients have been treated in this manner and their outcomes reported in the world literature [5]. The 30-day mortality rate was 6.7%, no patient has required early or late amputation and the prevalence of late re-infection was 15%. However, there is a growing consensus that this treatment modality is perhaps not the most appropriate if the underlying organism is MRSA. Unfortunately this cannot always be determined, reliably, before surgery.

In situ replacement with a silver coated prosthesis

Silver is a recognised antibacterial agent and the silver prosthesis is a polyester graft coated with Type I bovine collagen and silver acetate. The rationale is identical to that underpinning the use of a rifampicin-bonded graft for *in situ* replacement following TGE. The silver graft is not licensed for use in the USA, but recent legislation in the UK now allows it to be bonded with rifampicin. Few published series exist, but a prospective registry of 24 patients documented a 16.6% operative mortality rate and no early or late amputations [6]. One-year survival was 85% and the re-infection rate was low (3.7%).

In situ replacement with fresh or cryopreserved allografts

Unlike their counterparts in the UK, vascular surgeons in mainland Europe have access to fresh or cryopreserved allografts and these have emerged as yet another alternative for *in situ* revascularisation after TGE. In Kieffer's extensive series (179 patients), fresh allografts were associated with a high rate of early and late graft-related complications and the Paris group subsequently switched to cryopreserved allografts in 1996 [7]. Several North American and European registries have now published their experience with this strategy. Almost all document 30-day mortality rates of 15-20% and most report a 16-20% incidence of late allograft failure (rupture due to re-infection, fistula formation, thrombosis). Late allograft degeneration remains the main problem with this approach.

In situ replacement with superficial femoral vein

This mode of treatment is gaining increasing prominence around the world, but few surgeons have extensive experience [8-10]. This operative strategy (which takes 5-8 hours depending on whether one or two surgical teams are operating together) is to harvest the superficial femoral veins bilaterally. These are then reconstructed according to the needs of the patient. In most situations, a bifurcated venous conduit is fashioned (Figure 14), with the second commonest strategy being a unilateral aortofemoral bypass with a femoro-femoral extension. This strategy is, however, contra-indicated if the patient has a past history of deep venous thrombosis. From a practical point of view, it is essential to preserve the deep

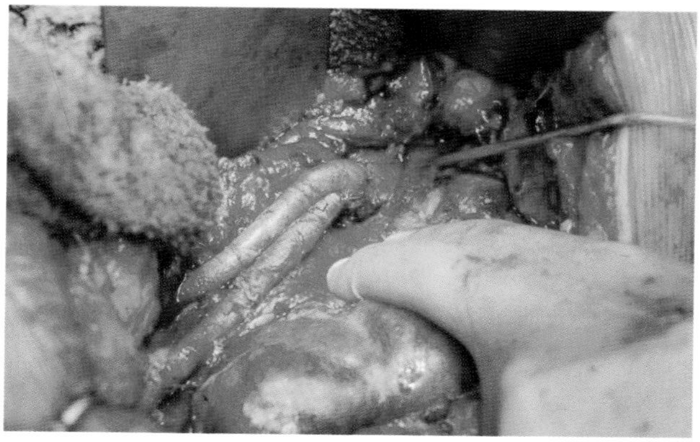

Figure 14. Total aortic graft excision for infection followed by *in situ* replacement using both superficial femoral veins reconstituted as a bifurcated graft. Courtesy of Mr. C Gibbons.

profundal vein or there is a much greater risk of limb swelling and acute compartment syndrome. The risk of the latter is increased if the long saphenous vein is harvested synchronously [8-10].

In view of the length of time taken to perform this type of reconstruction, it is clear that careful patient selection is vital. Most centres advocating this approach exclude patients with aorto-enteric fistulae. This is an important point to consider (when comparing results with other series), because these patients have the worst outcomes whatever operative technique is employed. Notwithstanding this observation, a number of reports have documented lower operative mortality rates (0-10%) and amputation rates (0-5%) One-year survival is typically over 75%, with extremely low rates of late amputation and re-infection. Despite having harvested both superficial femoral veins, remarkably few patients seem to develop leg swelling. Evidence suggests that only 6-10% of patients need to wear compression hosiery long term [8-10].

Summary of treatment strategies

Total graft excision and extra-anatomic bypass has historically been considered the standard against which all other modalities have been compared. One of the major changes in practice over the last decade has been the emergence of *in situ* reconstruction as an alternative, primarily because of the higher flow rates and the very low incidence of late graft failure and re-infection. The choice of management strategy must always be tailored to the individual patient. Although TGE and *in situ* replacement with superficial femoral vein might be viewed (by some) as being the new gold standard, many sick patients (especially those with an aorto-enteric fistula) will simply be too unfit to be treated by a procedure lasting 5-8 hours. Finally, the reader is advised to be cautious in making uncritical comparisons between published series. Remember that the worst outcomes are always seen in patients undergoing emergency surgery, particularly for aorto-enteric fistulae.

Key points

- Graft infection is the diagnosis that no-one wants to make.
- The treatment of graft infection is formidable; teamwork is the cornerstone to good practice.
- Never incise an abscess over a carotid wound without a vascular surgeon being present.
- There are a variety of endovascular innovations that can save lives in an emergency situation.
- Sometimes a bridging procedure may enable an unfit patient to undergo definitive surgery at a later date.
- There is no such thing as a gold standard for aortic graft infection. Management strategies need to be tailored to individual patients.
- Published results in the world literature are as good as they get. In the real world, early and late risks are inevitably much worse.

References

1. Naylor AR, Payne D, Thompson MM, *et al.* Prosthetic patch infection after carotid endarterectomy. *Eur J Vasc Endovasc Surg* 2002; 23: 11-6.
2. Rizzo A, Hertzer NR, O'Hara PJ, Krajewski LP, Beven EG. Dacron carotid patch infection: a report of eight cases. *J Vasc Surg* 2000; 32: 602-6.
3. Rockman C, Su WT, Domenig C, *et al.* Postoperative infection associated with polyester patch angioplasty after carotid endarterectomy. *J Vasc Surg* 2003; 38: 251-6.
4. Lazaris A, Sayers RD, Thompson MM, *et al.* Patch corrugation on duplex ultrasonography may be an early warning of prosthetic patch infection. *Eur J Vasc Endovasc Surg* 2005; 29: 91-2.
5. Naylor AR. Limitations in the use of rifampicin-gelatin grafts against virulent organisms. *J Vasc Surg* 2002; 35: 823-4.
6. Batt M, Magne J-L, Alric P, *et al. In situ* revascularisation with silver-coated polyester grafts to treat aortic infection: early and midterm results. *J Vasc Surg* 2003; 38: 983-9.
7. Kieffer E, Gomes D, Chiche L, *et al.* Allograft replacement for infra-renal aortic graft infection: early and late results in 179 patients. *J Vasc Surg* 2004; 39: 1009-17.
8. Gibbons CP, Ferguson CJ, Fligelstone L, *et al.* Experience with femoro-popliteal vein as a conduit for vascular reconstruction in infected fields. *Eur J Vasc Endovasc Surg* 2003; 25: 424-31.
9. Clagett GP, Valentine RJ, Hagino RT. Autogenous aorto-iliac/femoral reconstruction from superficial femoral-popliteal veins: feasibility and durability *J Vasc Surg* 1997; 25: 255-70.
10. Daenens K, Fourneau I, Nevelsteen A. Ten-year experience in autogenous reconstruction with the femoral vein in the treatment of aortofemoral prosthetic infection. *Eur J Vasc Endovasc Surg* 2003; 25: 40-245.

Case vignette

Aspergillus niger infection in aortic aneurysm

Frank CT Smith BSc MD FRCS FRCS (Ed) FRCS (Glas), Consultant Senior Lecturer, Bristol Royal Infirmary, UK

A 78-year-old lady underwent repair of a saccular 7cm aortic aneurysm (Figure 1). She had been taking 4mg of prednisolone daily for 1 year, for unconfirmed diagnosis of temporal arteritis. Chest X-ray revealed a few small dense nodules in the left lung apex with the appearance of inactive tubercle. Routine microscopy of aneurysm thrombus revealed dense infestation with *Aspergillus niger* (Figure 2). Postoperatively, she was treated with prolonged antifungal therapy with careful monitoring of hepatic and renal function and had no further complications at 1 year.

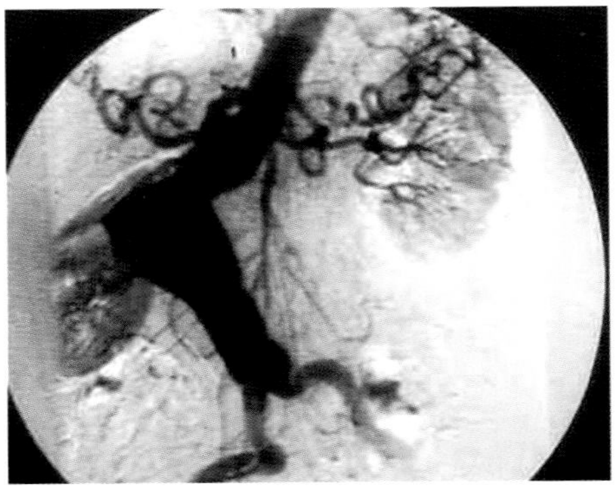

Figure 1.

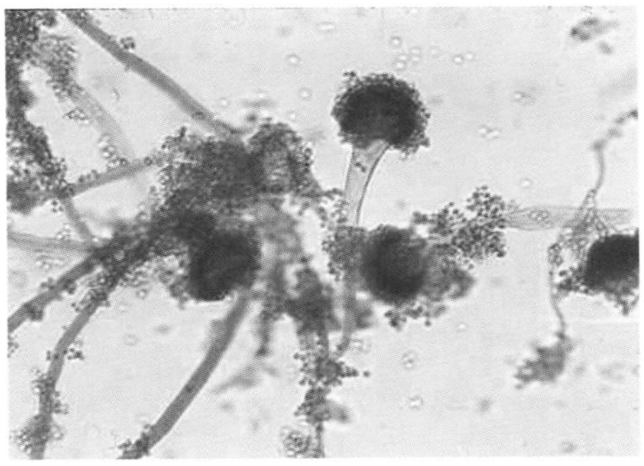

Figure 2.

Chapter 33

Mycotic aneurysms

Ravul Jindal MS DNB FRCS, Senior Registrar, Vascular Surgery
Michael Jenkins BSc MS FRCS, Consultant Vascular Surgeon
St. Mary's Hospital, London, UK

Introduction

Mycotic aneurysms are different from other aneurysms as they affect arteries in variable locations, require individual treatment and have a poorer outcome. They provide a diagnostic and therapeutic challenge and are associated with mortality rates of 16-75%, with morbidity rates as high as 60% [1].

History

One of the earliest reports of arterial infection was described by Ambroise Paré in the 16th Century, when he described a patient who ruptured a syphilitic aneurysm of the descending thoracic aorta [2]. Although the association between bacterial endocarditis and distal arterial disruption had already been noted by Koch, Osler was the first to use the term mycotic aneurysm in his Gulstonian lectures of 1884. He used this term to describe multiple aneurysms of the thoracic aorta laden with vegetations in a 30-year-old man with bacterial endocarditis. However, the term mycotic aneurysm is a misnomer, since a true fungal aetiology is rare [3].

Definition

Primary arterial infection is a condition in which infectious agents invade and destroy the wall of an artery, irrespective of its pre-existing state, resulting in disruption and pseudo-aneurysm formation. Typically, but not necessarily, the native artery contains atherosclerotic plaque or intimal damage; normal arteries are thought to be resistant to bacteraemia. Osler initially introduced the term mycotic aneurysm to signify infected aneurysms found in association with bacterial endocarditis. Currently, the term has come to imply an infected aneurysm of any type. Crane further classified primary mycotic aneurysm to denote an infective aneurysm not associated with endocarditis or infective focus, and secondary mycotic aneurysm where an aneurysm is secondary to endocarditis.

Pathogenesis

Although there are different mechanisms, the source of infection is either intravascular or extravascular.

Intravascular

- Septic embolisation - can be from any source, especially infective endocarditis. Septic emboli from valvular vegetations lodge within the lumen or arterial wall and result in suppuration and aneurysm formation. This can occur in normal and abnormal (atherosclerotic or aneurysmal) arteries. In the pre-antibiotic era, approximately 90% of all mycotic aneurysms were the result of septic emboli from endocarditis.
- Microbial arteritis - during a bacteraemia, blood in a normal or atherosclerotic artery allows infective material to lodge in the vasa vasorum.
- Infection of a pre-existing aneurysm - these aneurysms are mostly atherosclerotic and become infected by haematogenous spread, where bacteria settle within the intramural thrombus.

Extravascular

- After arterial puncture - injecting drug use, radiological procedures, trauma.
- Contiguous spread - from infected lymph nodes, osteomyelitis, abscesses.

If the destruction of the arterial wall by bacteria is gradual and accompanied by a vigorous inflammatory response, the arterial infection will result in pseudo-aneurysm formation. If the process is rapid, loss of arterial integrity can lead to rupture with arterial haemorrhage. Small vegetations can embolise to distal vessels, resulting in cutaneous necrosis or digital petechiae, whereas large septic emboli tend to lodge at arterial bifurcations and result in a mycotic pseudo-aneurysm.

Once established, the natural course of a mycotic aneurysm is to enlarge and eventually rupture in most cases. Occasionally, spontaneous thrombosis may occur with resolution of the septic process. However, the thrombosed aneurysm may serve as a continuing septic focus and emboli can arise from it resulting in miliary abscesses and septic arthritis.

Pathology

There has been a change in the bacteriology of mycotic aneurysms since the original description in the 1800s. The main reasons are the declining incidence of rheumatic fever (and thus infective endocarditis), a significant decrease in the prevalence of syphilis and more widespread antibiotic use. Moreover, iatrogenic and traumatic causes tend to involve different organisms. Syphilitic infection is now rare and occurs due to Treponema invasion of the vasa vasorum. It tends to involve the ascending aorta and results in aneurysmal dilatation. Fungal infections are rare and mainly occur in immunosuppressed patients. Most common fungal species are *Histoplasma capsulatum*, *Aspergillus* and *Candida*.

When bacterial endocarditis is the source, *Streptococcus* (*viridans* and *faecalis*), *Pneumococcus*, *Haemophilus* and *Staphylococcus* (*aureus* and *epidermidis*) prevail.

In non-endocarditis bacteraemia, Salmonella is the commonest pathogen isolated and, in some series, is reported to be present in up to 50% of aneurysms. The most virulent species, *Salmonella choleraesuis* and *Salmonella typhimurium*, account for over 60% of the reported cases of Salmonella arteritis. Other organisms commonly isolated are *Streptococcus*, *Bacteroides*, *Escherichia coli* and *Staphylococcus aureus*. Infection of an existing atherosclerotic plaque is the principal factor in the pathogenesis of microbial arteritis and it is therefore not surprising that the aorta is a common site.

In injecting drug users, a predominance of gram-positive bacteria such as *Staphylococcus* and *Streptococcus* are isolated, but occasionally, gram-negative species such as *E. coli* and *Pseudomonas* are seen. Staphylococcal species are usually associated with infected false aneurysms secondary to trauma.

Characterisation of the different bacteria is important, since gram-negative sepsis results in higher rupture rates than infection with gram-positive bacteria.

Anatomical location

Mycotic aneurysms secondary to septic emboli usually involve the large muscular and elastic arteries. They occur in virtually every named artery intracranially, in the great vessels, the thoraco-abdominal aorta, and the visceral, extremity, pulmonary and coronary arteries. The aorta is the most common site (Figure 1), due to the higher incidence of underlying atherosclerotic plaques and aneurysms, and also possibly due to relatively larger vasa vasorum where infected emboli may lodge.

Arterial infection as a result of drug misuse, trauma or vascular access involves arteries that are easily accessible and have minimal soft tissue coverage. The most common sites are femoral and brachial arteries.

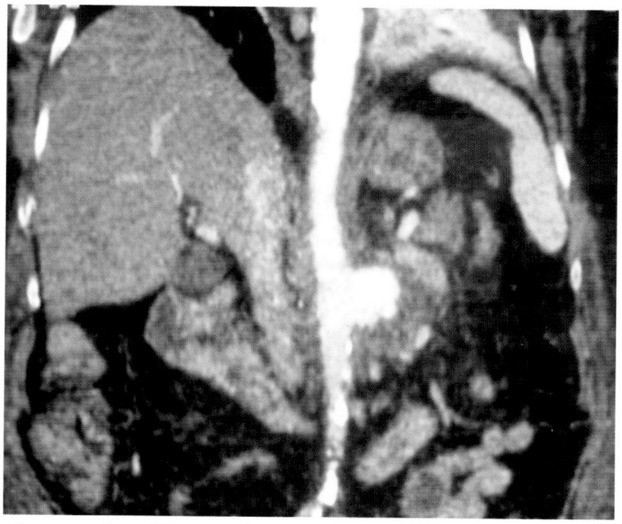

Figure 1. CT angiogram showing a mycotic aneurysm of the infrarenal aorta.

Clinical presentation

Patients present with a wide range of signs and symptoms depending on the pathophysiology, bacteriology and location of the involved artery. Typically the patient is febrile. Localised tenderness is the most readily recognised sign related to the inflammatory destruction of the arterial wall. As many as 40% of infected abdominal aortic aneurysms may not be palpable and go unrecognised until they rupture. Patients may also present with compression of surrounding structures and distal embolic phenomena: petechial skin lesions and septic arthritis are not uncommon. Presentation with a free rupture of a mycotic aneurysm involving a large artery is almost invariably fatal, and the diagnosis is usually made at post mortem.

Diagnosis

An astute surgeon should have a high index of suspicion on clinical history and examination sufficient to make an early diagnosis and to request appropriate investigations. The diagnosis should be suspected in a patient who presents unwell 2 weeks after Salmonella bacteraemia. Most patients have some combination of fever, malaise, weight loss, chills, night sweats, pain, leukocytosis, positive blood cultures and/or elevated inflammatory markers. Leukocytosis is a sensitive, but non-specific indicator of an infected aneurysm. The mainstays of investigation are radiological localisation and microbiological isolation.

Bacteria may be detected either by blood or tissue culture. There is a high incidence of negative blood cultures; in reported series only 50-60% of patients have positive pre-operative blood cultures [4]. Blood cultures may not detect the organism for several days or weeks, limiting their influence on clinical management. Asymptomatic patients, without evidence of sepsis, not surprisingly tend to have fewer positive blood cultures. In most cases, empirical antibiotic therapy has been commenced rendering microbiological analysis more difficult.

In the presence of negative venous blood cultures, downstream arterial puncture can sometimes yield a positive result. Intra-operative tissue culture is extremely important to guide further antibiotic treatment and long-term prophylaxis. In relatively asymptomatic patients (where blood cultures are often negative), tissue cultures are far more likely to result in an organism being detected. Intra-operative frozen section has been used to look for histological evidence of bacterial invasion where pre-operative antibiotic use has rendered cultures futile. Aneurysm wall cultures are most likely to produce a result and have been reported to be positive in 80-90% in some series [5].

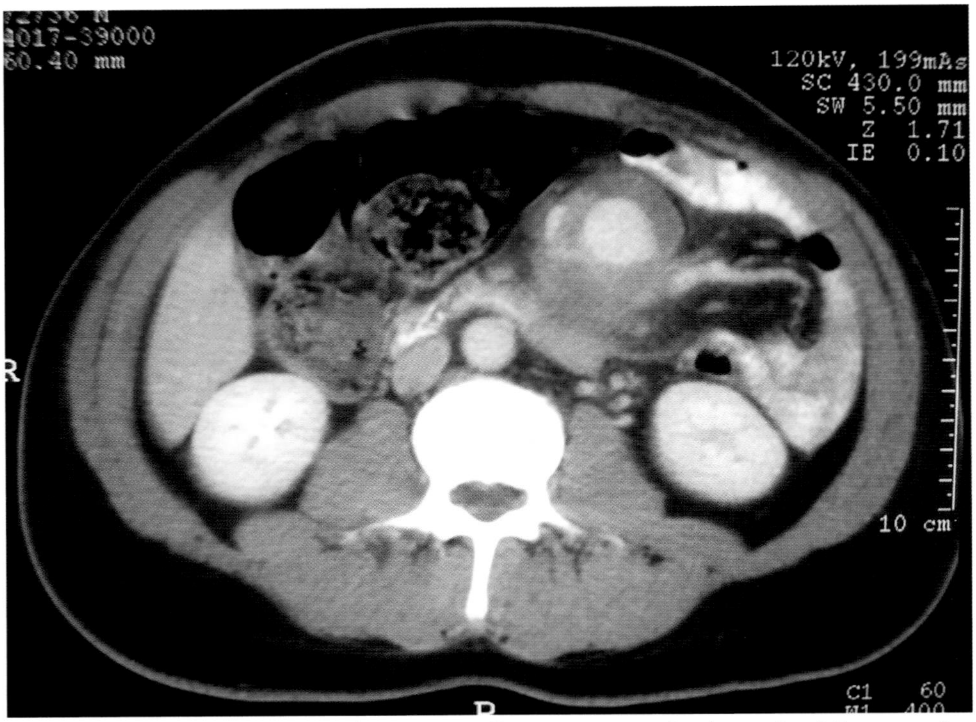

Figure 2. Abdominal CT showing a mycotic aneurysm of a branch of the superior mesenteric artery with surrounding infammation and oedema.

Radiology

Radiolabelled white cell imaging

This investigation takes advantage of the migration of defence cells to the site of inflammation. Correlation with CT findings allows organ localisation and facilitates the diagnosis of infected aneurysms.

Duplex imaging

This has the advantage of being non-invasive, but it can be painful in a tender peripheral aneurysm. It will reveal the presence of an aneurysm, but information regarding infection will depend on the technologist's experience.

CT and MRI scanning

Both CT and MRI are effective. The diagnostic features suggesting that the aneurysm is mycotic include saccular shape, tissue oedema and the presence of gas in peri-arterial tissue (Figure 2). MRI may have some advantages over CT, with better resolution, use of non-nephrotoxic contrast agents and better detection of tissue oedema.

Angiography

Angiography may be useful to define both the inflow and run-off anatomy when arterial reconstruction is planned. Good quality computer reconstructions following CT and MRI may soon make diagnostic angiography obsolete.

Treatment

The fundamental aspects of treatment are control of sepsis and establishment of arterial continuity.

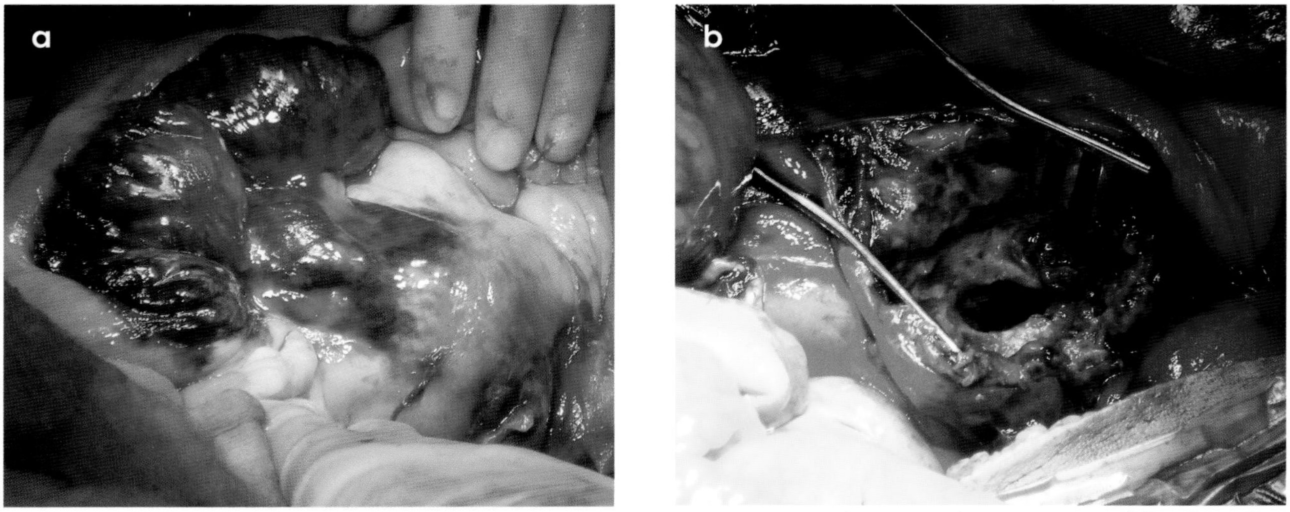

Figure 3. Intra-operative photograph of the same patient as in Figure 2. a) A mycotic aneurysm arising from the superior mesenteric artery. b) After debridement and ligation.

Control of sepsis

Antibiotics

After taking adequate blood cultures, all patients should be started on pre-operative broad-spectrum antibiotics. Antibiotics must be continued until the source of bacteraemia is removed. The duration of antibiotic treatment is controversial. Most clinicians recommend intravenous antibiotics for 6 weeks and oral antibiotics for another 6 weeks, depending on the contamination and cultures. The antibiotics can be discontinued provided there is no clinical, haematological or radiological evidence of ongoing sepsis. Some authors believe that patients with a prosthetic reconstruction should continue on low-dose antibiotics for life.

Debridement

All infected arterial tissue must be debrided up to the point where the arterial tissue is healthy. This helps to prevent subsequent recurrence of infection and disruption of the arterial suture line. Soft tissue adjacent to the infected artery should also be debrided. After debridement the whole area should be irrigated with antibiotic solution and normal saline.

Establishment of arterial continuity

The principles of surgery for mycotic aneurysm include: control of haemorrhage, debridement of infected tissue and arterial reconstruction to allow adequate distal perfusion. The methods available depend on the anatomical location and the effectiveness of any collateral circulation.

Surgical options include extra-anatomic bypass followed by aneurysm resection, aneurysm resection followed by extra-anatomic bypass (if required), aneurysm resection alone or aneurysm resection with *in situ* reconstruction.

Excision and debridement alone

When the collateral circulation is good, excision followed by proximal and distal ligation without reconstruction is the treatment of choice (Figure 3). Monofilament (rather than braided) sutures should be used for ligation because of lower risk of recurrent infection. If possible, the ligated arterial stump should be covered with healthy tissue. In the abdomen, omentum or prevertebral fascia may be used; in the periphery a muscle can be transposed. Sartorius is particularly useful in the groin.

Arterial reconstruction

The virulence of the organism and the severity and extent of the arterial infection are more important determinants than strict adherence to any single operative approach or method of arterial reconstruction. When there is gross contamination within the abdomen from a mycotic aortic aneurysm, excision and extra-anatomic bypass is the treatment of choice, athough this has a mortality rate ranging from 36-48% [1]. In addition, limb loss and late arterial stump dehiscence are not uncommon. Ideally, the reconstruction (e.g. axillobifemoral graft) should be performed before the infected cavity is approached and all wounds pertaining to the reconstruction carefully protected. When contamination is less severe, the aorta may be replaced *in situ*. In certain areas such as the aortic arch, thoracic and suprarenal aorta, this is the only feasible method of reconstruction. Arthur Blackmore in 1947 first employed a Vitallium tube to replace an infected artery. There are various types of *in situ* repair described: cryopreserved human arterial or venous allografts, arterial or venous homografts, prosthetic grafts, and animal xenografts. However, the published data are derived from series with a small number of patients and a large number of variables.

Synthetic grafts

Review of the literature shows rather poor results from direct replacement of mycotic aneurysms with prosthetic grafts. There is an approximately 25% early mortality and a similar incidence of aortic septic complications and vascular re-interventions. Moreover, *in situ* reconstruction with a prosthetic graft is associated with a 16-20% risk of recurrent infection, requiring late extra-anatomic reconstruction [6]. In order to improve these results, gelatin-coated dacron grafts have been soaked in rifampicin, or used in conjunction with application of gentamicin-releasing carriers. Neither of these antibiotic treatments is definitely effective, but they are employed by many surgeons [7].

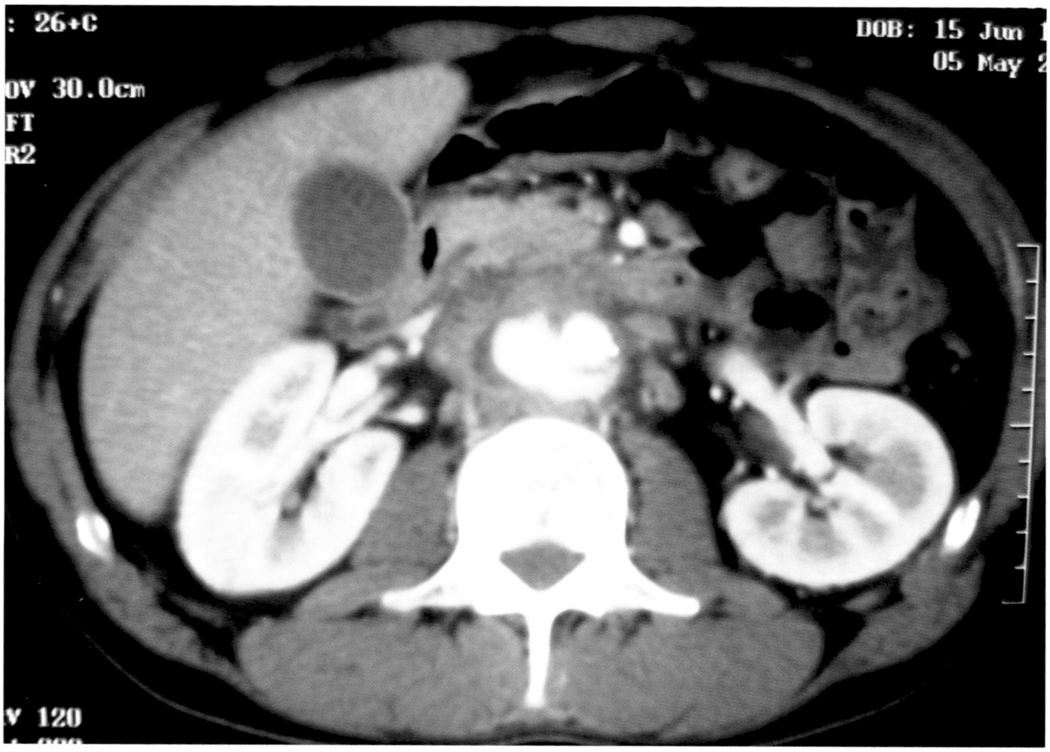

Figure 4. CT showing a saccular mycotic aneurysm of the aorta in a young patient that was treated by excision and *in situ* replacement with superficial femoral vein.

Autologous tissue

Vein grafts tend to be superior to synthetic grafts as they are more resistant to infection. Claggett *et al* reported the use of autogenous superficial femoropopliteal veins as a conduit for *in situ* reconstruction of infected aortic aneurysms (Figure 4). Their 5-year primary and secondary patency rates were 83% and 100%, respectively, with excellent limb salvage and minimal long-term lower extremity venous congestion [8]. They have reported peri-operative mortality rates similar to prosthetic graft repair with low amputation rates and recurrent infection. Size match between the superficial femoral vein and the aorta is good and there is no aneurysmal degeneration in the short and mid term. If the profunda vein is preserved, long-term limb swelling is not as marked as might have been predicted [9].

Allografts

There are various reports in the literature showing good short-term and mid-term results for reconstruction with cryopreserved arterial allografts [10]. The allografts may be more resistant to infection because they allow transfer of antibiotics and immunocompetent cells across the wall and also into the perigraft space. However, limited availability, high cost, lack of data on long-term storage, allograft quality and performance limit the widespread use of such grafts.

Endovascular treatment

Recently, use of endovascular stent graft and composite stent-autologous vein graft combinations have been reported with good short-term results. Long-term data are not available [11]. This treatment may have a role in treating patients who are surgically unwell and where open surgery has high morbidity and mortality, particularly for mycotic aneurysm of the thoracic aorta. There is a significant risk of re-infection if the mycotic aneurysm is not excised, and long-term antibiotic treatment is recommended. Vein-covered stents have proved to be non-thrombogenic with minimal intimal hyperplasia and a lower re-infection rate.

Key points

- Mycotic aneurysms have high mortality and morbidity rates.
- The aorta is a common site due to the presence of atherosclerosis there.
- A high index of suspicion is required for early diagnosis.
- Surgical options should be tailored to individual patients.
- New interventions such as *in situ* replacement with antibiotic-impregnated grafts and endovascular stenting remain unproven in the long term.

References

1. Patetsios PP, Shutze W, Holden B, *et al.* Repair of a mycotic aneurysm of the infrarenal aorta in a patient with HIV, using a Palmaz stent and autologous femoral vein graft. *Ann Vasc Surg* 2002; 16: 521-3.
2. Pare A. Of aneurismas. In: *The Apologie and Treatise of Ambroise Pare. Containing the Voyages Made into Divers Places with many of his Writings upon surgery.* The Classics of Medicine Library, Birmingham, Ala, USA, 1984.
3. Osler W. The Gulstonian lectures on malignant endocarditis. *BMJ* 1885; 1: 467.
4. Bennett DE. Primary mycotic aneurysms of the aorta: report of case and review of the literature. *Arch Surg* 1967; 94: 758-65.
5. Reddy DJ, Shepard AD, Evans JR, *et al.* Management of infected aortoiliac aneurysms. *Arch Surg* 1991; 126: 873.
6. Kyriakides C, Kan Y, Kerle M, *et al.* 11-year experience with anatomical and extra-anatomical repair of mycotic aortic aneurysms. *Eur J Vasc Endovasc Surg* 2004; 27: 585-9.
7. Earnshaw JJ. The current role of rifampicin-impregnated grafts: pragmatism versus science. *Eur J Vasc Endovasc Surg* 2000; 20: 409-12.
8. Claggett PG, Valentine JR, Hagino RT. Autogenous aortoiliac/femoral reconstruction from superficial femoro-popliteal veins: feasibility and durability. *J Vasc Surg* 1997; 25: 255-70.
9. Gibbons CP, Ferguson CJ, Fligelstone LJ, Edwards K. Experience with femoropopliteal vein as a conduit for vascular reconstruction in infected fields. *Eur J Vasc Endovasc Surg* 2003; 25: 424-31.
10. Teebken OE, Pichlmaier MA, Brand S, Haverich A. Cryopreserved arterial allografts for *in situ* reconstruction of infected arterial vessels. *Eur J Vasc Endovasc Surg* 2004; 27: 597-602.
11. Madhaven P, McDonell CL, Dowd MO, *et al.* Suprarenal mycotic aneurysm exclusion using a stent with a partial autologous covering. *J Endovasc Ther* 2000; 7: 404-9.

Chapter 34

Rare causes of arterial embolism

David A Ratliff MD FRCP FRCS, Consultant Vascular Surgeon
Northampton General Hospital, Northampton, UK

Introduction

Arterial emboli most commonly arise from thrombus in the heart, located in the left atrium or ventricle, and frequently in association with recent myocardial infarction, atrial fibrillation or mitral stenosis. Less commonly they arise from heart valves or a proximal source of atheroma from aortic, popliteal and femoral aneurysms or atheromatous plaque in the aorta. These will not be considered further here.

Rare causes of arterial embolism include cardiac myxoma and paradoxical embolism; this chapter focuses on these two conditions.

Myxoma

Myxoma is the most frequent primary cardiac tumour, accounting for 30-50% of all benign and malignant tumours, and approximately 75% of the tumours that are treated surgically. Although they are histologically benign, they may be lethal because of their location. Cardiac myxoma may present with diverse cardiac or systemic manifestations and the diagnosis should be considered in unexplained cardiac failure, suspected mitral valve obstruction, endocarditis with negative blood cultures, peripheral emboli in young patients and atypical connective tissue disease. Surgical removal of the tumour should be performed as soon as possible. The long-term prognosis is excellent and recurrence is rare.

A left atrial myxoma was first described in 1845, but before 1951 the diagnosis of intracardiac tumours was made only at post mortem examination. In that year a myxoma was recognised by angiography and the first atrial myxoma was excised using cardiopulmonary bypass in 1954. The subsequent introduction of echocardiography has greatly facilitated the diagnosis. Supplementary imaging methods include CT and MRI.

Myxomas occur at all ages from the very young to the very old, but are particularly frequent between the third and sixth decades; women predominate in most series. The large majority are sporadic, but some are familial with autosomal dominant inheritance or are part of the myxoma syndrome that involves a complex of abnormalities: cutaneous myxomas and skin pigmentation, adrenal hyperplasia, breast fibroadenomas and unusual testicular tumours.

Pathological findings

About 75% of myxomas originate in the left atrium and 15-20% in the right atrium. Most arise from the interatrial septum in the region of the fossa ovalis, but they can also originate from the posterior and anterior atrial walls and the atrial appendage. Some 3-4% of myxomas occur in the left or right ventricle, respectively, and approximately 5% are bilateral. They range in size from 1-15cm diameter (mean 5-6cm) and weigh from 15-180g (mean 37g) [1].

Myxomas are intracavitary tumours of endocardial origin, arising from multipotential mesenchymal cells that persist as embryonic residues during septation of the heart. Macroscopically, 85% are pedunculated with a smooth or gently lobulated surface, although they may be sessile. The mobility of the tumour depends on its consistency and varies with the extent of its attachment and the length of the stalk. Pedunculated tumours tend to be soft, friable and irregularly papillary or villous, while the sessile type tend to be firm and round or polypoid.

Histologically, papillary or villous myxomas have a surface that consists of multiple fine villous extensions that are gelatinous and fragile and have a tendency to fragment and embolise. Polypoid myxomas show little tendency towards spontaneous fragmentation. Microscopically, myxoma cells are embedded in a myxoid matrix rich in acid mucopolysaccharide and their surface is frequently covered by thrombus [2].

Clinical findings

The clinical features of myxoma are determined by the location, size and mobility. Most patients present with one or more of the triad of embolism, intracardiac obstruction and constitutional symptoms. Occasionally there are no symptoms, particularly with small tumours.

Embolism

Embolisation occurs in 30-40% of patients with a myxoma; the emboli are frequently large, multiple and catastrophic in severity. They may consist of tumour material, overlying mural thrombus, or both. Any arterial bed may be affected, leading to a great variety of symptoms and signs. Cerebral embolisation is most frequent and may present as unexplained stroke or recurrent strokes. Transient or permanent visual loss may result from involvement of the retinal arteries. Massive embolisation can occur to the abdominal aorta and its bifurcation, both in adults and children, causing saddle embolus or complete obstruction of the abdominal aorta and renal arteries by large tumour emboli. Embolisation to major branches of the aorta can cause spinal cord ischaemia and transient flaccid paraplegia. Multiple peripheral emboli may cause acute or acute on chronic limb ischaemia [3,4].

Sudden cardiac death from myxomas can occur as a result of either coronary embolism or obstruction of the mitral valve. Clinically evident embolic events are uncommon with right-sided tumours, although massive pulmonary embolism or multiple emboli causing pulmonary hypertension have been reported. Occasionally myxomas may become infected, and in this circumstance there is great danger of systemic embolisation. Uncommonly myxoma emboli may show a malignant behaviour by infiltrating and destroying the arterial wall of cerebral, pulmonary, coronary and other systemic vessels, giving rise to myxomatous pseudo-aneurysms that may be multiple and can become apparent years later [1].

Intracardiac obstruction

Myxomas commonly give rise to signs of obstructed filling of the left or right ventricle causing dyspnoea, recurrent pulmonary oedema and heart failure. These signs mimic the clinical picture of mitral or tricuspid stenosis. The extent of valvular obstruction may vary with body position. If the tumour is large enough and has a long stalk, temporary complete obstruction of the orifice of the mitral or tricuspid valve may occur, resulting in syncope or sudden death (Figure 1). The motion of a tumour back and forth between the atrium and ventricle may also damage the valve (the wrecking ball effect).

Constitutional symptoms

Myxomas may also present with any of several non-cardiac symptoms and signs including fever, weight loss, malaise, arthralgia, rash, clubbing and

Raynaud's phenomenon. Laboratory abnormalities include anaemia, polycythaemia, leucocytosis, elevated erythrocyte sedimentation rate and C-reactive protein, and hypergammaglobulinaemia. Not surprisingly myxomas may therefore mimic endocarditis, connective tissue disorder or non-cardiac tumour and are frequently misdiagnosed. The production and release of the cytokine interleukin-6 (IL-6) by the tumour itself may be responsible for the inflammatory and autoimmune manifestations, and the systemic symptoms and signs disappear after the tumour is removed [1].

Physical examination

Systolic or diastolic murmurs may be heard in more than half the patients with a myxoma, depending on the size, location and mobility of the tumour, and body position. Diastolic murmurs are due to obstructed filling of the left or right ventricle. Systolic murmurs occur if the myxoma interferes with the closure of the mitral or tricuspid valves, or narrows the outflow tract. A characteristic low-pitched sound called a tumour plop may be audible during early or mid-diastole, and is thought to result from the tumour stopping abruptly as it strikes the ventricular wall.

Diagnosis

The differential diagnosis of peripheral embolism in general should include myxoma, particularly in a young patient. Embolic material obtained at embolectomy should be sent for histological examination to confirm the diagnosis; intra-operative frozen section may be helpful.

Transthoracic echocardiography is the investigation of first choice and allows determination of the site, size, shape, attachment and mobility of the tumour (Figure 1). These are also important considerations in planning surgical excision. Transoesophageal echocardiography (TOE) provides unimpeded visualisation of the atria and interatrial septum and an even more accurate pre-operative assessment, without the risk of fragmentation and embolisation that may occur during cardiac catheterisation. This can also be carried out intra-operatively during embolectomy and establish the diagnosis if unexpected haemodynamic instability or unexplained pulmonary oedema is present.

In cases with equivocal or negative echocardiography, CT and particularly MRI may be useful and can identify tumours measuring as little as

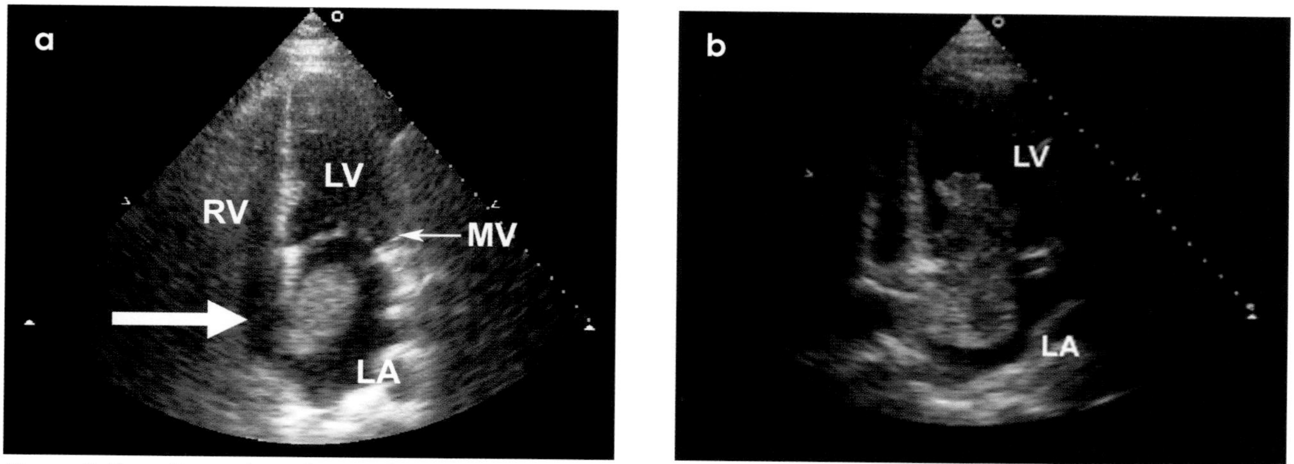

Figure 1. Transthoracic echocardiogram (apical four chamber view) of left atrial myxoma. a) Arising from the interatrial septum, 5cm in diameter. b) Prolapsing through the mitral valve into the left ventricle. Courtesy of Dr. P Davey and Dr. J Chambers. (LA=left atrium; MV=mitral valve; LV=left ventricle; RV=right ventricle).

0.5-1cm in diameter (Figure 2). Cardiac angiography is now performed less frequently before surgery, since adequate non-invasive information is usually available and other cardiac disease is unlikely. It may be appropriate, however, if coronary artery disease is suspected.

Treatment

Surgical exploration for embolisation may reveal white, grey or pale yellow gelatinous material or thrombus. This may be difficult to remove because of its viscous nature and difficulty may be experienced in passing a Fogarty catheter through it. Where there is saddle embolus or aortic occlusion the tumour may be solid and hard, and attempted removal from below by bilateral femoral embolectomy may be unsuccessful. In this event the abdomen should be opened and the aorta exposed to facilitate the passage of the embolectomy catheters. If this is still unsuccessful the aorta should be opened.

Once the diagnosis of myxoma has been made the patient should be referred for urgent surgical excision of the tumour using cardiopulmonary bypass; this is generally curative (Figure 3). Myxomas recur in 1-2% of sporadic cases and this may relate to inadequate resection. Recurrence occurs in approximately 12-22% of familial cases, probably due to multifocal lesions. There have been a small number of case reports of spontaneous cure of myxoma following embolisation, thought to be due to severance of the stalk [5].

Patients should be followed with echocardiography after surgery. Echocardiographic screening of first-degree relatives is appropriate because myxomas may be familial, particularly if the patient is young and has

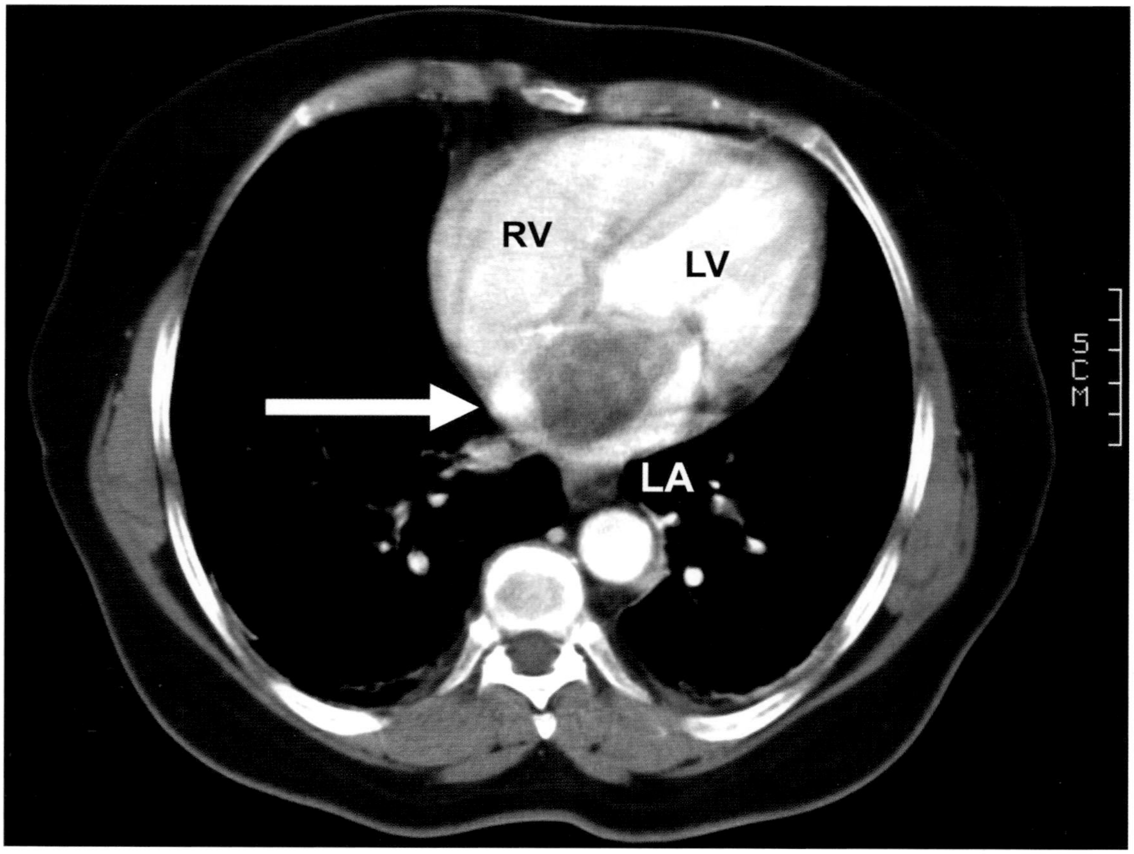

Figure 2. CT of the heart showing left atrial myxoma (arrow). Courtesy of Mr. SD Parvin. (LA=left atrium; LV=left ventricle; RV=right ventricle).

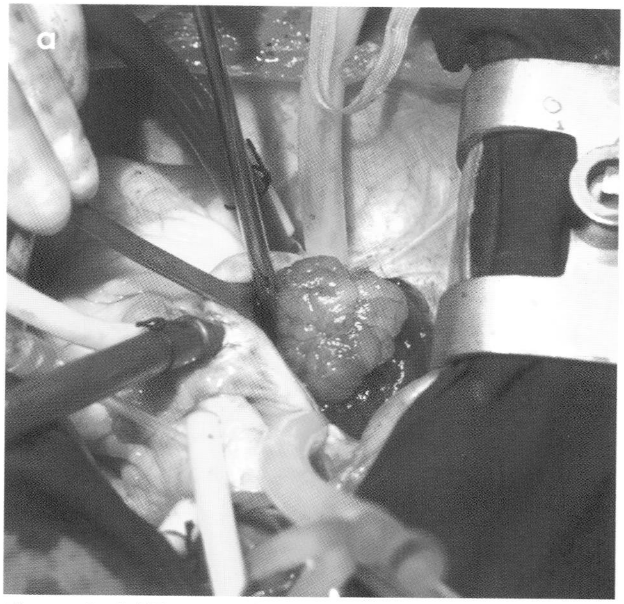

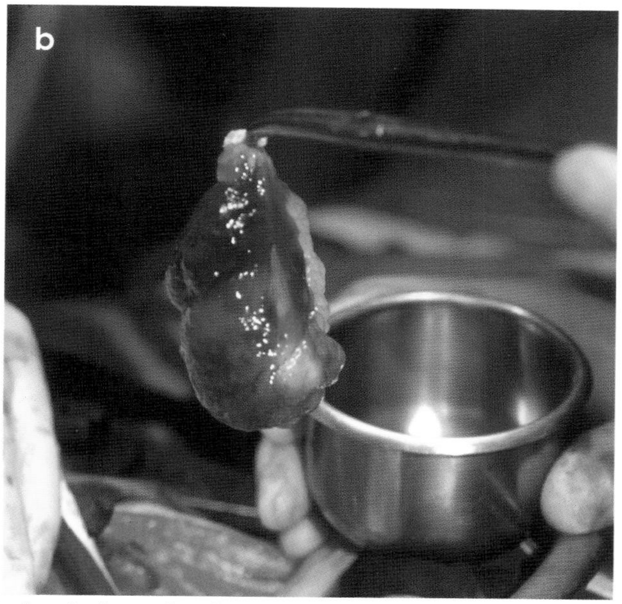

Figure 3. A 57-year-old lady presented with bilateral acute leg ischaemia of sudden onset with leg weakness, incontinence and abdominal pain. On examination she was in sinus rhythm and femoral and distal lower limb pulses were absent. There was a past history of possible vasculitis and she had recently been treated with steroids. A diagnosis of saddle embolus was made. Laparotomy revealed that the aorta was non-pulsatile, but there was no other abnormality. Synchronous bilateral femoral embolectomies were performed with additional external milking of clot from the aorta down the iliac arteries. Lower limb revascularisation was successful and she made a full recovery. Histology of the embolus confirmed myxoma and this was shown on CT scan (Figure 2). a & b) The myxoma was subsequently removed using cardiopulmonary bypass without complication and she remains well 5 years later, with no sign of recurrence. Courtesy of Mr. SD Parvin.

multiple tumours, or other evidence of myxoma syndrome.

Paradoxical embolism

Paradoxical embolism is a rare condition in which an arterial embolus originates in the venous circulation and passes into the arterial circulation through a right-to-left cardiac shunt. It is most likely to occur after deep vein thrombosis in a patient with a congenital cardiac lesion, most commonly a patent foramen ovale (PFO). Frequently the paradoxical embolus is preceded by pulmonary embolism causing pulmonary hypertension, inducing a right-to-left shunt.

The condition was first described by Cohnheim in 1877. The true incidence is unknown. Up to 40 years ago the diagnosis was most frequently made at post mortem. It is now more commonly made during life due to increased awareness and improved imaging, but it is likely that many cases are still not recognised.

Pathophysiology

The diagnosis should be considered whenever arterial and pulmonary emboli occur with no evidence of a cardiac source. The pathophysiology involves an embolic source, a patent foramen ovale or other abnormal communication between the right and left circulations and either an acute or chronic increase in right atrial pressure that favours right-to-left shunting, although this may be transient.

Venous thrombus originating in the pelvic or deep veins of the leg is the most common embolic source, but paradoxical embolisation of air, fat, thrombus from venous access catheters and cellular aggregates from the bone marrow have also been reported. Due to the anatomy of the heart emboli from the legs may preferentially be directed towards the PFO, whereas blood flow from the superior vena cava is directed preferentially into the tricuspid orifice in the right ventricle.

The foramen ovale normally closes in the first year of life, although it persists anatomically beyond this age in 25-30% of the general population [6]. It is not usually physiological active, however, and increased right heart pressures are necessary to facilitate opening of its valve-like mechanism and promote right-to-left blood flow. This may be caused by Valsalva-like manouevres, or any condition that increases pulmonary pressure such as pulmonary embolism, chronic obstructive airway disease, right ventricular infarction and obstructive sleep apnoea. Less frequently paradoxical embolism may occur through atrial and ventricular septal defects and pulmonary arteriovenous malformations.

Paradoxical embolism most frequently travels to the cerebral arteries; stroke has been reported to occur following injection sclerotherapy of varicose veins by this mechanism. It may also occur in the coronary arteries, aorta and limb arteries, commonly the arm, carotid bifurcation and superior mesenteric artery; it is

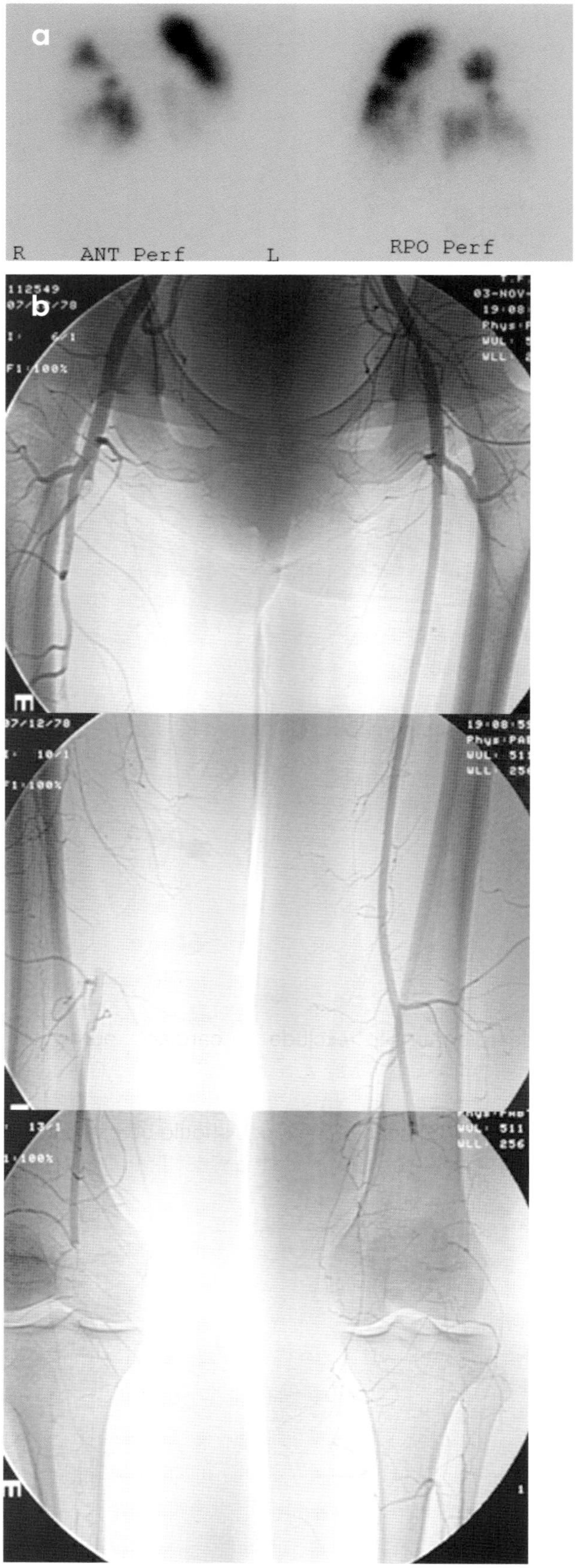

Figure 4. a) A 20-year-old lady was admitted to hospital as an emergency with dyspnoea. She had previously been fit and well with no significant past medical history, but was taking the oral contraceptive pill. A clinical diagnosis of pulmonary embolus was made. She was systemically anticoagulated with heparin and a ventilation-perfusion scan confirmed multiple pulmonary emboli. b) Three days after admission she developed bilateral acute leg ischaemia and emergency angiography confirmed multiple peripheral emboli. Bilateral femoral embolectomies were carried out under general anaesthesia with a successful result. Subsequent investigation revealed a patent foramen ovale and atrial septal aneurysm which was closed percutaneously with an Amplatzer device without complication. Courtesy of Mr. JJ Earnshaw.

frequently multiple. In a prospective study of 139 patients with pulmonary embolism, the presence of a PFO significantly increased the risk of stroke from 2.2% to 13% and peripheral arterial emboli from 0% to 15% [7].

Diagnosis

A paradoxical embolism has no pathognomonic symptoms or signs. The diagnosis is based on clinical suspicion whenever acute arterial occlusion and embolism presents with concomitant deep vein thrombosis or pulmonary embolism, or both. It should also be considered in any patient with arterial embolism when no embolic source is found.

If systemic and pulmonary arterial emboli occur simultaneously, the following should be considered in the differential diagnosis: paradoxical embolism, primary cardiomyopathy with bilateral mural thrombus, acute myocardial infarction with biventricular thrombus, bilateral atrial myxomas, mitral and tricuspid valvular disease, infective endocarditis of the right and left heart valves and bilateral valve vegetations or thrombi on prosthetic heart valves.

Investigation

The initial investigation of a patient with suspected paradoxical embolism should include a full blood count, coagulation profile, chest X-ray, ECG and echocardiogram to exclude a cardiac source for arterial emboli. If these are normal a venous duplex scan and/or venography of the legs and a ventilation-perfusion (VQ) scan of the lungs should be carried out to look for a source of deep venous thrombosis and pulmonary embolism. Angiography should be arranged before embolectomy (Figure 4).

The definitive diagnosis of paradoxical embolism requires the demonstration of a direct communication between the venous and arterial systems with a right-to-left shunt. Transoesophageal echocardiography with intravenous injection of echo-contrast (a bubble study) has become the investigation of choice for the identification of a cardiac right-to-left shunt [8], although positive results are frequently obtained by transthoracic echocardiography (Figure 5). Agitated saline containing tiny bubbles of air or a galactose-based agent may be used; the latter is a suspension of galactose microparticles with adherent tiny microbubbles smaller than human red cells. Transcranial Doppler is a useful alternative when TOE is unavailable [9]. Rarely the diagnosis may be made by imaging emboli lodged, or in transit through an intracardiac defect. Infrequently pulmonary angiography and/or right heart catheterisation may be necessary.

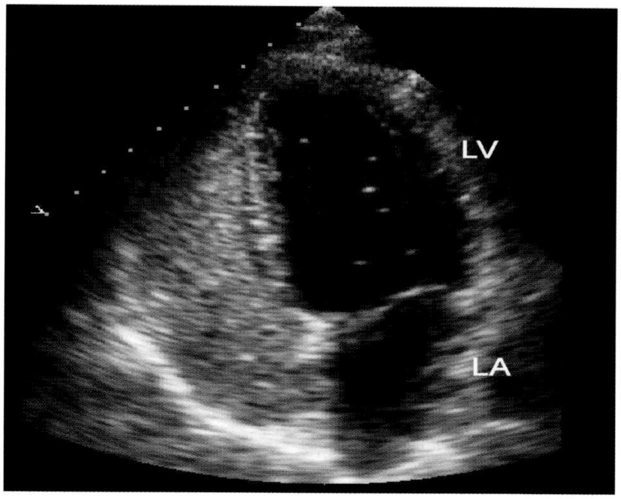

Figure 5. Transthoracic echocardiogram with injection of agitated saline showing right-to-left shunt (bubble study). Multiple air bubbles are seen in the left ventricle (LV). Courtesy of Dr. A Ryding.

Treatment

The management of paradoxical embolism requires both the treatment of the acute event and prevention of further embolisation. Nearly half of all patients who have had a paradoxical embolus present with cerebral ischaemia. Systemic anticoagulation with heparin should be commenced after the exclusion of a cerebral haemorrhage by CT. Emboli to the upper or lower limbs are likely to cause limb or life-threatening ischaemia and usually require treatment by embolectomy. Thrombolytic therapy may be an effective first approach, but this needs to be considered carefully in view of the risk of further embolisation, haemorrhage and stroke.

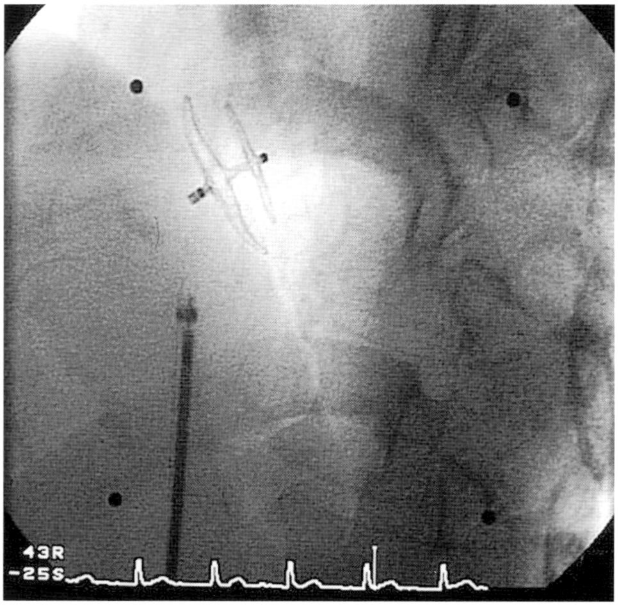

Figure 6. The Amplatzer device after release for percutaneous closure of a patent foramen ovale. Courtesy of AGA Medical.

There is no consensus as to optimal treatment to prevent recurrent events in the long term. Options include medical therapy with antiplatelet agents or anticoagulation, and surgical or percutaneous closure of the foramen ovale. No prospective, randomised trials have examined the efficacy of these different methods. Anticoagulation with warfarin does not seem to reduce the rate of recurrent stroke compared with antiplatelet therapy. Both surgical and catheter-based methods of foramen ovale closure have been shown to decrease the rate of subsequent embolic events substantially and avoid lifelong anticoagulation [10]. Surgical closure is safe and effective, but carries the morbidity of open heart surgery. Percutaneous PFO closure is an attractive alternative; it is a minimally invasive procedure that is safe and effective, with a high success rate [11]. The efficacy of percutaneous PFO closure compared with medical treatment in the prevention of recurrent embolic events is currently being examined in two randomised trials, one of which uses the Amplatzer device. This consists of a double disc made from nitinol wire mesh that sits closely against both sides of the atrial septum (Figure 6). Surgical and catheter-based methods of foramen ovale closure have not been compared directly.

Vena cava filters can also be considered for the prevention of recurrent pulmonary emboli, particularly if there is free-floating thrombus or a recurrent pulmonary or systemic embolus occurs during full anticoagulation. Their role in paradoxical embolism is limited, however, since they are not protective against emboli less than 3mm in diameter. Recurrent paradoxical embolism has been reported in a patient treated with a vena cava filter, due to its inability to capture small emboli [12]. These are unlikely to produce symptoms in the pulmonary circulation, but the consequences may be devastating if a single small embolus lodges in the brain.

Acknowledgement

The authors would like to thank Dr. P Davey and Dr. A Ryding, Northampton General Hospital, Dr. J Chambers, Guy's Hospital, London, Mr. SD Parvin, Royal Bournemouth Hospital, Mr. JJ Earnshaw, Gloucestershire Royal Hospital and AGA Medical for kindly providing the Figures.

Key points

- The differential diagnosis of peripheral embolism should include myxoma in young patients.
- Histological examination of the embolus is diagnostic and intra-operative frozen section may be helpful.
- Difficulty with lower limb revascularisation for saddle embolus by bilateral femoral embolectomy may be helped by opening the abdomen and exposing the aorta directly.
- Paradoxical embolism should be considered in patients with arterial emboli and deep vein thrombosis or pulmonary embolism, and no obvious cardiac source.
- Transoesophageal echocardiography with injection of an echo-contrast agent is the best way to identify cardiac right-to-left shunt.

References

1. Pinede L, Duhaut P, Loire R. Clinical presentation of left atrial cardiac myxoma. A series of 112 consecutive cases. *Medicine* 2001; 80: 159-72.
2. Burke A, Virmani R. Cardiac myxoma. A clinicopathologic study. *Am J Clin Pathol* 1993; 100: 671-80.
3. Val-Bernal J, Acebo E, Gomez-Roman J, *et al.* Anticipated diagnosis of left atrial myxoma following histological investigation of limb embolectomy specimens: a report of two cases. *Pathology International* 2003; 53: 489-94.
4. Wilson Y G, Thornton M J, Prance S, *et al.* Embolisation from atrial myxomas: a cause of acute on chronic limb ischemia. *Eur J Vasc Endovasc Surg* 1997; 14: 502-4.
5. Schweiger MJ, Hafer JG, Brown R, *et al.* Spontaneous cure of infected left atrial myxoma following embolisation. *Am Heart J* 1980; 99: 630-4.
6. Hagen PT, Scholz DG, Edwards WD. Incidence and size of patent foramen ovale during the first 10 decades of life. An autopsy study of 965 normal hearts. *Mayo Clin Proc* 1984; 59: 17-20.
7. Kostantinides S, Geibel A, Kasper W, *et al.* Patent foramen ovale is an important predictor of adverse outcome in patients with major pulmonary embolism. *Circulation* 1998; 97: 1946-1951.
8. Chen W, Kuan P, Lien W, *et al.* Detection of patent foramen ovale by contrast transoesophageal echocardiography. *Chest* 1992; 101: 1515-20.
9. Droste D, Kriete J, Stypmann J, *et al.* Contrast transcranial Doppler ultrasound in the detection of right-to-left shunts. Comparison of different procedures and different contrast agents. *Stroke* 1999; 30: 1827-32.
10. Horton S, Bunch T. Patent foramen ovale and stroke. *Mayo Clin Proc* 2004; 79: 79-88.
11. Holmes D, Cohen H, Katz W, *et al.* Patent foramen ovale, systemic embolisation and closure. *Curr Probl Cardiol* 2004; 29: 56-94.
12. Dahlman R, Kohler T. Cerebrovascular accident after Greenfield filter placement for paradoxical embolism. *J Vasc Surg* 1989; 9: 452-4.

Case vignette

Late presentation of a tibial false aneurysm with compartment syndrome

Michael Jenkins BSc MS FRCS, Consultant Vascular Surgeon, St. Mary's Hospital, London, UK

A 15-year-old girl presented with a swollen tender left calf. Following exclusion of a deep vein thrombosis, a diagnosis of ruptured Baker's cyst was made on ultrasound imaging. Over the next 24 hours the leg deteriorated and developed neurovascular compromise. Angiography revealed a large false aneurysm of the tibioperoneal trunk as a result of a forgotten injury with a letter opener two months previously. At operation, a large amount of thrombus was removed and the tibioperoneal trunk reconstructed with a vein patch. The anterior tibial artery origin was merely compressed and became patent spontaneously on decompression.

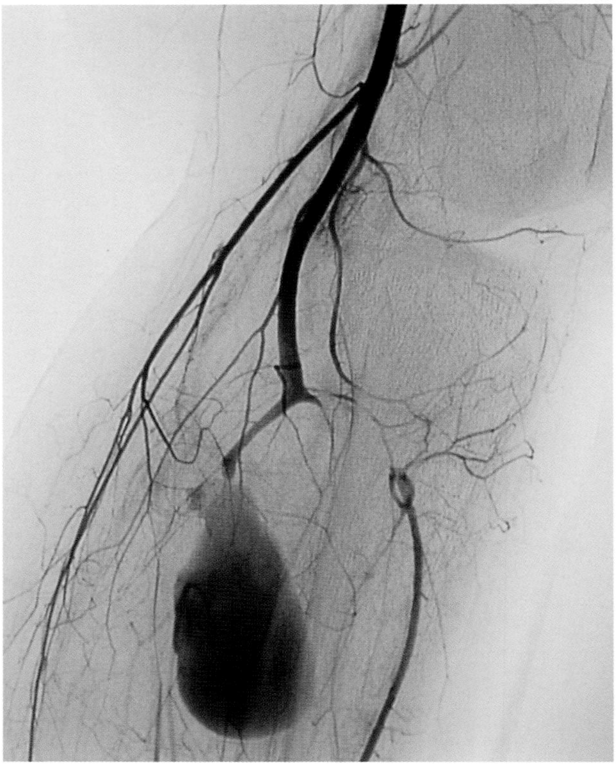

Chapter 35

Vascular involvement in limb sarcoma

Mohan Adiseshiah MA MS FRCS FRCP, Consultant Vascular & Endovascular Surgeon
University College Hospital, London, UK

Justin Cobb M Chir FRCS, Consultant Orthopaedic Surgeon
London Bone Tumour Service, University College Hospital, London, UK

Introduction

Malignant disease at any site in the body can involve arterial and venous structures. The involvement may be a primary tumour of the artery (aorta usually) [1] or vein (vena cava usually) [2]. Direct invasion is common in other tumours such as renal carcinoma, where the renal vein and inferior vena cava can be infiltrated. From time to time, proximity of a tumour to the vascular sheath is such that adequate tumour clearance is impossible without excising the artery and vein. Examples of the latter include gynaecological malignancy [3] and cancer of the head and neck [4]. This chapter is concerned with challenge of vascular involvement in cases of limb sarcoma, particularly osteogenic sarcoma.

Osteosarcoma is a rare malignancy affecting young people aged 10-25 years. Fewer than 200 new cases are diagnosed in the UK per year. The incidence in the USA is two per million population where, of 900 new cases per year, 600 are children or teenagers [5]. Over the last 40 years, standard treatment has moved away from major limb amputation, to local excision with prosthetic joint replacement (usually the knee), together with chemotherapy. Results have improved from this approach, and 5-year survival has increased from 20% to 70%, although another 5% die from disease between 5 and 10 years postoperatively [6]. Limb salvage with massive replacement was developed in the UK by Professor John Scales, and the Centre for Biomedical Engineering at University College London, with the surgeons from the Bone Tumour Services of London and Birmingham [7]. The alternatives of amputation, rotationplasty, or resection arthrodesis all still have their advocates, but in the developed world, massive replacement is now the reconstruction method of choice [8]. In the London Bone Tumour service, the incidence of limb salvage surgery continues to increase, at the expense of amputation (Figure 1).

Osteosarcoma of the limb

Approximately 3% of patients present with a tumour that is deemed inseparable from the neurovascular bundle of the limb. If the tumour shrinks with chemotherapy, the vessels may be saved; however, the risk of local recurrence is as high as 30% if the tumour is resistant to chemotherapy and radiotherapy [9]. Local recurrence seems to be strongly independently predictive of poor outcome [10]. In such cases, an orthopaedic surgeon and a vascular surgeon may collaborate to excise the lesion locally, along with the artery and vein, and maintain limb

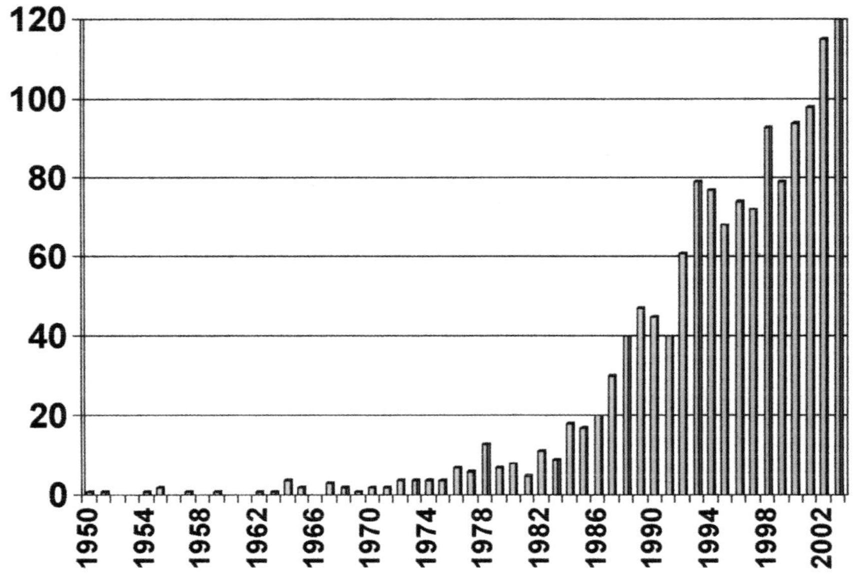

Figure 1. Limb salvage surgery in the London Bone Tumour Service.

perfusion by constructing an arterial bypass, usually from contralateral long saphenous vein. The deep veins are not usually reconstructed if there is adequate superficial venous drainage.

Management

Tumour imaging is usually undertaken using CT or MRI. These techniques can rule out distant metastases, but also assess local involvement of the vascular bundle with the tumour. It is usually possible to resect an osteosarcoma together with the knee joint, but preserving the popliteal artery and vein. If the tumour surrounds the artery and vein, radical local resection with preservation of the artery and vein is not possible. In this circumstance, the vascular sheath should be excised with the tumour and an arterial bypass carried out. The vein may also be bypassed, but the patency rate of vein bypass is disappointingly low and if the superficial veins are patent and competent, there is usually no lasting venous problem. If there has been previous venous damage, then there is a significant risk of chronic limb oedema as a result of venous (and lymphatic) interruption, though the problem usually eases over a year or two. Treatment is by limb elevation, when possible, and the use of graduated compression hosiery during the daytime when the patient is ambulant.

A typical patient with osteosarcoma

A 33-year-old woman presented with a low-grade parosteal osteosarcoma of the distal right femur (Figure 2). Pre-operative imaging showed that the tumour was intimately related to the femoral artery in the adductor canal, and it was judged impossible to obtain adequate tumour clearance without excising the femoral vessels. An orthopaedic bone tumour surgeon and a vascular surgeon conducted the operation jointly. The lower end of the femur containing the tumour was excised, together with the femoral artery and vein. A femoral prosthesis was inserted and a femoropopliteal reversed vein graft constructed. Check X-rays were satisfactory (Figures 3 and 4). The postoperative course was complicated by anterior compartment syndrome that was treated successfully by anterior tibial fasciotomy. The patient remains well 4 years after surgery.

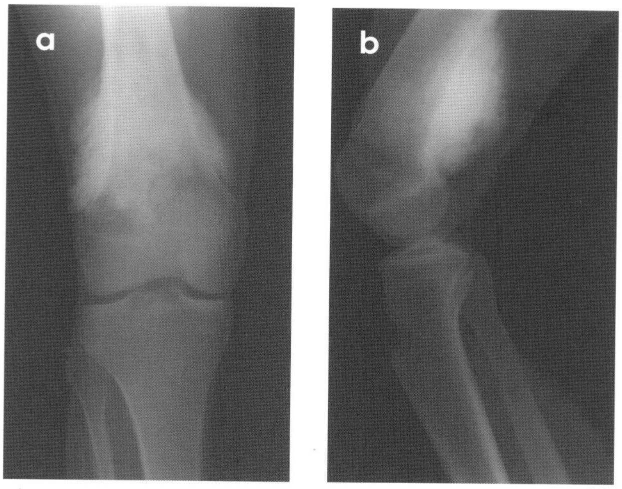

Figure 2. a) Plain anteroposterior and b) lateral X-ray of the femur showing the typical appearance of a parosteal osteosarcoma.

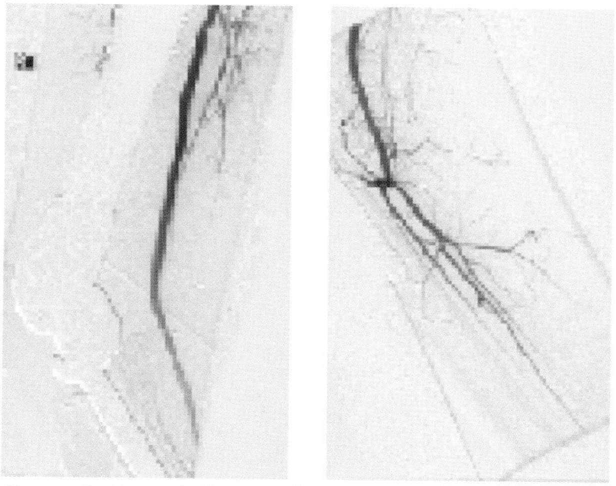

Figure 3. Completion angiogram confirming patency of a femoropopliteal reversed vein graft with good run-off into the calf arteries.

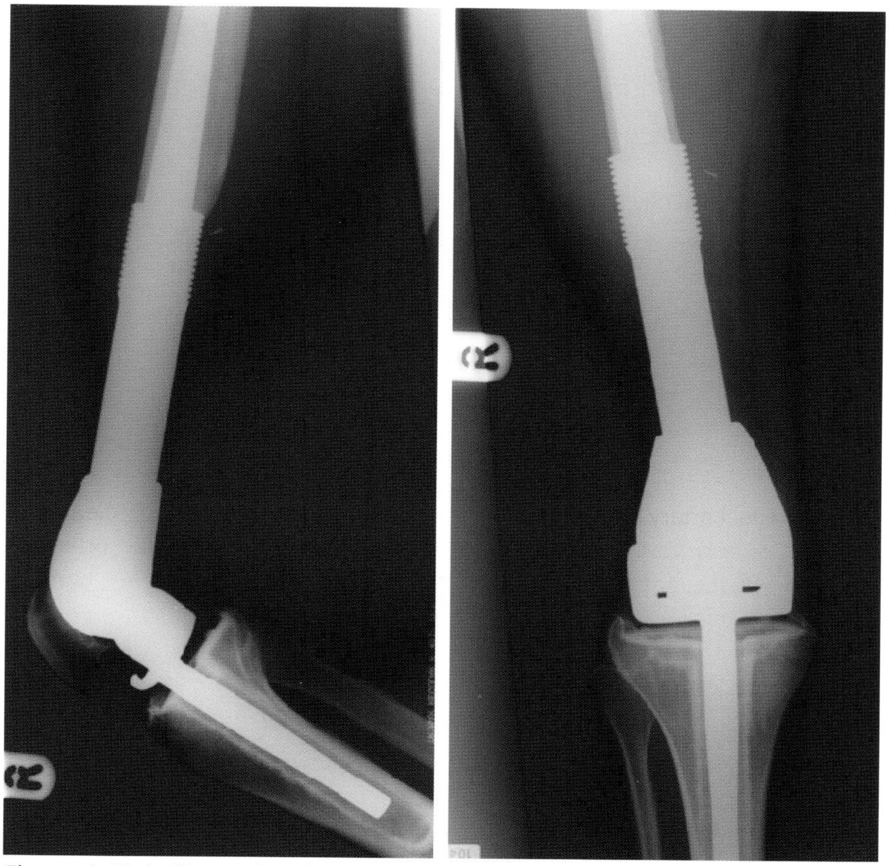

Figure 4. Plain X-ray showing good position of the knee prosthesis.

Key points

- **MRI is used to determine vascular involvement by osteosarcoma of the long bones.**
- **If the neurovascular bundle is involved, surgery should involve radical local tumour resection together with the artery and vein.**
- **The first stage in reconstruction is prosthetic joint replacement to stabilise the limb, followed by arterial reconstruction, usually with contralateral long saphenous vein.**

References

1. Majeski J, Crawford ES, Majeski EI, Duttenhaver JR. Primary aortic intimal sarcoma of the endothelial cell type with long-term survival. *J Vasc Surg* 1998; 27: 555-8.
2. El Mahi O, Bourhroum A, Alaoui M, *et al.* Two cases of malignant tumours of the inferior vena cava. *Arch Mal Coeur Vaiss* 2004; 97: 362-5.
3. Nabi G, Sheikh N, Greene D, Marsh R. Therapeutic transcatheter arterial embolisation in the management of intractable haemorrhage from pelvic urological malignancies: preliminary experience and long-term follow-up. *BJU Int* 2003; 92: 245-7.
4. East CA, Adiseshiah M, Grant HR. Resection of the extra cranial carotid artery in head and neck cancer. *J Otolaryngol* 1989; 18: 298-302.
5. Osteosarcoma Menu. www.cancerindex.org/ccw/guide2o.htm.
6. Bielack S, Kempfe-Bielack B, Schwenzer D, *et al.* Neoadjuvant therapy for localized osteosarcoma of extremities. Results from the Co-operative Osteosarcoma Study Group (COSS) of 925 patients. *Klin Paediatr* 1999; 211: 260-70.
7. Unwin PS, JP Cobb, Walker PS. Distal femoral arthroplasty using custom-made prostheses. The first 218 cases. *J Arthroplasty* 1993; 8: 259-68.
8. Blunn GW, Briggs TW, Cannon SR, *et al.* Cementless fixation for primary segmental bone tumour endoprostheses. *Clin Orthop* 2000; 372: 223-30.
9. Enneking WF, Springfield D, Gross M. The surgical treatment of parosteal osteosarcoma in long bones. *J Bone Joint Surg Am* 1985; 67: 125-35.
10. Bacci G. Predictive factors for local recurrence in osteosarcoma: 540 patients with extremity tumors followed for minimum 2.5 years after neoadjuvant chemotherapy. *Acta Orthop Scand* 1998; 69: 230-6.

Chapter 36

Profunda femoris aneurysms

Dan R Titcomb MRCS, Specialist Registrar, Vascular Surgery
Simon Ashley MS FRCS, Consultant Vascular Surgeon
Derriford Hospital, Plymouth, UK

Introduction

Reports of isolated aneurysmal dilatation of the profunda femoris artery (PFA) are scattered throughout the medical literature as interesting case studies. Aneurysms of the common femoral artery (CFA) and popliteal artery are much more common [1], whereas aneurysms of the PFA account for only 1-2.6% [2, 3] of all femoral artery aneurysms seen in clinical practice. Therefore, no guidelines exist for the investigation and management of this condition.

Background

True atherosclerotic PFA aneurysms were first described as a distinct entity in 1964 [2]. Since then, fewer than 70 case reports on this condition have been produced. Early treatments included control of haemorrhage with ligation of the aneurysmal neck and preservation of branching tributaries, aneurysm-orrhaphy or insertion of a dacron bypass graft. No studies documenting investigation, treatment or follow-up exist since most concentrate on disorders of the CFA. Interestingly, it would appear that PFA aneurysms are more common in Denmark [4], although there is no epidemiological or pathological explanation for this.

A proposed classification of PFA aneurysms is shown in Table 1. True aneurysms are extremely rare; more common are false aneurysms especially after trauma, and including iatrogenic causes. Most are found after a fracture of the femoral neck or develop later after orthopaedic intervention in the same area. They have also been described after therapeutic catheterisation of the PFA, and after blunt, penetrating or high velocity trauma. Mycotic aneurysms of the PFA can develop as unusual sequelae of bacterial endocarditis.

There are several hypotheses concerning the pathogenesis of true PFA aneurysms. True aneurysms of the CFA are attributed to atherosclerosis of the arterial wall. It would therefore seem logical to extrapolate this pathological process to include the PFA. Other possible causes include proximity to arteriovenous malformations, genetic disorders and autoimmune disease [5]; however, no such cases have been described in the literature. Discussion of the low incidence of PFA aneurysms is almost as rare as the aneurysm itself, although it has been stated that due to the confines of the adductor compartment in the upper thigh, aneurysmal dilatation of the artery is less likely to occur due to anatomical constraints [2, 6].

Table 1. A classification of profunda femoris artery aneurysms.

True aneurysms		
	Isolated profunda aneurysm	
	Involving common femoral artery bifurcation	
	Post-graft anastomosis	
False aneurysms		
	Anastomotic	
		Failure of graft/host vessel
	Traumatic	
		Iatrogenic - especially orthopaedic
		Blunt or penetrating
		Self inflicted
	Septic	
		Mycotic
	Mitotic	
		Tumour emboli

Clinical presentation

Most patients with true atherosclerotic aneurysm of the PFA are asymptomatic, although symptoms such as groin or thigh pain and/or thigh swelling have been described. A history of previous trauma to the site, including orthopaedic or radiological intervention should be sought. In the acute setting, patients may present with sudden onset of groin or thigh pain, cardiovascular collapse secondary to acute rupture, or acute leg ischaemia. Embolic phenomena are usually masked due to the anatomy of the vascular territory supplied by the PFA. Patients can also present after the aneurysm has been found incidentally on colour flow duplex imaging, digital subtraction arteriography or CT. Examination commonly reveals a painless pulsatile mass in the groin or upper thigh. There may be a thrill and/or a bruit overlying it. Distal pulses will be preserved unless there is concomitant occlusion of the superficial femoral artery (SFA).

Management

A high index of clinical suspicion of the potential diagnosis is required if a pulsatile groin or upper thigh mass is found. Imaging with colour flow duplex is quick and non-invasive, but the results may be confusing (Figure 1). Arteriography may be needed for definitive diagnosis and to plan treatment.

Subsequent management depends on the aetiology. All reported cases of true PFA aneurysm have been treated surgically. There have been reports of false PFA aneurysm treated by ultrasound-guided compression and/or injection of thrombin or angiographically-guided coil embolisation (see Chapter 40, False aneurysms). Surgical management depends on the viability of the leg and the aetiology of the aneurysm. In the presence of a patent SFA, the option is available simply to ligate the aneurysm. If the SFA is occluded, there is a threat to leg viability and reconstruction must be considered. Most cases are dealt with by excision of the aneurysm and insertion of an interposition graft, although the aneurysm can be ligated both proximally and distally, particularly after rupture. Immediate reconstruction with prosthetic material is questionable if the aneurysm is known or suspected to be due to infection. If primary ligation is performed, subsequent revascularisation may be required if the patient develops critical leg ischaemia.

In the patient shown in Figure 1, the authors ligated the aneurysm, with oversewing of all collateral branches. Tissue was sent for microbiology and histology. Immediate reconstruction was not carried out as there was concern regarding the possibility of infection. Although the leg remained immediately viable, 3 months later the patient developed critical leg ischaemia and underwent successful femorodistal bypass grafting.

Conclusions

False aneurysms of the PFA are more common than true PFA aneurysms. No attempt has previously been made to classify this disorder and all evidence for treatment is anecdotal. The goal of surgical and radiological intervention is control of haemorrhage (after rupture) and limb salvage. Acute rupture is a

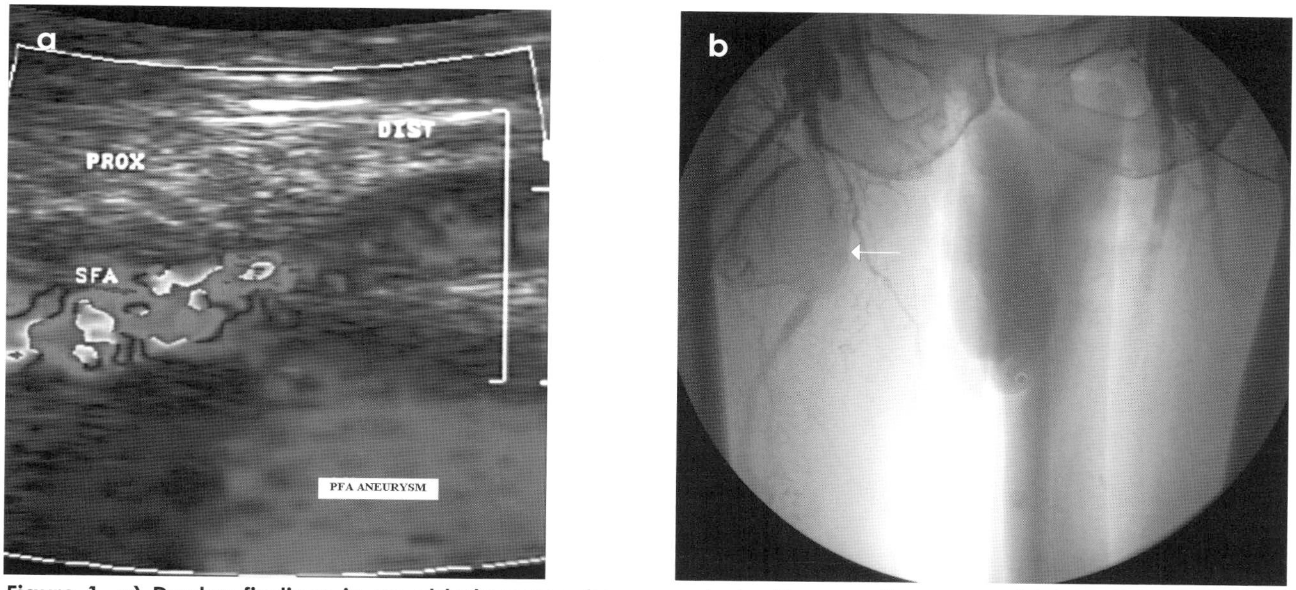

Figure 1. a) Duplex findings in an elderly man who presented with a swollen upper thigh. He had become shocked and a ruptured SFA aneurysm was thought to be the diagnosis. The scan was reported as showing a 7cm aneurysm of the SFA. b) Arteriography was performed via the contralateral CFA and the SFA was noted to be occluded from its origin; the diagnosis was established of PFA aneurysm arising 2cm from its origin (arrow).

common presentation. In this setting, the authors believe that if technically favourable and in the absence of infection, immediate reconstruction of the PFA is the most appropriate course of action. If necessary, ligation of a ruptured PFA aneurysm without immediate reconstruction does not automatically lead to loss of limb, even if the SFA is occluded. This approach can be used in the acute setting to stabilise the patient and allow further treatment at a later date. Historically, PFA aneurysms have been associated with a high amputation rate but this is almost certainly not the case.

Key points

- **False profunda aneurysms are more common than true profunda femoris artery aneurysms.**
- **A pulsatile groin/thigh swelling should arouse a high index of suspicion.**
- **Duplex ultrasonography and arteriography should be performed to make the diagnosis and plan management.**
- **Ligation of a PFA aneurysm without immediate reconstruction is acceptable if the leg remains viable, particularly after rupture.**

References

1. Cutler BS, Darling RC. Surgical management of arteriosclerotic femoral aneurysms. *Surgery* 1973; 74: 764-73.
2. Pappas G, Janes JM, Bernatz PE, *et al.* Femoral aneurysms. *JAMA* 1964; 190: 489-93.
3. Dent TL, Lindenauer SM, Ernst CB, *et al.* Multiple arterioscelrotic arterial aneurysms. *Arch Surg* 1972; 105: 338-44.
4. Levi N, Schroeder TV. Atherosclerotic femoral artery aneurysms: increase in deep femoral aneurysms? *Panminerva Med* 1996; 38: 164-6.
5. Roseman JM, Wyche D. True aneurysm of the profunda femoris artery. Literature review, differential diagnosis, management. *J Cardiovasc Surg* 1987; 28: 701-5.
6. Levi N, Schroeder TV. Arteriosclerotic femoral artery aneurysms. A short review. *J Cardiovasc Surg* 1997; 38: 335-8.

Case vignette

Fractured calcaneum secondary to diabetic foot infection

Jonothan J Earnshaw DM FRCS, Gloucestershire Royal Hospital, Gloucester, UK

50-year-old diabetic man with open neuropathic ulcer on his heel treated with popliteal angioplasty. Whilst the ulcer was healing he suddenly developed a pathological fracture of his calcaneum secondary to the infection. A below knee amputation was required.

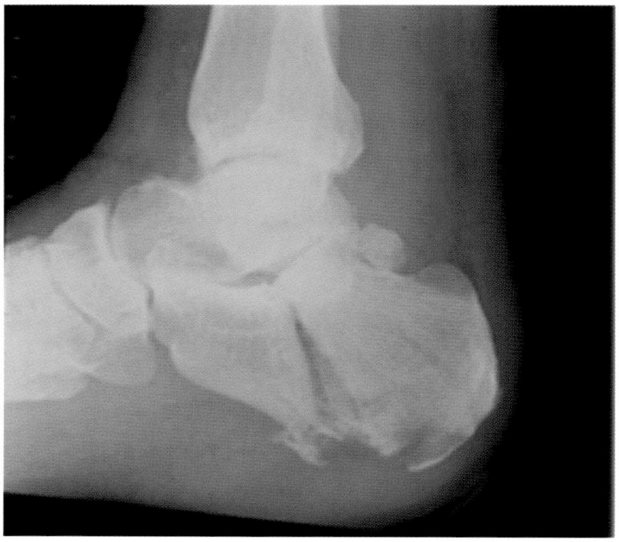

Chapter 37

Popliteal aneurysm

Robert B Galland MD FRCS, Consultant Vascular Surgeon
Royal Berkshire HospitaL, Reading, UK

Introduction

Popliteal artery aneurysm (PA) is the commonest peripheral artery aneurysm. In men aged 65-80 years the prevalence is approximately 1% [1]. PA is defined as a localised dilatation of the popliteal artery greater than 2cm in diameter, or greater than 150% of the normal arterial calibre. True PA are mostly atherosclerotic in origin; other rare causes include mycotic aneurysm, or those associated with Marfan's or Behcet's disease. Only atherosclerotic aneurysms will be considered here. PA can be single or multiple and can occur at any point along the popliteal artery. When examining for PA it is important not only to palpate the popliteal fossa posteriorly but also the lower part of the inner thigh where a PA in the upper part of the popliteal fossa will be apparent.

Historical perspective

Antyllus, a Greek surgeon (3rd Century AD), advocated treatment of aneurysms by proximal and distal ligation followed by opening the sac and evacuating its contents. For a popliteal aneurysm, the technique was to open and evacuate the aneurysm under tourniquet. The tourniquet was then released so that the popliteal artery entering and leaving the sac could be identified and the vessels ligated immediately above and below the aneurysm. Identification and control of haemorrhage were often difficult. Wilmer, a London surgeon, stated in 1779 that he "did not know a single case upon record where that operation had succeeded". Indeed, Percival Pott (1714-1788) advocated amputation as being the best treatment for popliteal aneurysms that had become symptomatic.

John Hunter (1728-1793) was the first to emphasise the importance of the development of a collateral circulation in terms of limb survival. He advocated proximal ligation remote from the aneurysm, which was not exposed. The aneurysm was thus allowed to thrombose as a collateral circulation developed. This procedure, perhaps combined with sympathectomy, was the treatment of choice well into the 20th Century. Rudolph Matas (1860-1957) advocated exposing and opening the aneurysm under tourniquet and suturing from within the sac all vessels entering and leaving it. The sac was then obliterated by successive layers of sutures; this he called obliterative endo-aneurismorrhaphy. Restorative endo-aneurismorrhaphy was applied to saccular aneurysms: once the sac had been opened and the contents evacuated, the connection between the main vessels was sutured so as to restore flow. Reconstructive endo-aneurismorrhaphy was used for fusiform aneurysms where continuity of the main artery was restored by making a new channel by suturing the walls of the sac together over a catheter. In 1906, Matas described the results of 19 popliteal aneurysms treated by endo-aneurismorrhaphy. One patient died. There were no cases of secondary haemorrhage and none of gangrene. Two patients ultimately required late amputation.

Restoration of circulation following isolation of the aneurysm using the popliteal vein was described by Goyanes in 1905 and using reversed saphenous vein by Pringle in 1913.

Despite these potential reconstructive measures, occlusion of the aneurysm by compression was frequently carried out through the latter part of the 19th Century. This comprised compression of the thigh so as to occlude the superficial femoral artery. By applying two compressors one could be released and the other tightened to avoid skin damage. This treatment was often required over many days and successful thrombosis of the aneurysm was achieved in about two thirds of patients.

Clinical details

Popliteal aneurysms tend to occur in older men who have significant comorbidity and a reported life expectancy of about 60% at 5 years [2]. These facts need to be borne in mind when planning treatment.

In the Reading series (1988-2004) of 112 PA in 71 patients there were only two women. The median age was 69 years (range 46-89 years). Significant comorbidity included hypertension in 31, ischaemic heart disease in 19, previous stroke in 12, diabetes in five and other non-cardiovascular comorbidity in 29 patients.

In 41 patients the aneurysms were bilateral. Other associated aneurysms included abdominal aortic aneurysm (AAA) in 35, iliac aneurysms in six and femoral aneurysms in five. In any patient who presents with an acutely ischaemic leg due to a thrombosed PA, the other leg should be examined for an asymptomatic PA and an AAA should be excluded.

Natural history of PA

In the Reading series, 43 (38%) PA were asymptomatic at the time of initial diagnosis. PA become symptomatic at a rate of about 14% per year (range 5-24%). Symptoms include pain or discomfort behind the knee, intermittent claudication either from thrombosis, repeated micro-emboli or combined stenotic arterial disease (25%), and leg swelling with, or without a deep venous thrombosis secondary to compression of the popliteal vein (3.6%). Rupture is very rare. It occurred in only one PA in this series. A 75-year-old man ruptured a previously asymptomatic PA when having intravenous heparin for a thrombosed PA on the contralateral side. The most feared complication of PA, however, is sudden development of acute ischaemia (33%) which prompted the description of popliteal aneurysm as a "sinister harbinger of sudden catastrophe". Paradoxically it was inducing this event, albeit in a controlled way, that was the mainstay of treatment until the 20th Century.

When should elective repair be undertaken?

Elective repair of asymptomatic PA is not without risk. Death and limb loss are both occasionally reported and about 1% of patients will be left with residual symptoms [2]. At 5 years, limb salvage and graft patency rates are approximately 90% and 80%, respectively.

Inevitably, patients will be made worse in the short term following operation on an asymptomatic PA. Using a Markov decision analysis, where the average rate of developing of symptoms was 14% per year, it was 16 months before a break-even point was reached such that the patient benefited from the operation [2]. Clearly, identifying patients who are at high risk of developing serious symptoms would shorten the time to the break-even point. Factors that may predispose to thrombosis and acute ischaemia are described below.

Size

It has been suggested that elective repair should be considered once a popliteal aneurysm reaches 2cm in diameter. There is little evidence to support this. Size does seem to relate to symptoms; in a multicentre study of 125 PA, asymptomatic PA had a mean diameter of 2cm, whereas those with limb-threatening ischaemia were 3cm in diameter [3]. In Reading patients there were no significant differences in the size of symptomatic or asymptomatic PA, or those that were thrombosed or patent. However, PA that caused acute ischaemia either due to thrombosis or distal embolisation were larger than PA that were asymptomatic. Similarly, PA that caused compression were significantly larger.

There is little information on rates of growth of PA. The authors followed 24 aneurysms with serial ultrasound scans [4]. The rate of expansion rose with increased aneurysm size. PA 2-3cm in diameter grew by an average of 3mm per year. Hypertension was associated with more rapid growth. Since most surgeons rely on size as a determinant of when to operate, the upper 95% confidence interval for expansion of PA less than 2cm in diameter was 3mm. If 2cm is the indication for surgery, PA less than 17mm could be imaged annually and those greater than 17mm should be imaged at 6-monthly intervals. Similarly, if 3cm is the size chosen for operation, annual scans would be required for PA less than 2.4cm diameter, with 6-monthly scans for larger PA.

Distortion

As the popliteal artery dilates it also lengthens. Since the upper and lower ends of the artery are relatively fixed the artery becomes distorted. There appears to be a direct correlation between diameter and degree of distortion (unpublished data). More importantly, distortion correlates with symptoms. There was a median distortion of 60° in patients with acutely thrombosed PA compared with none in patients with asymptomatic PA. Distortion was greater in symptomatic than asymptomatic PA, and in thrombosed compared with patent PA. Size alone did not differentiate these two groups.

The combination of size greater than 3cm and distortion was present in 13 of 15 thrombosed popliteal aneurysms from Reading described in 1993 [5]. Since then, in the absence of symptoms or significant distortion, the policy has been to monitor PA less than 3cm in diameter with 6-monthly ultrasound scans. Operation is advised for fit patients with PA greater than 3cm [6].

To date, 17 PA 2-3cm in diameter have been monitored. These would all have been considered for surgical treatment if a cut-off of 2cm had been adopted. Four developed symptoms, consisting of discomfort behind the knee, and underwent operation. None has so far thrombosed (median follow-up 26 months). These results are no worse than the results of 27 elective bypass procedures (median follow-up 38 months). In the operative series, there was no mortality, no amputation and a 5-year patency of 82%. Seven patients had PA greater than 3cm in diameter who refused or were unfit for operation; all PA became symptomatic and three thrombosed.

Thrombus

It is often stated that thrombus within a PA is an indication for elective operation. In the JVRG study, 83 PA underwent ultrasound imaging, and 70% contained thrombus [3]. PAs with thrombus were significantly larger than those with none. There is no evidence that the presence of thrombus is an independent risk factor for subsequent thrombosis.

Run-off

Thrombus from within the PA can embolise into the calf arteries. Large emboli usually produce an obvious clinical picture. Small emboli, for example those blocking only one crural artery might be silent but result in loss of run-off. Micro-emboli can produce the acute blue toe syndrome or digital gangrene. It is clear that once embolisation occurs, the aneurysm cannot truly be regarded as being asymptomatic and therefore surgical repair should be considered. Poor run-off, postulated as being due to embolisation, has been suggested as an indication for early repair, but there is little evidence to support this.

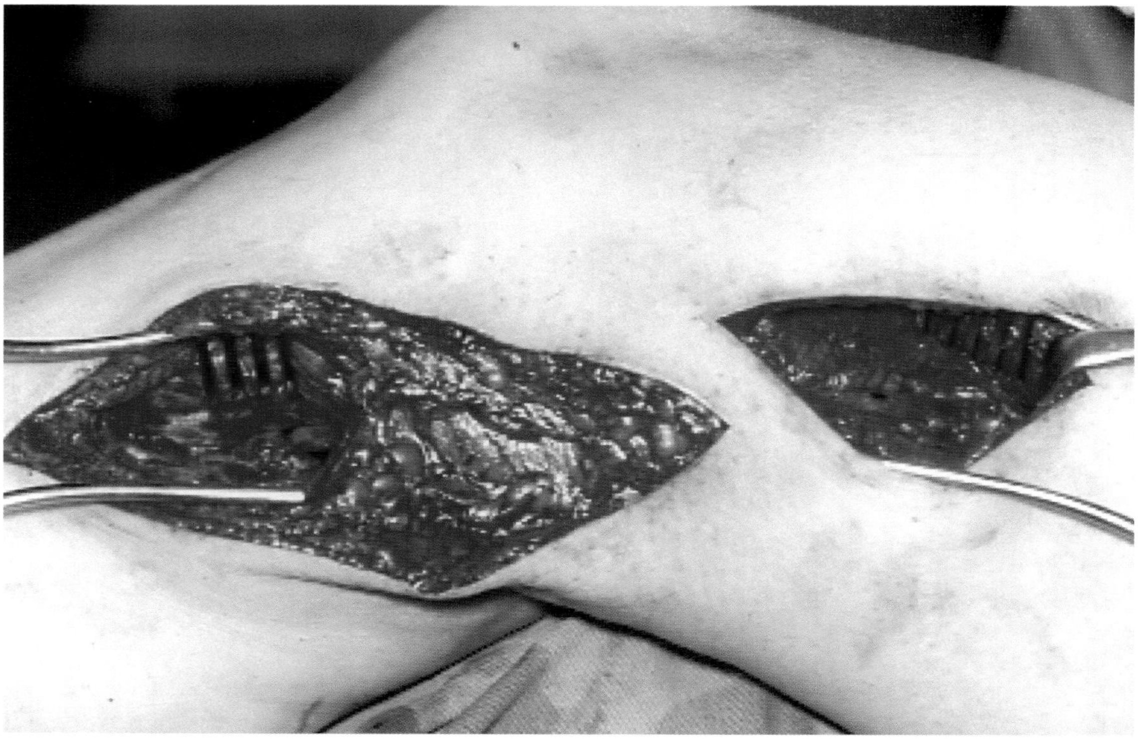

Figure 1. Medial approach to right popliteal aneurysm. The popliteal arteries are exposed above and below the aneurysm in the same way as for a femoropopliteal bypass. The lower incision has been extended to harvest the vein. The vein (marked in blue) has been reversed and anastomosed end-to-side to the popliteal arteries. The popliteal aneurysm has been excluded by proximal and distal ligation with a non-absorbable suture.

Elective repair

Bypass

The standard way of dealing with PA is proximal and distal ligation combined with either popliteal-popliteal bypass or femoropopliteal bypass using vein or a synthetic graft. This is usually carried out through a medial approach (Figure 1). Vein grafts generally provide better results then synthetic grafts with an overall 5-year patency of about 80% (range 70-94%).

The fate of the excluded PA

A number of studies have examined the status of the PA following ligation and bypass. In 12 of 36 patients who had undergone elective or acute bypass, duplex imaging at a median of 48 months later showed intrasac flow [7]. An increase in size was seen in eight of these aneurysms and six developed symptoms including one that ruptured and one that produced distal embolisation. However, not all of these PA had proximal and distal ligation. In another study, flow was seen in 12 of 16 PA following bypass and ligation [8]. This flow within the aneurysm did not always correlate with increase in size of the aneurysm postoperatively. Another report with mean follow-up of 46 months, showed that of 36 PA, seven either remained patent or there were arteries that communicated with an apparently thrombosed PA [9]. Approximately one third of the PAs enlarged significantly compared with pre-operatively. The results of popliteal-popliteal bypass with proximal and distal ligation of the aneurysm were better than either femoropopliteal bypass with proximal and distal ligation where the proximal ligation was at the origin of the superficial femoral artery, or exclusion of the aneurysm with a single proximal ligature. Thus, if femoropopliteal bypass is to be carried out, the proximal ligation should be as close as possible to the

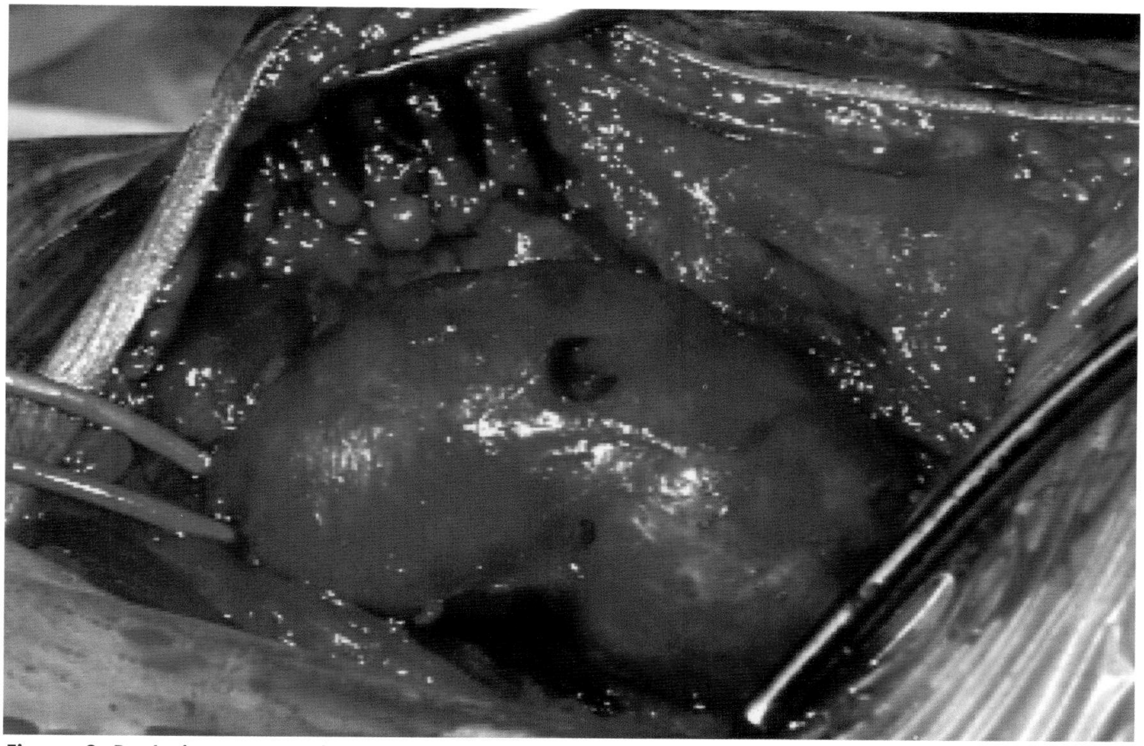

Figure 2. Posterior approach to a large popliteal aneurysm that was causing compression of the popliteal vein. The patient is supine and the PA approached using a "lazy S" incision. In the mid part of the popliteal fossa the artery is crossed posteriorly from lateral to medial by the tibial nerve. With a posterior approach the nerve lies between the aneurysm and the popliteal fascia and should carefully be dissected free and preserved.

popliteal aneurysm. Consideration should also be given to packing a patent PA with thrombogenic foam at the time of bypass.

It is clear that postoperative surveillance (looking for the equivalent of Type II endoleaks following endovascular treatment of aortic aneurysm) is worthwhile. If the PA increases in size, intervention should be considered. This might take the form of further surgery or percutaneous injection of thrombogenic agents such as thrombin or glue.

Inlay procedures

Though less commonly carried out, an inlay procedure is useful for a large PA causing pressure symptoms. It is carried out through a posterior approach (Figure 2) and has the advantages that all vessels arising from the aneurysm can be ligated and the sac removed, if necessary. The disadvantages are that it can be a difficult procedure when the PA extends into the superficial femoral artery and it may not be possible to find a suitable vein through the same incision.

Endovascular treatment

Use of a covered stent to deal with PA has been shown to be feasible in selected cases. The procedure can be carried out under local anaesthetic which would be an advantage in an unfit patient. However, patency is only of the order of 50-60% at 1 year. This compares unfavourably with operative results and the technique cannot be recommended for routine use.

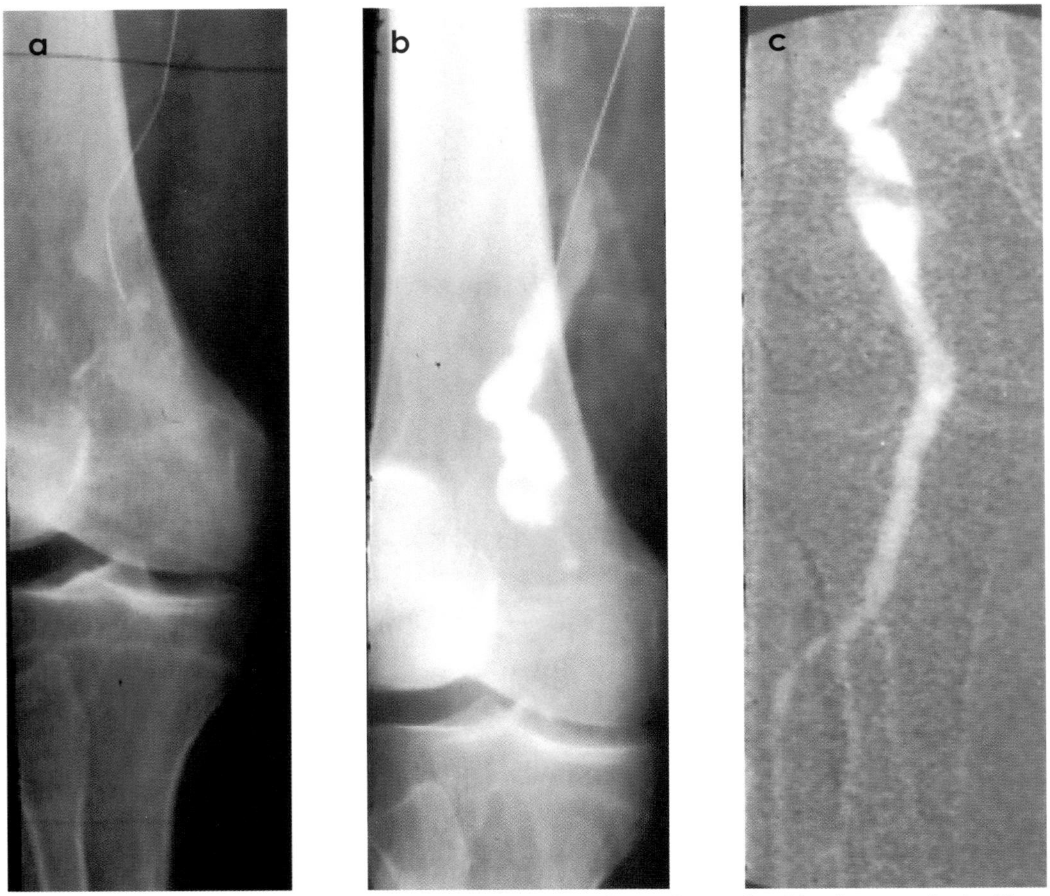

Figure 3. Intra-arterial thrombolysis for a thrombosed PA. The patient had presented with a 6-week history of a painful swollen leg which had been diagnosed as being due to a deep venous thrombosis. a) Shows an infusion catheter in the popliteal artery. b) Shows the popliteal aneurysm starting to be cleared by streptokinase. c) Shows clearance of the aneurysm and run-off. There is some residual thrombus in the popliteal aneurysm. Note distortion of the popliteal aneurysm.

Treatment of thrombosed PA

In contrast to the relatively good results following elective repair, results following PA thrombosis are poor. Mortality is approximately 5% with amputation rates of 20%, or even higher in some series. The surviving leg will have residual symptoms in 10% of patients and 5-year graft patency is about 65% [2].

In Reading, serious complications developed in 13 of 36 PA that presented with thrombosis (including one death and four major amputations) compared with no significant complications following 19 elective repairs [6].

Clearly, if the leg is not viable, primary amputation is indicated. Controversy centres around the use of intra-arterial thrombolysis for acute thrombosis of a PA. There is no doubt that intra-arterial thrombolysis, using such agents as streptokinase, urokinase or recombinant tissue plasminogen activator can clear acute thrombus (Figure 3). However, there are a significantly greater number of complications in patients undergoing pre-operative thrombolysis and operation, compared to those who simply had an operation with, or without on-table thrombolysis. In addition to the common complications of bleeding (and in particular, intracranial bleeding which can be fatal), acute deterioration of the leg during

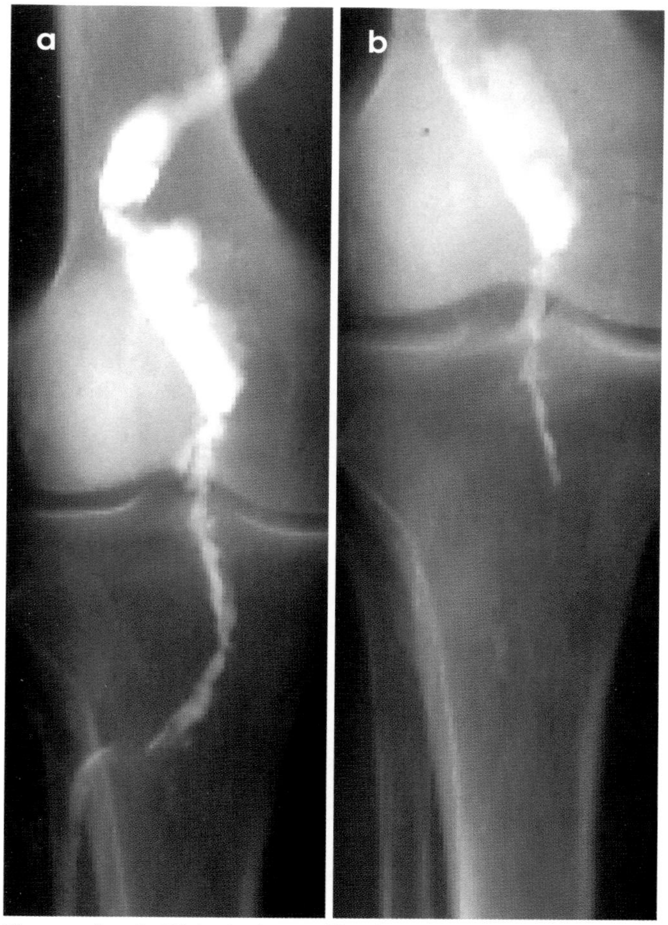

Figure 4. a) Distorted popliteal aneurysm with acute thrombosis being cleared with t-PA. b) Shows that run-off is worsening despite the infusion continuing. This coincided with increased ischaemia of the leg.

thrombolysis seems to be a particular problem when dealing with PA (Figure 4). In a multicentre study involving 866 patients, it was found that 13% of patients undergoing intra-arterial thrombolysis for a thrombosed popliteal aneurysm experienced acute deterioration compared with 1.5% of those undergoing thrombolysis of a thrombosed native artery [10].

Since the aim of thromboylsis is to clear the run-off, not to open the aneurysm, on-table lysis is a better option than pre-operative lysis. The lytic agent can be infused into the calf vessels while the upper dissection and anastomosis are being performed [11].

Key points

- Asymptomatic popliteal aneurysms less than 3cm in diameter and without significant distortion can be managed by ultrasound surveillance with no greater risk of thrombosis than that following elective bypass of a patent popliteal aneurysm.
- Proximal and distal ligation of the popliteal aneurysm should be carried out as close as possible to the sac.
- Following ligation and bypass, duplex surveillance of the excluded aneurysm is useful.
- Intra-arterial thrombolysis of an acutely thrombosed popliteal aneurysm is associated with a significant risk of limb deterioration. Lysis is best reserved for intra-operative use to clear the run-off vessels.

References

1. Trickett JP, Scott RAP, Tilney HS. Screening and management of asymptomatic popliteal aneurysms. *J Med Screen* 2002; 9: 92-3.
2. Michaels JA, Galland RB. Management of asymptomatic popliteal aneurysms: the use of a Markov decision tree to determine the criteria for a conservative approach. *Eur J Vasc Surg* 1993; 7: 136-43.
3. Varga ZA, Locke-Edmunds JC, Baird RN. A multicenter study of popliteal aneurysms. *J Vasc Surg* 1994; 20: 171-7.
4. Pittathankal AA, Dattani R, Magee TR, Galland RB. Expansion rates of asymptomatic popliteal artery aneurysms. *Eur J Vasc Endovasc Surg* 2004; 27: 382-4.
5. Ramesh S, Michaels JA, Galland RB. Popliteal aneurysm: morphology and management. *Br J Surg* 1993; 80: 1531-3.
6. Galland RB, Magee TR. Management of popliteal aneurysm. *Br J Surg* 2002; 89: 1382-5.
7. Kirkpatrick UJ, McWilliams RG, Martin J, *et al.* Late complications after ligation and bypass for popliteal aneurysm. *Br J Surg* 2004; 91: 174-7.
8. Ebaugh JL, Morasch MD, Matsumura JS, *et al.* Fate of excluded popliteal artery aneurysms. *J Vasc Surg* 2003; 37: 954-9.
9. Jones WT, Hagino RT, Chiou AC, *et al.* Graft patency is not the only clinical predictor of success after exclusion and bypass of popliteal artery aneurysms. *J Vasc Surg* 2003; 37: 392-8.
10. Galland RB, Earnshaw JJ, Baird RN, *et al.* Acute limb deterioration during intra-arterial thrombolysis. *Br J Surg* 1993; 80: 1118-20.
11. Thompson JF, Beard J, Scott DJ, *et al.* Intra-operative thrombolysis in the management of thrombosed popliteal aneurysm. *Br J Surg* 1993; 80: 858-9.

Case vignette

Popliteal aneurysm bypass

John F Thompson MS FRCS (Ed) FRCS, Consultant Surgeon, Royal Devon and Exeter Hospitals, Exeter, UK

This 80-year-old man presented to the DVT clinic with a swollen calf. Examination revealed a huge popliteal aneurysm, with good run-off on angiography. Since it has been suggested that simple ligation and bypass risks continued expansion due to persistent inflow from the geniculate vessels, the aneurysm was explored using the posterior approach (Figure 1). There was no usable long saphenous vein, so a 6mm PTFE graft was used to restore the arterial circulation (Figure 2).

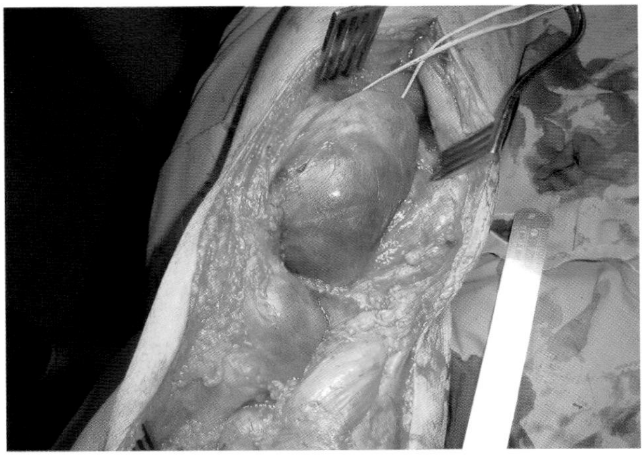

Figure 1.

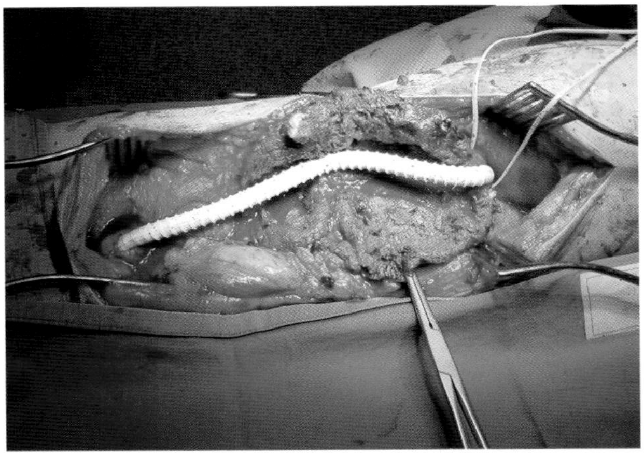

Figure 2.

Chapter 38

Popliteal artery entrapment syndrome

Ahmed Assar FRCS, Specialist Registrar, Vascular Surgery
Shane MacSweeney MA MChir FRCS, Consultant Vascular Surgeon
Queen's Medical Centre, Nottingham, UK

Introduction and history

Popliteal artery entrapment syndrome (PAES) typically arises in young athletic men and may result in claudication, arterial occlusion, and rarely critical ischaemia. It occurs when an abnormal anatomical relationship between the popliteal artery and the surrounding musculotendinous structures causes symptoms resulting from arterial compression. It is second only to atherosclerosis as the most common surgically correctable cause of leg claudication in young adults. In 1879, an Edinburgh medical student, TP Anderson Stuart, described an anatomical variant of the popliteal artery which he had dissected from a gangrenous limb [1]. The significance of this anomaly was not recognised until 1959 when Hamming and Vink in the Netherlands described the clinical syndrome that is associated with entrapment of the popliteal artery. Isolated cases were reported subsequently but the term popliteal artery entrapment syndrome did not appear until the mid-sixties [2].

Incidence

The true incidence of PAES is unknown but congenital anomalies are found in 3.5% in post mortem studies [3], whereas the clinical syndrome was present in only 0.165% of 20,000 military recruits [4]. Most individuals with PAES are young active men, often athletes or undergoing military training. More recent publications suggest that the condition is commoner in women than previously thought, with a male: female ratio of 2:1. At presentation, 80% are younger than 30 years of age and fewer than 10% are over 50. In a large series of patients under the age of 50 years presenting with claudication, more than half were subsequently demonstrated to have popliteal artery entrapment syndrome as the cause of their symptoms. Moreover, in a series of 140 legs studied, if PAES presented with unilateral symptoms, an entrapment abnormality was detected on the contralateral side in two thirds of subjects.

Embryology of the popliteal artery

The popliteal artery is formed from a combination of elements derived from the primitive ischiadic artery and the external iliac artery, that create the femoral artery. In addition, during this process the medial head of gastrocnemius migrates medially and cranially [5]. Errors in the timing and extent of these complex processes can produce a number of anatomical variants.

Table 1. Classification of PAES (after Whelan) [6].

- Type I. If the definitive distal popliteal artery has formed by premature fusion of the newly developed anterior and posterior tibial vessels prior to the medial migration of the medial head of the gastrocnemius, the newly formed artery may as a result be swept medially by the migrating muscle. Here, the popliteal artery passes medial to the normally inserted medial head of the gastrocnemius muscle.
- Type II. Occurs if the prematurely formed distal popliteal artery partially arrests the migration of the medial head of the gastrocnemius. The artery is in normal position but passes medial to an abnormal medial head of the gastrocnemius muscle, which is inserted too far laterally on the distal femur.
- Type III. Where any remnants of the migrating medial head persist, or the popliteal artery develops within the migrating muscle mass. This is characterised by a normally located artery that is either compressed by an aberrant slip of the medial head of gastrocnemius or passes through the muscle head.
- Type IV. Should the axial artery persist as the definitive distal popliteal artery, it will lie in the primitive position i.e. deep to the popliteus muscle. This leads to compression of the posterior aspect of the popliteal artery irrespective of the position of the medial head of gastrocnemius.
- Type V. Rich and colleagues added Type V PAES which is typified by involvement of both the popliteal artery and vein. Any of the types of entrapment, with the possible exception of Type I, may include the tibial nerves.
- Type VI or Type F popliteal entrapment has been described in symptomatic individuals who demonstrate compression of the popliteal artery with stress manoeuvres, but in whom no apparent anatomic abnormality is present. This condition has been termed functional entrapment, as the mechanism remains unclear.

Anatomical variants

It is possible to classify popliteal artery entrapment syndrome by the mechanism of the underlying anatomical developmental abnormality. This widely used modification of Whelan's classification [6] is shown in Table 1. While this is helpful in understanding the pathogenesis of the condition, practical use is limited because of its complexity. Several abnormalities may co-exist and it can be difficult to define them fully even at operative exploration. The important practical issues to appreciate are that while the artery is often displaced medially by involvement with the medial head of gastrocnemius, it may lie in a normal position, with compression occurring due to atypical muscle insertions or fibrous bands. The popliteal vein and or the tibial nerve may also be involved causing venous and neurological symptoms.

Clinical picture

The clinical diagnosis of popliteal entrapment relies upon recognition of a history of calf claudication in the young and often athletic individual, which is sometimes accompanied by paraesthesiae of the foot. The symptoms are often sudden, precipitated by an episode of intense physical activity e.g. running a marathon. Claudication may be most prominent when walking and less so when running. This is probably because gastrocnemius contraction is more sustained during walking than running, which may result in a greater period of relative ischaemia due to popliteal compression. Other symptoms include tiredness or cramping in the calf and the foot, leg swelling and pain at rest. Patients may also report numbness, blanching, coldness, or cramps of the leg in a variety of postures, that usually resolve with a change of position [5].

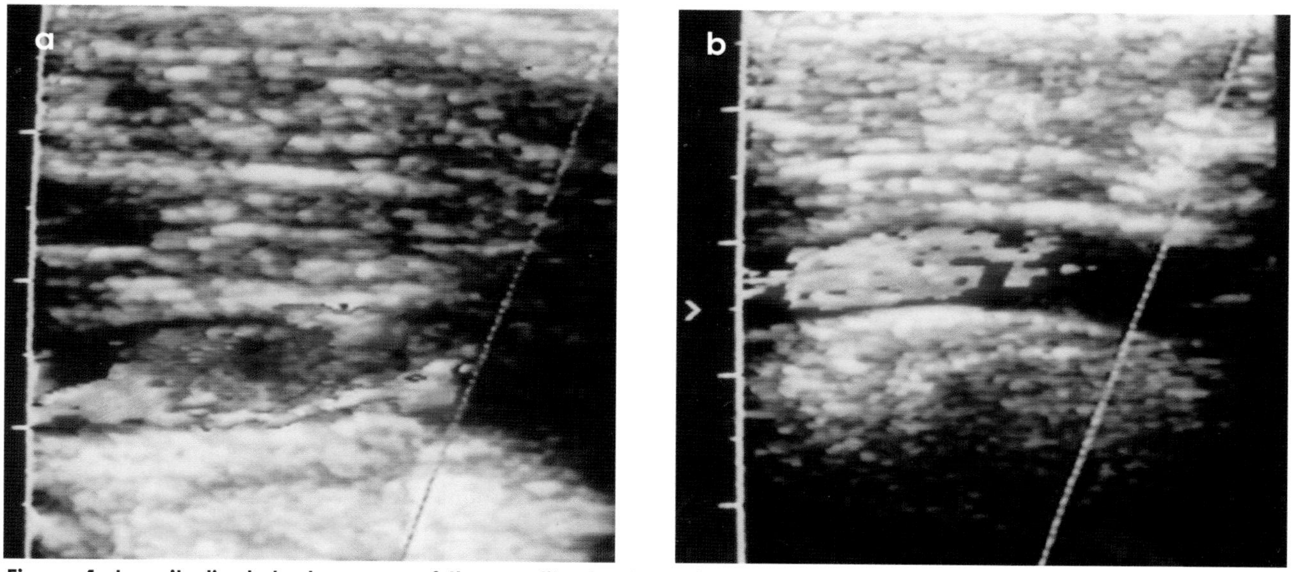

Figure 1. Longitudinal duplex scan of the popliteal artery of a young man who presented with short distance claudication. a) A thrombus can be seen within the lumen of the popliteal artery with blood (orange) flowing around it. b) For comparison, his contralateral popliteal artery is shown. This appeared normal at rest but resisted plantar flexion caused compression both on duplex scanning and at angiography (see Figure 3). Reproduced with permission from WB Saunders, © 1992. MacSweeney S, Cumming R, Greenhalgh RM. Diagnosis and management of popliteal artery entrapment syndrome. In: *Emergency Vascular Surgery*. Greenhalgh RM, Hollier LH, Eds. WB Saunders, 1992: 449-58.

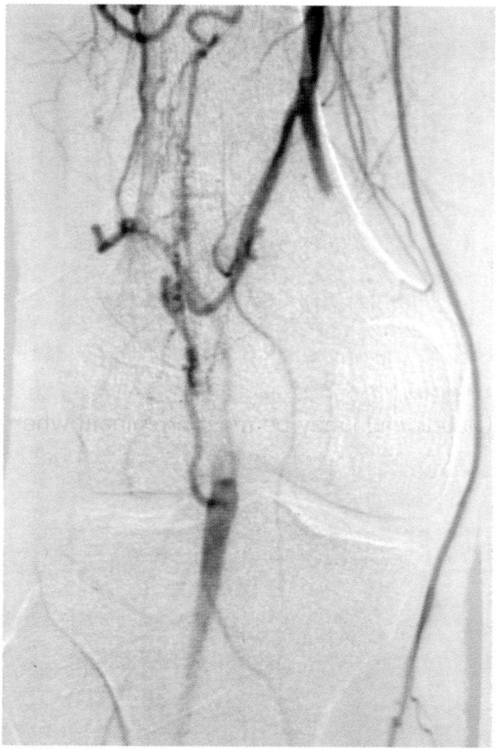

Figure 2. Angiogram in an 18-year-old man who presented with an occluded popliteal artery due to PAES. Courtesy of Mr. JJ Earnshaw.

In the early stages of the condition the artery is normal and only compressed during muscular contraction; therefore, peripheral pulses are normal. Plantar flexion against resistance may cause the foot pulses to diminish or disappear but this is common in normal subjects and so is suggestive, but not diagnostic [7]. Repeated low-grade arterial trauma may eventually cause thrombosis, aneurysm formation, or embolisation (Figure 1). At this stage, missing pulses may occur and ischaemia becomes obvious. About 50% of patients will present with arterial occlusion, but clearly the objective should be early diagnosis before arterial complications occur (Figure 2).

The differential diagnosis includes atherosclerotic vascular disease, Buerger's disease, trauma, popliteal aneurysm, adventitial cystic disease, and extrinsic mass compression. Rarely, entrapment has been described due to tight fibrous bands at the adductor hiatus, a condition named the adductor canal outlet or compression syndrome. This site warrants inquiry if investigating the popliteal fossa does not reveal a cause for the presenting symptoms.

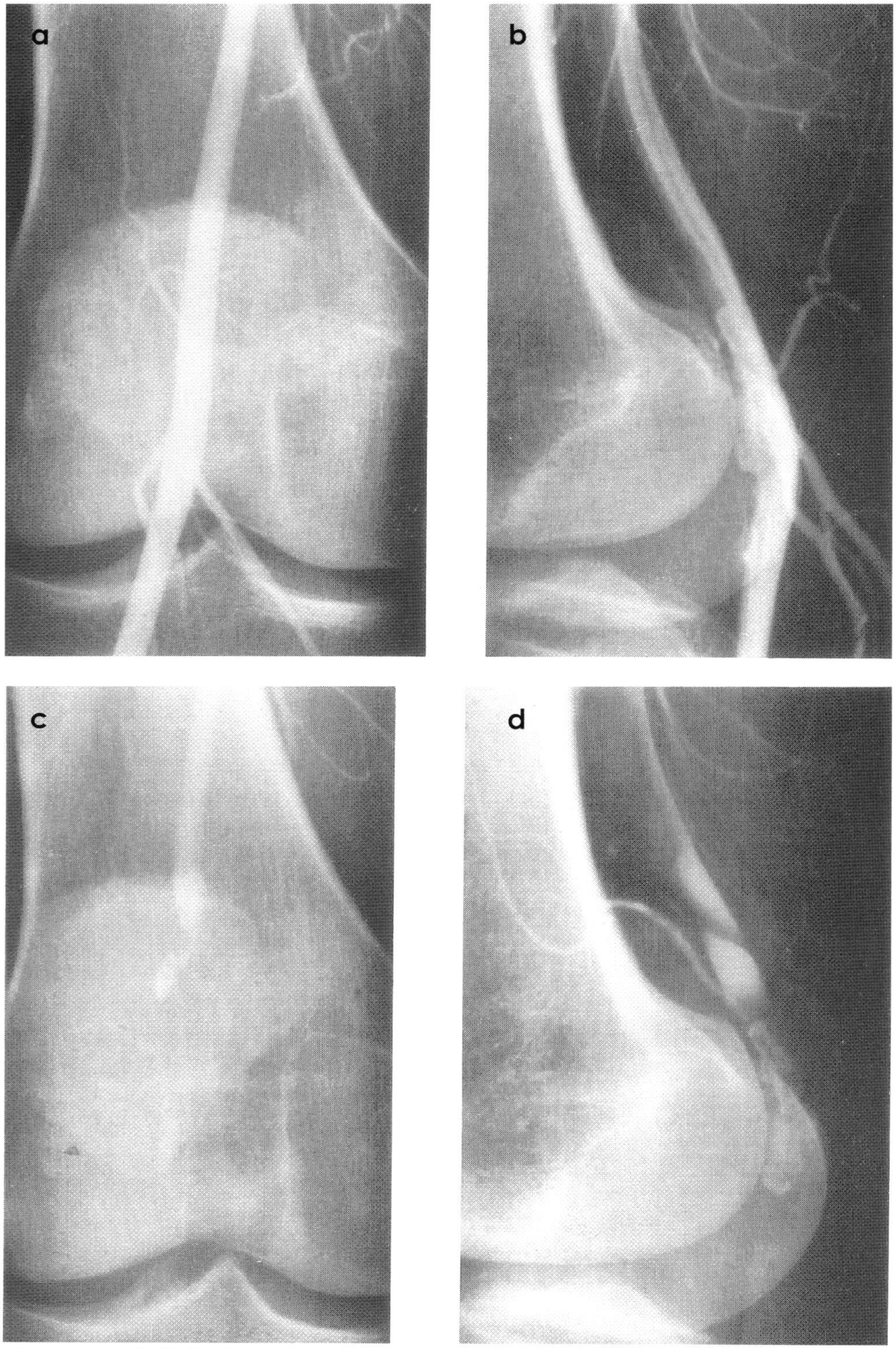

Figure 3. AP (left side) and lateral (right side) angiograms of a patient with PAES. a & b) The angiograms appear normal at rest. c & d) But resisted plantar flexion causes the artery to occlude. Reproduced with permission from WB Saunders, © 1992. MacSweeney S, Cumming R, Greenhalgh RM. Diagnosis and management of popliteal artery entrapment syndrome. In: *Emergency Vascular Surgery*. Greenhalgh RM, Hollier LH, Eds. WB Saunders, 1992: 449-58.

Investigation

The major diagnostic challenge is to detect entrapment before it has led to arterial complications. Since the artery may be normal at rest it is essential to demonstrate popliteal artery compression, with reduced, or abolished popliteal artery blood flow occurring with forced active plantar flexion or dorsiflexion of the foot against resistance [7]. If the possibility of PAES is not raised when the investigation is requested, standard imaging techniques may miss the diagnosis (Figure 3). Once arterial complications have occurred, then abnormalities will also be present at rest. The diagnosis may be supported by Doppler ankle pressure measurement, extended treadmill testing, colour duplex imaging, CT, MRI or magnetic resonance angiography [5]. The most widely used diagnostic method continues to be contrast angiography, particularly to plan surgery when degeneration, aneurysm, or occlusion of the popliteal artery is suspected. MRI has an increasingly important role in demonstrating an abnormal relationship between the popliteal artery and the medial head of the gastrocnemius muscle. Gorres and colleagues demonstrated the superiority of MRI over duplex and CT in defining the exact anatomical abnormality of the syndrome. It is important to remember that approximately 50% of normal people will demonstrate extrinsic compression of the popliteal artery on flexion/extension manoeuvres so the diagnosis is often based on the combination of history, signs and investigations rather than a single definitive test.

Treatment

Based on the current literature and the natural history of the anatomically entrapped artery, all patients with Types I to V entrapment should probably be offered surgical treatment once diagnosed. If the vessel remains undamaged, simple release of the popliteal artery by division of the medial head of gastrocnemius or other abnormal slips of muscle and tendon may be all that is required (Figure 4). Reconstruction of the divided muscles does not appear to be necessary. Excellent results with up to

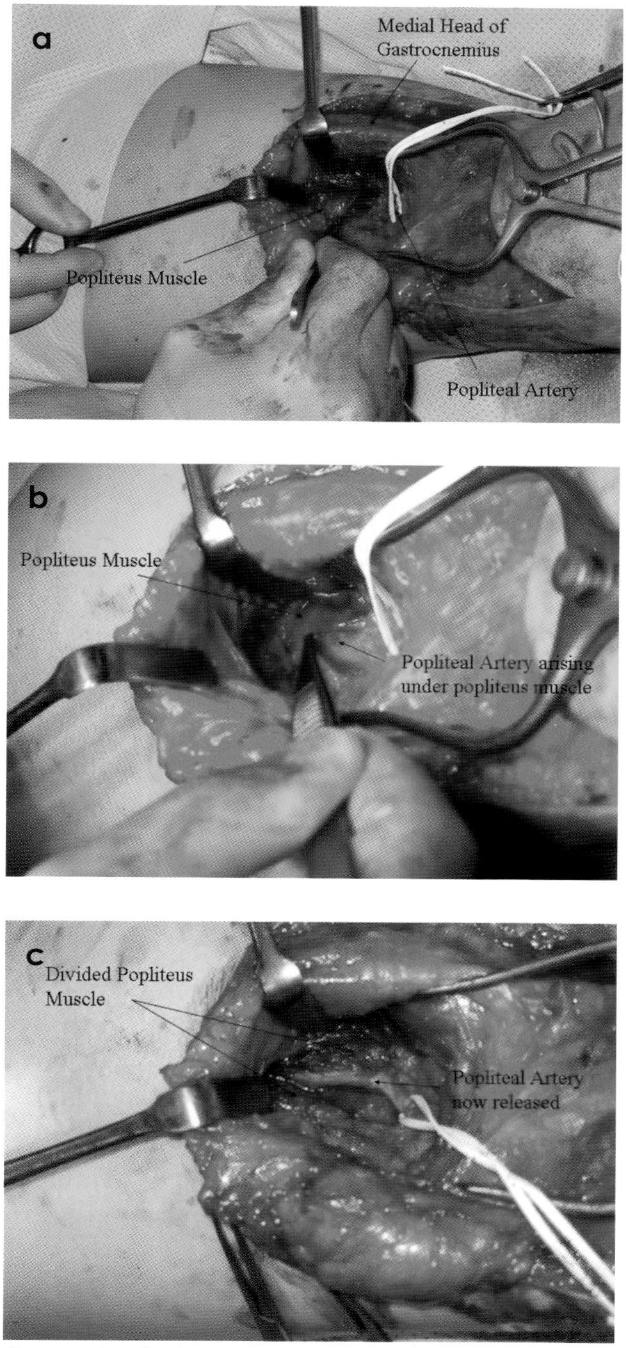

Figure 4. a) Operative photographs showing the popliteal fossa exposed by a posterior approach. b) The popliteal artery is shown by the white sling, passing deep to the popliteus muscle (an example of Type IV entrapment, see Table 1). c) The popliteus has been divided, freeing up the popliteal artery. Courtesy of Mr. B Braithwaite.

10 years follow-up are reported for such treatment. On the other hand, patients with popliteal artery abnormalities such as luminal irregularities on angiography, marked thickening and nodularity of the wall at the entrapment site, aneurysm formation, thrombo-embolic problems, or thrombosed arteries are best treated by replacement of the diseased artery with a saphenous vein graft after division of the entrapment mechanism. Thrombo-endarterectomy and vein patching may seem an attractive option but excellent 10-year patency is reported with saphenous vein grafts for popliteal entrapment. Stenting produces poor results as the underlying compression continues.

From a technical standpoint, a short popliteal occlusion is best approached posteriorly with the patient in the prone position (Figure 4). This provides good access to the popliteal fossa and enables the surgeon to use a suitable short length of saphenous vein as an interposition graft. For longer occlusions, the medial approach to the popliteal artery is preferred as a femoropopliteal bypass may be required. A disadvantage of this approach, however, is that complete exposure of the popliteal artery and its relationship to the surrounding muscle is difficult. This can lead to the underlying entrapment being missed.

Functional entrapment

This is a poorly understood entity. Compression of the popliteal artery during flexion/extension manoeuvres is extremely common in healthy asymptomatic people. In some this occurs readily and is associated with symptoms, despite there being no evident anatomical abnormality. A few of these have severe symptoms and cases of popliteal artery thrombosis have occurred. Surgical decompression of the popliteal artery has been reported to produce durable relief of symptoms [7]. In the absence of any demonstrable anatomical abnormality, a careful search for an alternative explanation of symptoms is required if unrewarding exploration of the popliteal fossa is to be avoided.

Perhaps PAES is best regarded as a continuum. At one extreme are those with major anatomical abnormalities, who develop extreme compression of the artery with minimal effort and are bound to develop severe complications at an early age if the condition is unrecognised. At the other extreme are normal subjects who have compression of the artery during flexion/extension manoeuvres but who will never develop symptoms. In between are those with lesser anatomical abnormalities who may or may not develop symptoms, depending on factors such as how much exercise they take and whether their muscles hypertrophy.

Key points

- **The diagnosis of popliteal artery entrapment syndrome is often delayed or missed causing avoidable deterioration.**
- **The possibility of popliteal artery entrapment syndrome should be considered in a fit young adult with arterial symptoms.**
- **Peripheral pulses and ankle pressures are often normal at rest.**
- **Special manoeuvres are required to ensure that the artery is imaged while compression is occurring if the diagnosis of popliteal artery entrapment syndrome is not to be missed.**

References

1. Stuart TP. Note on a variation in the course of the popliteal artery. *J Anat Physiol* 1879; 13: 162.
2. Love JW, Whelan TJ. Popliteal artery entrapment syndrome. *Am J Surg* 1965; 109: 620-4.
3. Gibson MHL, Mills JG, Johnson GE, *et al.* Popliteal entrapment syndrome. *Ann Surg* 1977; 185: 341-8.
4. Bouhoutsos J, Daskalakis E. Muscular abnormalities affecting the popliteal vessels. *Br J Surg* 1981; 68: 501-6.
5. Levien LJ. Popliteal artery entrapment syndrome. *Semin Vasc Surg* 2003; 16: 223-31.
6. Whelan TJ, Haimovici, Eds. *Vascular Surgery: Principles and Techniques,* 2nd Edition. McGraw-Hill, New York, 1984: 557-67.
7. Levien LJ, Veller MG. Popliteal artery entrapment syndrome: more common than previously recognised. *J Vasc Surg* 1999; 30: 587-98.

Chapter 39

Cystic adventitial disease

Peter Lewis MD FRCS, Consultant Vascular Surgeon
South Devon Health Care Trust, Torquay, UK

Introduction

Cystic adventitial disease (CAD), as its name indicates, is a disease complex caused by a cystic lesion of the arterial adventitia. The lesion appears as an isolated discoloured swelling involving a variable length of part, or the entire vessel circumference. The disease is unifocal and the popliteal artery is the most commonly affected artery by far. The resultant luminal narrowing causes ischaemic symptoms and may progress to arterial occlusion.

Historical perspective

The first case of CAD was reported in 1947 [1]. The patient, a 40-year-old policeman, presented with calf and thigh claudication and had a palpable mass in the groin. Surgical exploration confirmed that the mass was arising from the posterior aspect of the external iliac artery. The lump was dissected off the artery with difficulty, and was described as "a typical ganglion containing myxomatous tissue".

Hiertonn described the first case involving the popliteal artery [2] and the term "cystic adventitial degeneration" arose after collaboration between Hiertonn and Rob [3]. The more modern term cystic adventitial disease has developed because of uncertainty about the disease aetiology. Knowledge of CAD has been gleaned from a plethora of case reports and two publications [4, 5] that summarise most of the available literature.

The natural history of CAD has not been studied directly, but is becoming clearer with greater experience of the condition. The diagnosis of CAD was historically based on angiography, but is now possible using non-invasive diagnostic techniques such as duplex imaging.

The original report by Atkins and Key [1] pointed to a difference in the operative approach to CAD compared with atheromatous peripheral vascular disease and this principle has persisted. The merits of resectional versus non-resectional techniques continue to be debated and there is increasing awareness of the place of more conservative intervention.

The debate about aetiology

Four principle aetiological theories have been advanced. The microtrauma and systemic disorder theories are self-descriptive, but have little supporting evidence.

The developmental theory suggests that adventitial cysts are formed by condensations of mesenchymal tissue laid down during embryological development. This theory is supported by the distribution of CAD in non-axial blood vessels close to joints [6]. Although CAD can occur in children, this theory fails to explain the more common appearance of CAD in middle-aged men.

The synovial theory is arguably the most plausible aetiology of CAD. The basis of the synovial theory is that herniation of the synovial membrane through the capsule of a joint involves the adventitia of an adjacent artery. The connection between joint and artery may be an articular branch of the artery. Communications between an artery involved with CAD and the adjacent joint have been demonstrated radiologically and at operation [7]. This theory would also explain the common sites of arterial involvement in CAD.

Paradoxically, the most important part of the aetiological debate may be the lack of evidence for the systemic theory. CAD is not associated with a systemic disorder, and there is no report of involvement of a second vessel in the same patient. In practice this indicates that patients with CAD do not require additional investigations or life-long surveillance.

Pathology

Macroscopically, CAD appears as a swelling on the outside of an artery, often blue grey in colour but sometimes reddish when it has been likened to a hotdog. The extent of the lesion is variable and it can be circumferential, or involve long segments of the artery. It is important to realise that the lesion may contain multiple non-communicating cysts.

The adventitial lesion is a true cyst in that it has an epithelial lining. The lining is often discontinuous and the cells themselves are often described as pseudosynovial, since they may not take up histochemical markers for synovium. Analysis of adventitial cyst fluid shows amino acids and hyaluronic acid. However, the concentration of hyaluronic acid (the ground substance of connective tissue) is much higher in adventitial cyst fluid than synovial fluid.

Although the cystic lesion in CAD has been likened to a ganglion, these features prove that the comparison is not exact and casts doubt on the synovial theory of development [8].

Natural history

There is no natural history study of CAD; however, certain features may be deduced from the literature. There are no reports of CAD discovered co-incidentally in asymptomatic patients. This is surprising given the widespread use of non-invasive imaging of the knee joint. A small proportion of reported patients have an occluded artery and a minority present with limb-threatening ischaemia. Most, however, have symptoms of claudication. These findings indicate that CAD probably presents with ischaemic symptoms early in its natural history, but has the potential to cause limb loss. CAD should therefore be regarded as a progressive vascular disorder that benefits from early recognition and intervention. If the condition is recognised early during duplex imaging investigation for vascular symptoms, non-resectional surgical treatment of the stenosed, but patent popliteal artery can be undertaken.

Incidence

CAD is rare. In Glasgow Royal Infirmary in the 1960s the condition was found once in approximately every 1000 angiograms performed [9]. Even this statistic is probably an overestimate, since only 323 cases were reported in the world literature in the 50 years from 1947 to 1997. Only four surgeons have reported a case to the Rare Diagnosis and Operations Register of the JVRG (see Chapter 1). It is safe to say that the average vascular surgeon will therefore only see a few cases in their career.

Clinical presentation

The patient is classically a man aged 40 to 50, the male to female ratio is 5:1. Despite the characteristic age at presentation the reported age range is wide (10 to 77 years). Patients almost invariably present with ischaemic symptoms although rest pain is

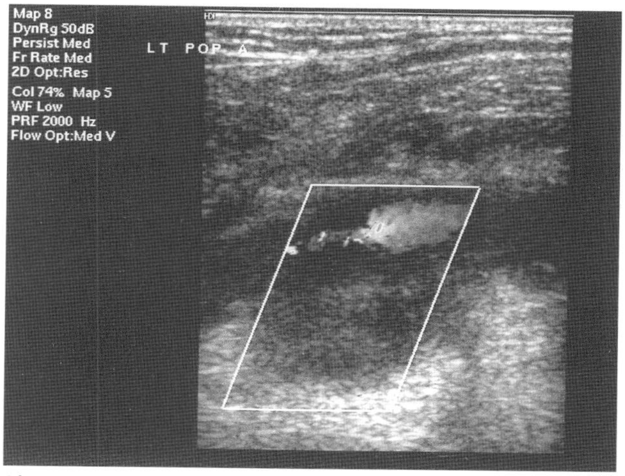

Figure 1. A duplex scan of a popliteal artery affected by CAD. The scan shows the cyst involving the wall of the artery and the hour-glass effect on the colour flow pattern.

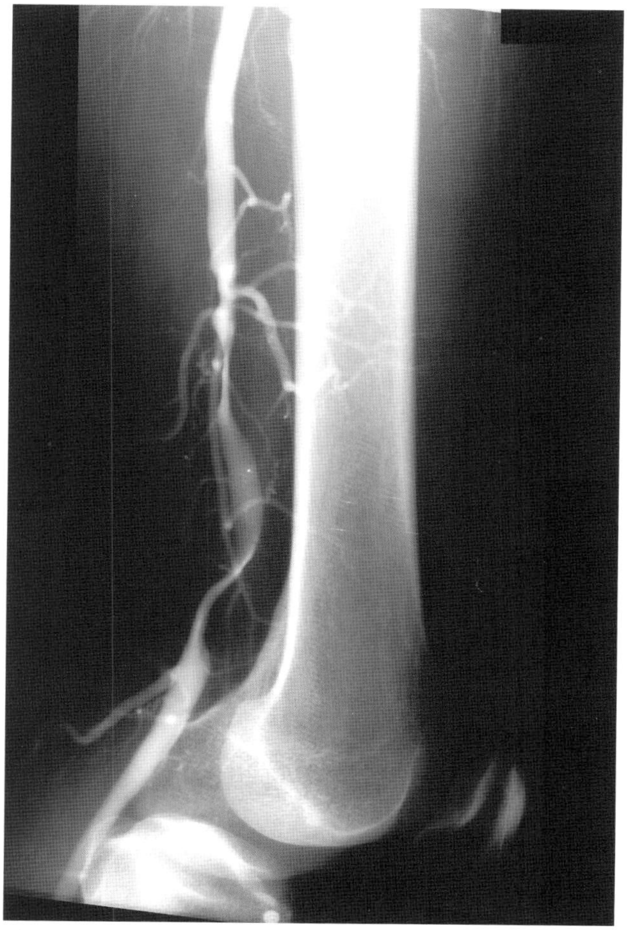

Figure 2. An angiogram of the below knee popliteal artery that shows smooth stenoses due to extrinsic compression from an extensive adventitial cyst.

uncommon. Neurological symptoms have been reported; they are likely to be due to involvement of the lateral popliteal nerve by pressure from the cyst itself and/or peri-arterial adhesions.

In the past, the diagnosis of CAD was dependent on angiography. Consequently, much was made of the physical signs associated with the disease. These signs are, however, largely unreliable. For example, a lump is rarely palpable in the popliteal fossa. Abolition of foot pulses by forced knee flexion can occur in normal subjects. Detection of a bruit in the popliteal fossa may only indicate the presence of a stenosis rather than the underlying cause.

Physical examination should therefore be regarded as unreliable and non-invasive imaging should be considered in all young patients who present with ischaemic symptoms.

Investigation

Young patients with claudication should undergo duplex imaging, since it is an accurate diagnostic tool for all disorders of the peripheral arteries. In CAD, duplex imaging shows the stenosis as a deformity of the colour flow pattern and also simultaneously demonstrates the cyst in the vessel wall (Figure 1). Angiography used to be the gold standard investigation and shows characteristic hourglass (Figure 2) or scimitar signs due to extrinsic compression of the popliteal artery.

Little is currently known about the role of CT angiography, but the use of MRI and magnetic resonance angiography (MRA) have also been described. MRI provides a non-invasive method of demonstrating both the cyst and the extent of the arterial stenosis or occlusion (Figure 3).

There are no comparative data on the relative sensitivities of duplex, angiography and MRI for the investigation of CAD. The fact that duplex imaging is not regarded as the definitive investigation is probably a reflection of surgical tradition requiring anatomical clarity rather than the sensitivity of the technique.

It would appear that MR is a reasonable balance between duplex and angiography, providing clear

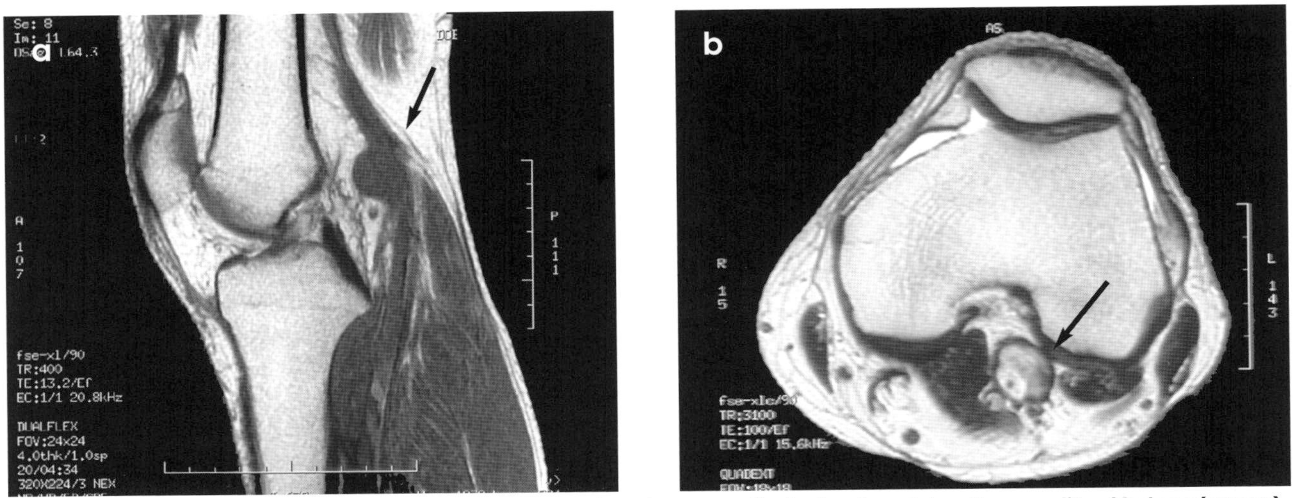

Figure 3. a) A T1 sagittal MRI of the popliteal fossa showing a cystic lesion involving the popliteal artery (arrow). b) An axial T2 MRI of the popliteal region showing a patent popliteal artery surrounded by a complex cystic lesion (arrow).

anatomical information using a non-invasive technique.

It is therefore fair to conclude that duplex imaging should be used to screen for CAD and MR imaging should be regarded as the definitive investigation [10].

Treatment

Although there are case reports of spontaneous resolution [11], what little natural history evidence there is suggests that CAD with a patent politeal artery should be an absolute indication for surgery. This is contrary to the modern principle of conservative treatment for claudication. Open surgery provides definitive treatment for CAD. Treatment options that do not involve open surgery are not curative and are at best temporising measures. The choice between reconstructive surgery and cyst excision depends on the patency of the popliteal artery. Patch angioplasty should be avoided since arteriotomy is unnecessary and patch aneurysms can occur [9].

CAD with a patent popliteal artery

When the affected popliteal artery is patent, the preferred surgical option is excision of the adventitial cyst. The advantage of this procedure is it preserves the native vessel and avoids the early and late complications of interposition or bypass grafting.

A variety of procedures have been described, varying from open evacuation of cyst contents to circumferentional adventitial resection. Recurrence can follow cyst drainage, though this is probably a failure to recognise multiple cysts rather than inadequacy of cyst drainage. Fears about aneurysm development after adventitial resection do not seem to have been justified.

Treatment of popliteal artery occluded by CAD

When the popliteal artery is occluded, surgical reconstruction using autologous vein is the procedure of choice. Many of the case reports describe excision of the affected segment of artery with vein interposition rather than simple bypass. There is little explanation of this choice of surgical procedure, but interposition grafting has the advantage of using a short vein bypass and excision of the affected segment of artery allows the vein to lie in an optimal position.

There are no follow-up data on what happens if the residual adventitial cyst is left *in situ* after bypass.

However, many authors report that exploration of the segment of popliteal artery affected by CAD is technically demanding due to perivascular inflammation and fibrosis. It could be speculated that failure to remove the adventitial cyst may predispose to protracted symptoms due to involvement of adjacent structures. There is no report of CAD causing a deep vein thrombosis; however, there are reports of associated neurological symptoms. Therefore, neurological symptoms, possibly caused by cyst pressure or peri-arterial inflammation, may be a relative indication for excision of the affected artery.

Percutaneous procedures

Percutaneous drainage of the adventitial cyst is technically feasible and is an attractive option; however, there is abundant evidence that aspiration alone is usually followed by recurrence. Aspiration cannot therefore be regarded as a definitive treatment for CAD.

There are sporadic reports of an apparently occluded popliteal artery becoming patent after drainage of the adventitial cyst. It is tempting to aspirate a cyst when the popliteal artery is apparently occluded, since this procedure may uncover a patent vessel and thus avoid the need for excision and reconstruction.

Percutaneous angioplasty does not work in CAD. This is probably because the affected artery is compliant and springs back after balloon inflation. There are no reports of endoluminal stenting but in general, the place of stenting across the knee joint remains controversial.

Key points

- **It is important to recognise cystic adventitial disease because it is a progressive disorder.**
- **It is most common in men in their 40s and 50s who present with claudication.**
- **The diagnosis is made by duplex imaging, but MR scans are useful for planning treatment.**
- **The treatment of choice in patients who present with a patent popliteal artery is open surgical excision of the cyst.**
- **In the minority of patients with an occluded popliteal artery, excision and interposition vein grafting should be performed, when possible.**

References

1. Atkins HJB, Key JA. A case of myxomatous tumour arising in the adventitia of the left external iliac artery. *Br J Surg* 1947; 34: 426-7.
2. Ejrup B, Hiertonn T. Intermittent claudication; three cases treated by free vein grafts. *Acta Chir Scand* 1954; 108: 217-30.
3. Hiertonn T, Lindberg K, Rob C. Cystic degeneration of the popliteal artery. *Br J Surg* 1957; 44: 348-51.
4. Flanigan DP, Burnham SJ, Goodreau JJ, Bergan JJ. Summary of cases of adventitial cystic disease of the popliteal artery. *Ann Surg* 1979; 189: 165-75.
5. Ishikawa K. Cystic adventitial disease of the popliteal artery and of other stem vessels in the extremities. *Jpn J Surg* 1987; 17: 221-9.
6. Levien LJ, Benn C-A. Adventitial cystic disease: a unifying hypothesis. *Vasc Surg* 1998; 28: 193-205.
7. Shute K, Rothnie NG. The aetiology of cystic arterial disease. *Br J Surg* 1973; 60(5): 397-400.
8. Leaf G. Amino-acid analysis of protein present in a popliteal artery cyst. *Br Med J* 1967; 3: 415.
9. Lewis GJT, Douglas DM, Reid W, Kennedy Watt J. Cystic adventitial disease of the popliteal artery. *Br Med J* 1967; 3: 411-5.
10. Miller A, Salenius, J-P, Sacks BA, Gupta SK, Shoukimas GM. Noninvasive vascular imaging in the diagnosis and treatment of adventitial cystic disease of the popliteal artery. *J Vasc Surg* 1997; 26: 715-20.
11. Pursell R, Torrie EPH, Gibson M, Galland RB. Spontaneous and permanent resolution of cystic adventitial disease of the popliteal artery: ten-year follow-up. *J Roy Soc Med* 2004; 97: 77-8.

Case vignette

Transection of the popliteal artery

Kenneth R Woodburn MD FRCSG (Gen), Consultant Vascular Surgeon & Honorary Clinical Lecturer
Peninsula Medical School & Royal Cornwall Hospitals Trust, Truro, Cornwall, UK

A 17-year-old female sustained a traumatic anterior knee dislocation while trampolining. Popliteal and pedal pulses were absent before and after reduction under GA, although there was only minor sensory disturbance and no calf tenderness. CT angiography (inset, Figure 1) confirmed a traumatic occlusion of the popliteal artery at the knee joint. A posterior approach using a lazy-S incision was used to explore the popliteal fossa and the vessel was found to be completely transected (arrows, Figure 1). After resection of the damaged ends, an interposition reversed vein graft was used to reconstruct the popliteal artery (Figure 2). The ipsilateral short saphenous vein was of inadequate calibre, and the ipsilateral long saphenous vein was therefore isolated and harvested at the level of the knee joint. Subcutaneous dissection from the medial edge of the popliteal wound in the direction of the vein gave adequate exposure and avoided any additional skin incisions.

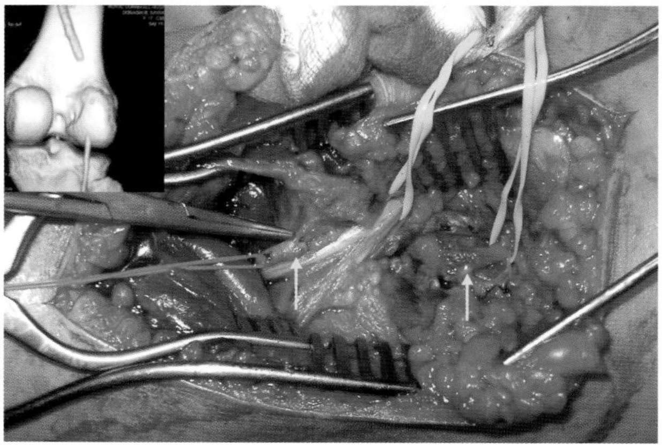

Figure 1.

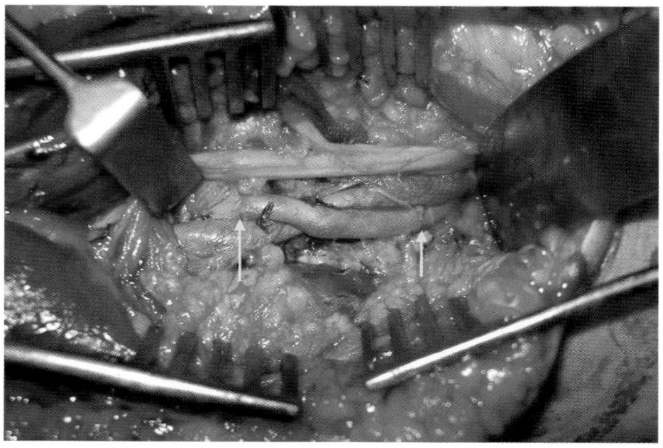

Figure 2.

Chapter 40

False aneurysms

Kenneth R Woodburn MD FRCSG (Gen), Consultant Vascular Surgeon & Honorary Clinical Lecturer
Peninsula Medical School & Royal Cornwall Hospitals Trust, Truro, Cornwall, UK

Definition

An aneurysm is a sac filled with blood in direct communication with the inside of an artery. Whereas a true aneurysm is due to dilatation of the artery and has a wall consisting of all three layers of the vessel, a false aneurysm is more accurately described as a "pulsatile haematoma" that is not contained by the vessel wall, but by a fibrous capsule. Arising as a consequence of disruption of a vessel wall or vascular anastomosis, the subsequent haemorrhage is contained by surrounding tissue, the contents of the sac communicating directly with the arterial lumen. Lacking elastic tissue in the fibrous capsule, the persisting communication with the arterial lumen results in gradual expansion of the aneurysm, which may eventually rupture. As the aneurysm exists outside the arterial lumen, embolic and occlusive phenomena are rarely associated with false aneurysms, although symptoms may be produced as a result of pressure on surrounding structures such as nerves. Distal ischaemia is occasionally caused by arterial compression. Infection of false aneurysms can also occur, and as up to one quarter of false aneurysms are not pulsatile, the infected false aneurysm may be mistaken for an abscess, with potentially disastrous results when incision and drainage is attempted!

Venous false aneurysm

While false aneurysms are almost exclusively arterial, venous false aneurysms have been reported in association with injecting drug misuse [1]. The only reports of venous false aneurysm are in the common femoral vein where they present as an infected groin mass, most likely caused by an infected haematoma leading to secondary venous disruption. The diagnosis is usually made at operation and surgery consists of excision and ligation of the infected common femoral vein and pseudo-aneurysm. Appropriate broad-spectrum antibiotic cover should be initiated at surgery, and continued pending results of microbiological investigation.

Arterial false aneurysms

Aetiological factors

False aneurysms are usually traumatic or anastomotic. Traumatic aneurysms are commonly iatrogenic, associated with arterial puncture undertaken for diagnostic purposes, or interventional procedures such as cardiac catheterisation and indwelling arterial lines. The incidence of false aneurysm formation following percutaneous arterial puncture is reported to be as high as 7% [2], and is more common following interventional procedures where larger catheters are employed. Other factors associated with the development of post-catheterisation false aneurysms include concurrent anticoagulation, female sex, and the presence of peripheral vascular disease. The increase in percutaneous arterial interventional procedures in recent years has meant that the management of iatrogenic false aneurysms represents a significant patient burden for vascular services. In one recent single-centre series, more than 50% of the false aneurysms had arisen after arterial catheterisation and a further one third were anastomotic false aneurysms [3].

Anastomotic aneurysms develop following vascular grafting procedures. They are caused by a disruption of the anastomosis between the vascular prosthesis and the native vessel. The fibrous tissue capsule around the vessel and prosthesis maintains vascular continuity but, with time, it stretches and becomes aneurysmal. Anastomotic false aneurysms arise as a consequence of:

- suture failure which is usually secondary to damage to polypropylene monofilament sutures at the time of surgery;
- graft infection with destruction of the adjacent artery allowing the suture line to disrupt;
- haematoma communicating with the vessel lumen through a small defect between sutures;
- shallow placement of sutures in the arterial wall allowing suture loops to pull through the edge of the artery;
- excessive tension on the anastomosis due to joint motion or the elastic tendency of crimped grafts to return to their crimped configuration following stretching.

Arterial puncture (usually inadvertent) is also the underlying cause of false aneurysms reported in injecting drug misusers, the majority developing in the femoral artery [4]. Commonly, these false aneurysms are infected by a variety of organisms inoculated at the time of injury [5]. The infected arterial false aneurysm thus becomes an "aneurysmal abscess" with secondary destruction of the arterial structures involved in the infective process.

Traumatic false aneurysms also occur as a late complication of partial arterial transection, commonly the result of sharp injury such as a stab wound, where the arterial injury is not apparent at the time of initial presentation. They can also develop following blunt trauma that produces complete disruption of the arterial wall, the resulting haematoma being contained by the adventitial tissue (Figure 1).

False aneurysms rarely arise from spontaneous rupture of an ulcerated atherosclerotic plaque through the arterial wall. When the rupture is contained by surrounding tissue and the communication with the arterial lumen persists, a false aneurysm exists. Although rare, they more commonly arise from the thoracic aorta, but have also been reported in the abdominal aorta [6].

Anatomical considerations

Iatrogenic false aneurysms most often involve the common femoral artery, although they can occur at any site of arterial puncture, and may be seen following removal of upper limb arterial lines in intensive care (Figure 2). Anecdotal evidence suggests that common femoral false aneurysms following percutaneous procedures are more common in obese patients, where accurate compression of the arterial puncture at the time of sheath removal is often compromised.

Anastomotic false aneurysms can occur at any suture line, although they are most commonly encountered in groin anastomoses. This may reflect ease of detection at this site, as anastomotic aneurysms elsewhere may not be apparent to the patient, or on clinical examination.

Traumatic false aneurysms can occur at any site of arterial injury, although those arising as a consequence of blunt trauma and deceleration injury typically occur at those parts of the vascular tree where a relatively fixed portion of the vessel is in continuity with a more mobile portion. This is typified by the thoracic aortic disruption encountered following high-speed motor vehicle accidents. In the few patients who survive this injury the aortic disruption is contained by adventitia and a false

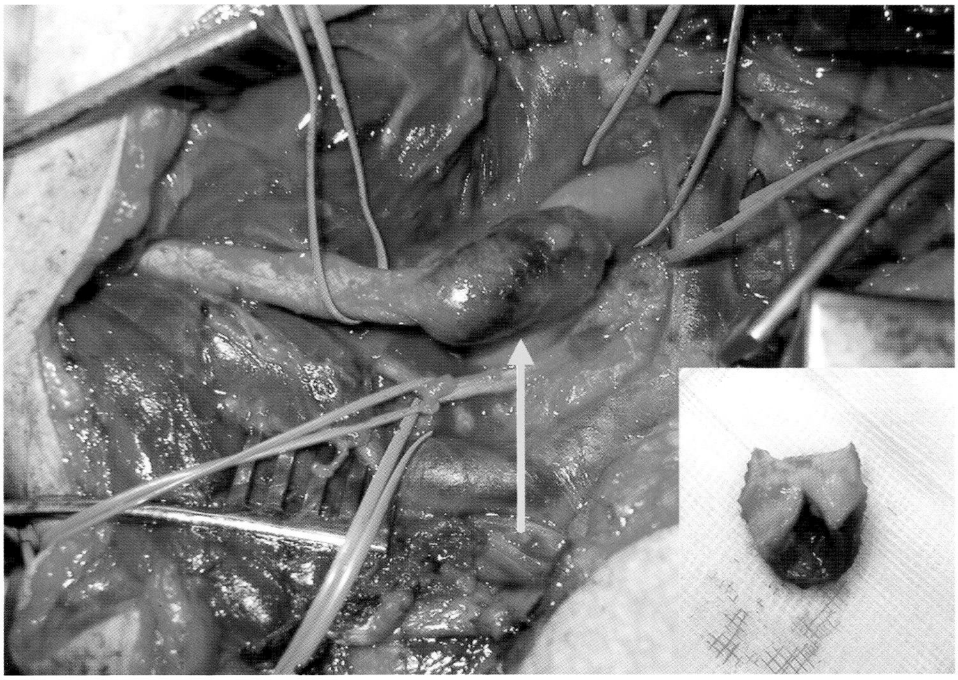

Figure 1. Traumatic false aneurysm (arrowed) arising from the origin of the right common carotid artery due to a deceleration injury in a high speed road traffic accident. The innominate vein and artery can be seen immediately to the right of the aneurysm. The resection specimen (bottom right) shows the upper extent of the split in the common carotid arterial wall giving rise to the aneurysm.

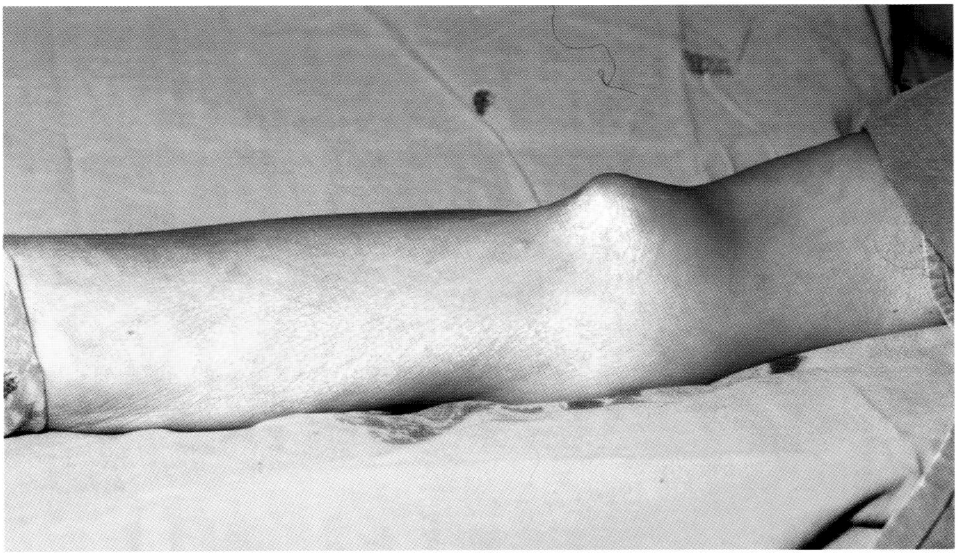

Figure 2. Right brachial artery false aneurysm following long-term arterial cannulation in intensive care.

aneurysm develops which, if left untreated, may rupture days or even months later.

Clinical presentation

Iatrogenic false aneurysms often present soon after arterial catheterisation and are usually associated with common femoral artery cannulation. Frequently, they are associated with considerable haematoma around the puncture site and present with a tender, palpable groin mass (Figure 3). The presence or absence of pulsation in the mass is not a reliable indicator of the likelihood of a false aneurysm, and clinical examination is often impaired by pain associated with the haematoma. On occasion, compression of the femoral vein by a femoral false aneurysm leads to leg swelling, and arterial compression can lead to ischaemic symptoms. More common, however, is ischaemic change in the overlying skin, secondary to pressure from a large false aneurysm.

Late presentation with a painless pulsatile mass is common in traumatic false aneurysms arising at other sites, either secondary to arterial catheterisation (Figure 2) or to traumatic arterial injury. Similarly, anastomotic false aneurysms tend to present as a painless groin swelling in a patient with a history of arterial surgery involving a groin anastomosis (Figure 4). Some may have clinical features suggestive of infection and this should always be borne in mind when treating anastomotic aneurysms. In general, the incidence of anastomotic false aneurysms increases with the time after the original surgery. False aneurysms (traumatic, anastomotic, and iatrogenic) arising from major vessels such as the aorta or its arch vessels are often asymptomatic until they become large enough to produce pressure effects on surrounding structures. Symptoms then vary with the surrounding structures involved and are often non-specific.

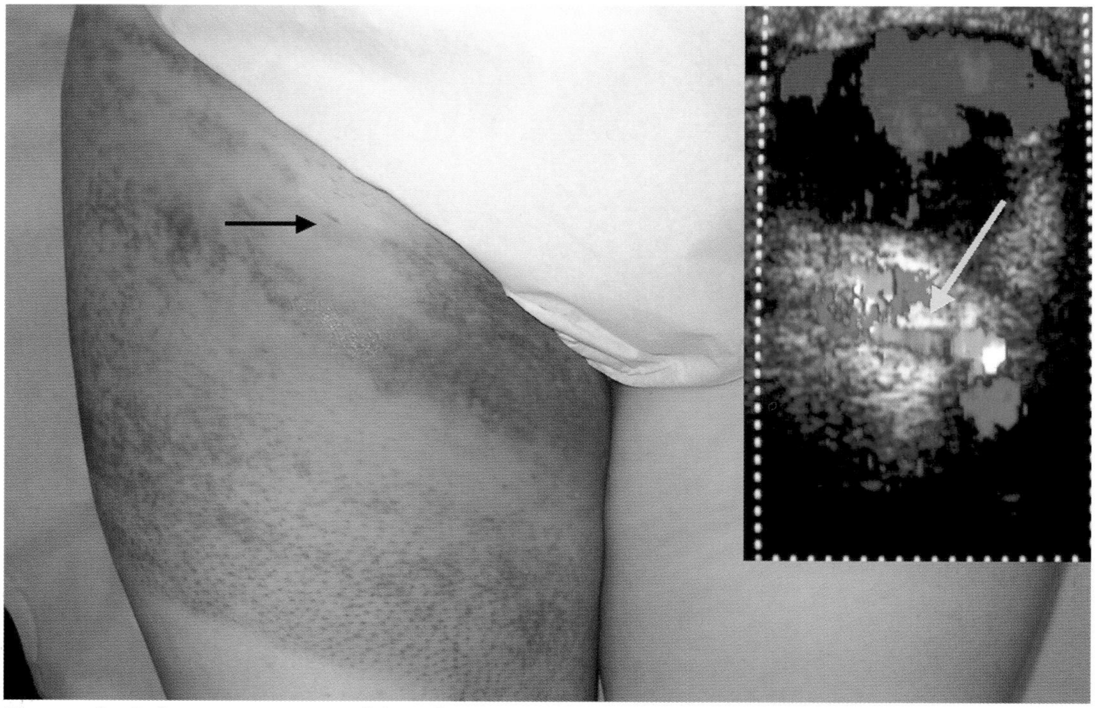

Figure 3. False aneurysm arising from the common femoral artery following cardiac catheterisation. Clinical appearance with resolving haematoma is typical and the puncture site can clearly be seen (black arrow). Colour duplex of this false aneurysm shows the communicating tract (yellow arrow) from the native vessel (bottom right of image) to the false aneurysm sac (top of image).

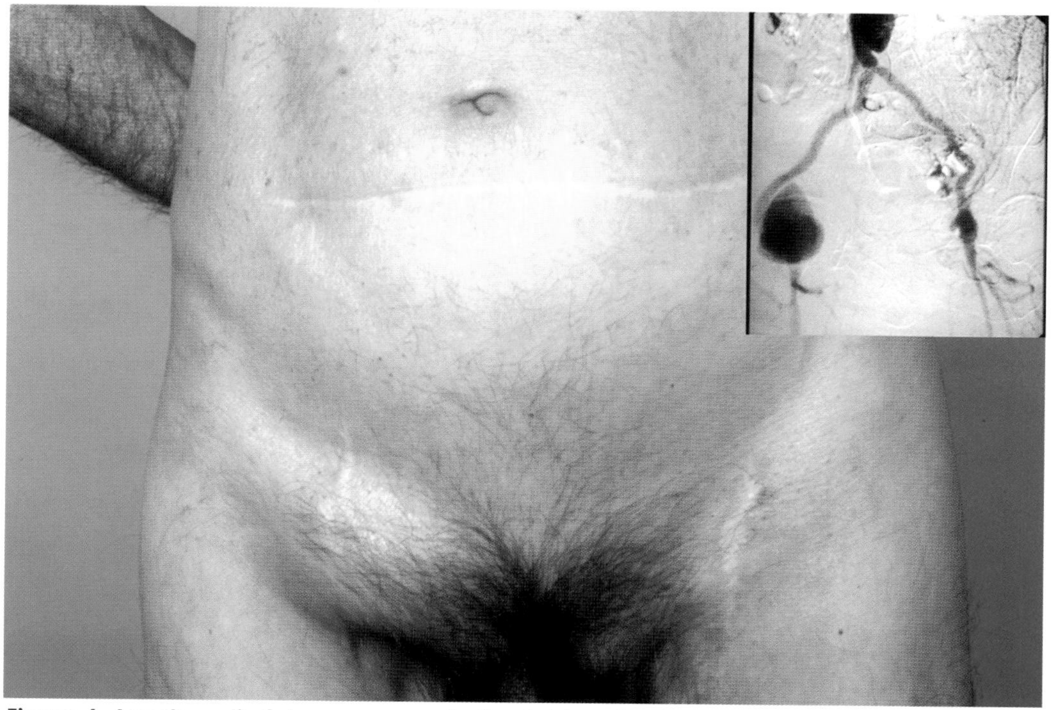

Figure 4. Anastomotic false aneurysm in the right groin. The scars are from aortobifemoral grafting and the angiogram appearance confirms the presence of false aneurysms at all the anastomoses.

Haemorrhage from false aneurysms can occur as the aneurysm expands; it is more often associated with infected false aneurysms, or occult traumatic false aneurysms arising from vessels such as the aorta, where the aneurysm can reach a considerable size without detection.

Diagnosis

While history and clinical examination may point to the diagnosis of an arterial false aneurysm, colour duplex ultrasound imaging is the ideal investigation to confirm the diagnosis (Figure 3), identify the site of underlying arterial injury, the patency of inflow and outflow vessels, and also the morphology of the false aneurysm. The latter will influence the treatment options available. Unless the false aneurysm is associated with limb ischaemia, arteriography is only recommended prior to reconstructive surgery for anastomotic false aneurysms. While some surgeons are happy to proceed on the basis of duplex imaging alone, a formal angiogram may assist operative decision-making in what can become complex revision surgery.

False aneurysms arising from the abdominal aorta or pelvic vessels are best imaged by CT, where they are often found incidentally on scans undertaken in the investigation of other abdominal symptoms (Figure 5).

Clinical management

Some iatrogenic aneurysms will thrombose spontaneously, although predicting which will resolve without intervention is unreliable [7]. Small false aneurysms (less than 2cm) can be followed-up with weekly ultrasound surveillance until either thrombosis or expansion takes place. Drawbacks of this course of action include the resource implications and the length of time until resolution. Spontaneous resolution is unlikely in patients on anticoagulant or antiplatelet

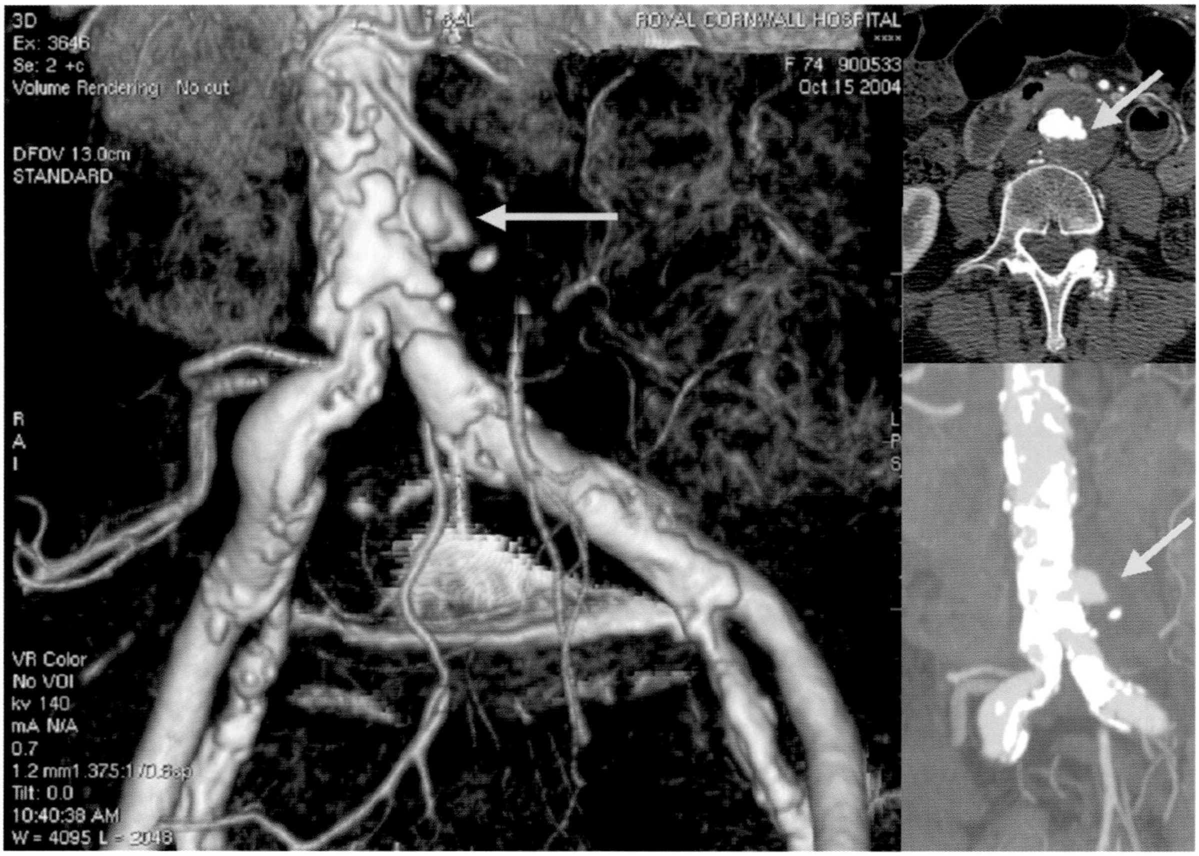

Figure 5. CT with multiplanar colour reconstruction showing an aortic false aneurysm (arrowed) arising from a ruptured atherosclerotic plaque. The false aneurysm and surrounding haematoma is shown more clearly (arrowed) on the coronal and axial images (right).

therapy, where the false aneurysm is over 3cm in diameter, and when there is continued expansion of the aneurysm following initial diagnosis.

If circumstances preclude spontaneous thrombosis, ultrasound-guided compression may be used in an attempt to induce thrombosis in false aneurysms following catheterisation. First described in 1991 [8], this technique aims to occlude the communication between the true arterial lumen, and the false aneurysm sac, by direct compression of the tract. Direct pressure is maintained for 10 minutes (20 minutes in those on anticoagulants), then released slowly. The process is repeated until no flow is observed in the sac. This can, however, take over 2 hours to achieve! The technique is contra-indicated when there is suspected infection, overlying skin necrosis, pressure symptoms on the femoral artery or nerve, limb ischaemia, a puncture site above the inguinal ligament, severe tenderness preventing adequate compression and injuries more than 1 month old. Success rates between 63-88% [2] have been reported. Current anticoagulation, presence of arteriovenous fistula, aneurysm diameter over 4cm and a site other than the common femoral artery are all associated with a high failure rate. If successful, however, the recurrence rate at 24 hours is under 5%, and few complications of the technique have been reported.

Recently, percutaneous thrombin injection has been advocated as a means of successfully occluding false aneurysms resulting from catheterisation [2,7]. The various techniques used are described elsewhere [2], but in essence involve the direct inoculation of between 500-1000 IU of thrombin into the false aneurysm sac. Although bovine thrombin can be used, there is a risk of anaphylaxis, so reconstituted human thrombin is preferred. Technical success is in the region of 90-100% for this technique, and does not seem to be affected adversely by concurrent anticoagulant therapy. Procedure times are considerably shorter than for ultrasound-guided compression. Complications arise from the escape of thrombin into the native circulation. This results in distal embolisation in up to 2% of procedures, although this is rarely clinically significant.

Operative management

Ultimately, a number of false aneurysms will require operative surgery. Clear indications for operative intervention are:

- a rapidly expanding aneurysm;
- haemodynamic instability or proven rupture;
- an infected false aneurysm;
- distal ischaemia due to pressure on the femoral artery;
- neuropathy caused by local pressure on the femoral nerve;
- failed percutaneous treatment; or
- skin necrosis over the false aneurysm.

Ideally, surgery should be undertaken as an elective procedure, although urgent surgery may occasionally be required for rupture. The surgical treatment of most false aneurysms follows standard vascular techniques, with control of proximal and distal vessels (inflow and outflow vessels) being obtained before approaching the false aneurysm. This gives controlled incision into the aneurysm sac and is followed by interposition grafting or direct repair to reconstruct the vessel. Variations in this technique depend on the underlying aetiology of the aneurysm, the most important factor in decision-making being the presence or absence of infection.

Infected false aneurysms

Infected false aneurysms require aggressive antibiotic therapy based on the results of blood cultures. In injecting drug users, broad-spectrum therapy is required [5], while in others therapy should be directed against the commonest pathogens: *Staphylococcus aureus* and *Salmonella* species. In all cases therapy should continue for at least 6 weeks. At operation, control of healthy proximal and distal arteries is required, then the infected aneurysm sac should be excised, along with surrounding infected and necrotic tissue. The risks inherent in then placing an interposition graft into an infected field is such that only autologous vein (preferably passed through healthy tissue remote from the site of infection) should be employed to minimise the risks of anastomotic disruption and postoperative haemorrhage. Because of this risk, a policy of excision and ligation of the infected false aneurysm, with subsequent revascularisation where there is postoperative threat to the limb, is justified [5]. Patients with infected false aneurysms due to drug injection who undergo common femoral artery ligation alone have a low rate of subsequent amputation, whereas ligation of all three groin vessels (common, superficial and deep femoral) carries a greater threat to the leg. In this group of patients, only a small minority require revascularisation, although most will develop claudication. The overall risk of limb loss following surgery for an infected femoral pseudo-aneurysm is approximately 10-20%, although when triple femoral vessel ligation is required this may be as high as 33% [5]. While the literature concentrates on infected femoral false aneurysms, the principles outlined can be applied to any infected false aneurysm.

Traumatic and post-catheterisation aneurysms

As with most false aneurysms, obtaining proximal and distal control early in the procedure will greatly assist in the operative management of traumatic false aneurysms. Thereafter, the surgeon can pursue the dissection of the aneurysm sac with impunity. For large femoral aneurysms, this may require control of the external iliac artery through a small incision above the inguinal ligament with an extraperitoneal dissection. Once isolated, the sac is opened and any thrombus removed. At this stage it may be possible to repair the underlying arterial defect (Figure 6) with a couple of sutures. These must be placed longitudinally to avoid creating a stenosis. In situations where the underlying arterial defect is too large, or the vessel is damaged too severely to allow primary closure, then

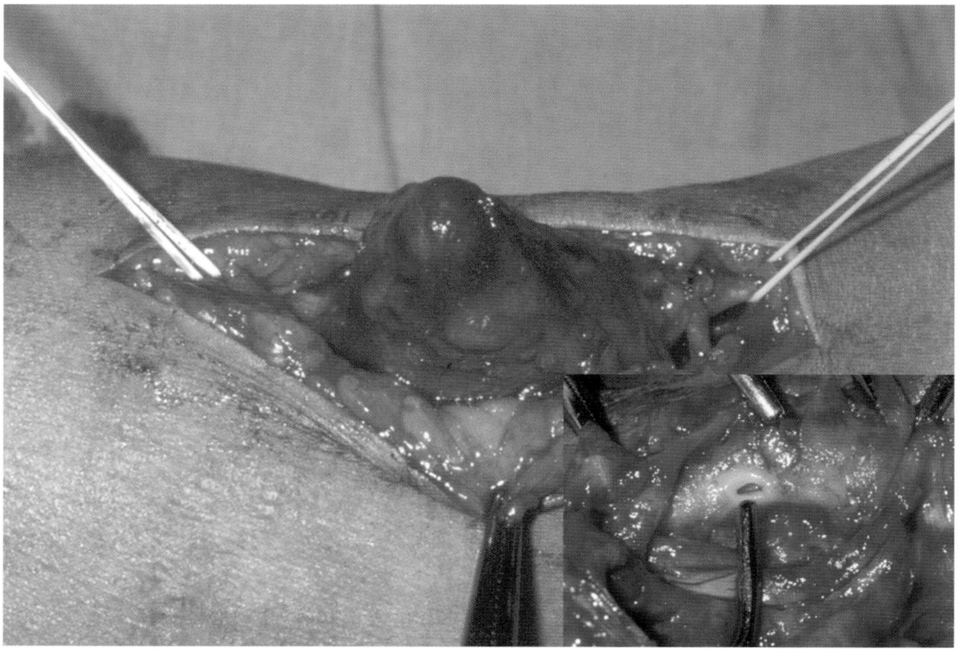

Figure 6. Dissection of the longstanding brachial false aneurysm shown in Figure 2, with proximal and distal control enabling the sac to be opened and the longstanding defect in the arterial wall to be visualised and repaired.

patch repair with either a synthetic or vein patch would be appropriate after performing an arteriotomy and resection of the damaged artery. In cases where the vessel has been completely transected or where the underlying cause has been a blunt or deceleration injury, then resection of the damaged segment with interposition grafting may be required. Blunt injury often damages the artery quite extensively, and all the intimal damage should be resected, with anastomosis to healthy artery. Prosthetic material or autologous vein can be employed as a graft in these situations where the risk of infection is deemed to be minimal, and with appropriate attention to technique the results should be extremely good.

As an alternative to the (sometimes) extensive dissection required to obtain proximal and distal control of a false aneurysm, a more direct technique can be employed, whereby the dissection is taken right down onto the false aneurysm from the outset, the sac opened, and direct digital pressure used to control the defect in the artery before placing the necessary sutures. This technique works best for false aneurysms after arterial catheterisation, where the bleeding point is usually easily sutured. It is still advisable to have an assistant present to occlude arterial flow while sutures are placed. Alternatively, a balloon occlusion catheter can be placed through the arterial defect and inflated against the vessel wall to occlude the bleeding point while it is sutured. For larger defects, occlusion catheters placed proximally and distally will ensure a bloodless field while arterial repair is undertaken.

Anastomotic aneurysms

The operative management of anastomotic false aneurysms is the same as for any other false aneurysm, with proximal and distal control obtained by approaching the vessels through fresh tissue immediately adjacent to the operative scar. In end-to-side anastomoses, both the native vessel and graft limb need to be isolated to obtain proximal control. As tissue planes are often absent around the false aneurysm and prosthetic graft, early control is advised. Once the aneurysm is dissected out the sac should be opened after applying clamps to proximal and distal vessels. Occlusion catheters placed from within the sac can then control any back bleeding vessels. This step is often required to control the profunda femoris artery, which can be difficult to identify and isolate in the postoperative groin; in multiple re-do procedures this method may be the only way to identify and control all the vessels involved in the false aneurysm.

No attempt should be made to repair the defect giving rise to an anastomotic aneurysm. The recommended course of action is to excise the old anastomosis and insert a new interposition graft between the limb of the old graft and the femoral artery. It is not necessary to excise the sac, as there is a risk of damage to the adjacent femoral nerve. The excised anastomosis should be sent for microbiological examination, as infection may have been the cause of the aneurysm developing. This method has a 90% cure rate for anastomotic aneurysms. For the 10% that recur, re-operation using the same principles also has a 90% cure rate, as long as infection has been excluded.

Endovascular methods

Endovascular techniques offer a method of treating more complex false aneurysms without the need for major surgery. They can be valuable for the treatment of post-traumatic thoracic pseudo-aneurysms, as well as anastomotic [9] and other aortic false aneurysms (Figure 7). Endovascular techniques will doubtless be employed to treat an increasing range of false aneurysms in the near future, but there remain considerable concerns about their use where there may be an infective component to the false aneurysm, particularly where alternative operative therapy that doesn't involve introducing prosthetic material is available.

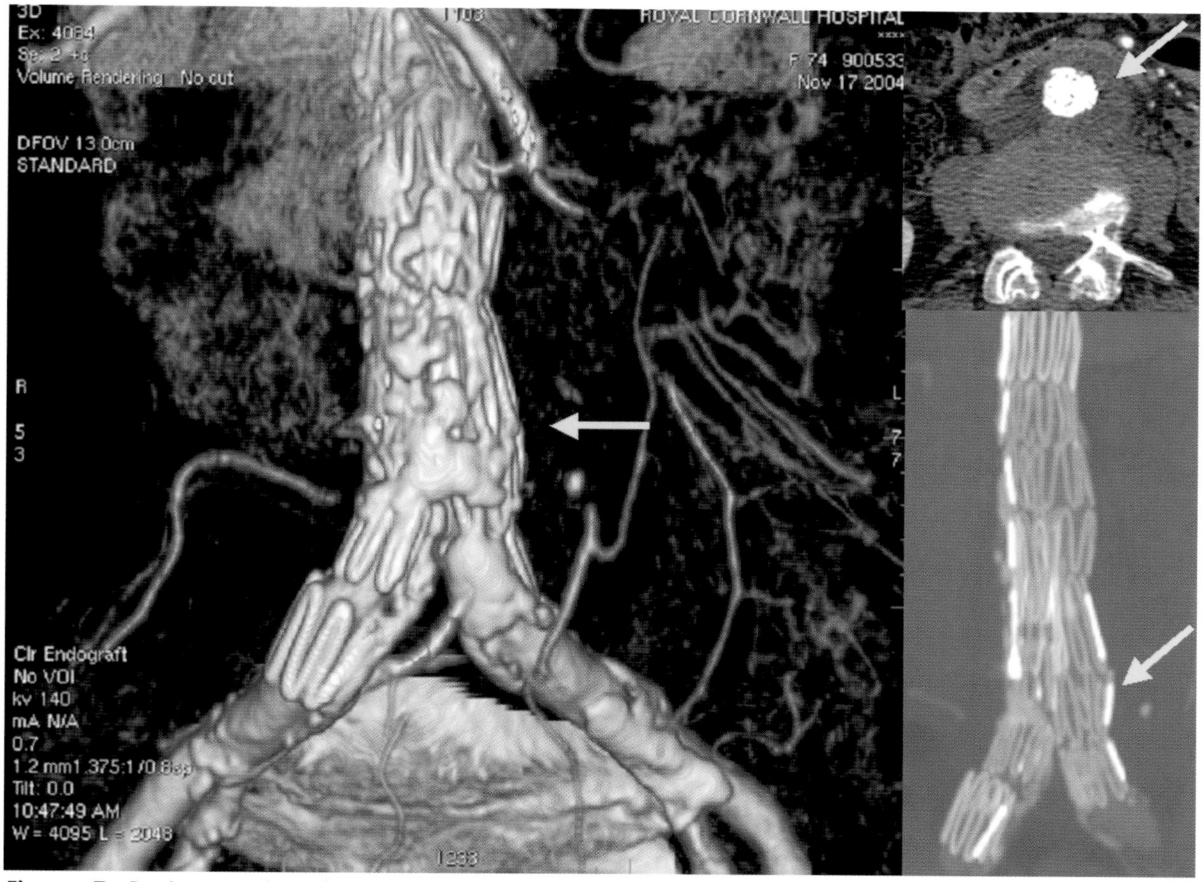

Figure 7. Post-procedure images from the patient illustrated in Figure 5, showing a bifurcated endovascular aortic prosthesis placed to occlude the aortic false aneurysm. The haematoma associated with the false aneurysm is shown on the coronal and axial images (arrowed).

Acknowledgements

The author would like to thank Dr Simon Travis, Dr John Hancock, Consultant Vascular Radiologists, and Daniella Bond, Vascular technologist (all Royal Cornwall Hospitals Trust) for their assistance in obtaining a number of the images used to illustrate this chapter.

Key points

- **Colour duplex imaging is the investigation of choice for false aneurysms, as up to 25% are non-pulsatile on clinical assessment.**
- **Most false aneurysms that occur after femoral artery catheterisation can be treated radiologically with ultrasound-guided therapies, or injected thrombin.**
- **Anastomotic aneurysms should be treated by resection and bypass. Specimens from the operation should be sent for microbiological examination to exclude an infective cause. Balloon occlusion catheters are valuable to control the vessels around the aneurysm.**
- **Infected aneurysms, particularly in drug injecters, can be treated by vessel ligation alone. Reconstruction is only required if the limb becomes critically ischaemic.**
- **Endovascular methods are increasingly used for the treatment of a variety of false aneurysms, although long-term follow-up is not yet available.**

References

1. Woodburn KR, Murie JA. Vascular complications of injecting drug misuse. *Br J Surg* 1996; 83: 1329-34.
2. Morgan R, Belli A-M. Current treatment methods for postcatheterisation aneurysms. *J Vasc Intervent Radiol* 2003; 14: 696-710.
3. Norwood MGA, Lloyd GM, Moore S, *et al.* The changing face of femoral false aneurysms. *Eur J Vasc Endovasc Surg* 2004; 27: 385-8.
4. Benitez PR, Newell MA. Vascular trauma in drug abuse: patterns of injury. *Ann Vasc Surg* 1986; 1: 175-81.
5. Reddy DJ, Smith RF, Elliot JP, *et al.* Infected femoral artery false aneurysms in drug addicts: evolution of selective vascular reconstruction. *J Vasc Surg* 1986; 3: 718-24.
6. Vasquez J, Poultsides GA, Lorenzo AC, *et al.* Endovascular stent-graft placement for nonaneurysmal aortic rupture: a case report and review of the literature. *J Vasc Surg* 2003; 38: 836-9.
7. Franklin JA, Brigham D, Bogey WM. Treatment of iatrogenic false aneurysms. *J Am Coll Surg* 2003; 197: 293-301.
8. Fellmeth BD, Roberts AC, Bookstein JJ, *et al.* Postangiographic femoral artery injuries: nonsurgical repair with US-guided compression. *Radiology* 1991; 178: 671-5.
9. Magnan PE, Albertini JN, Bartoli JM, *et al.* Endovascular treatment of anastomotic false aneurysms of the abdominal aorta. *Ann Vasc Surg* 2003; 17: 365-74.

Chapter 41

Buerger's disease

Denis W Harkin MD FRCS (Gen Surg) EBSQ-VASC, Consultant Vascular Surgeon
Royal Victoria Hospital, Belfast, Northern Ireland

Introduction

Buerger's disease (thrombo-angiitis obliterans) is a non-atherosclerotic segmental inflammatory disease of medium and small-sized arteries and veins, principally affecting the upper and lower extremities. In 1908, Leo Buerger described the pathology of "a strange endarteritis and endophlebitis with gangrene of the feet" in 11 amputated legs, coining the term "thrombo-angiitis obliterans" for the disease that now bears his name [1]. von Winiwarter may have described the same process some 29 years earlier. This non-atherosclerotic occlusive disease is commonest among young men, were it is strongly associated with tobacco smoking. The disease has a geographical predisposition for the southeast Mediterranean and the Middle and Far East; it is becoming increasingly rare in western countries. It remains the most prevalent vascular disease in some Asian countries and has a high incidence among the Jewish population [2] (Figure 1).

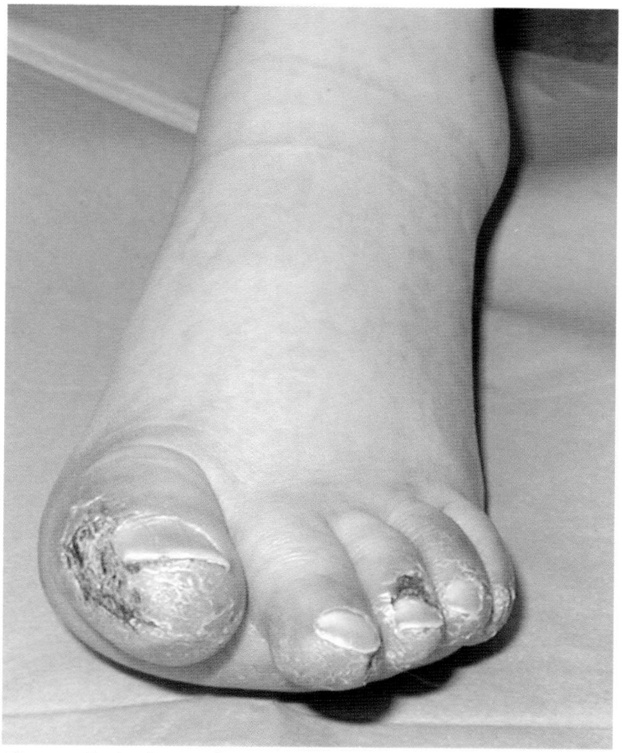

Figure 1. Ischaemic ulcers on the toes in a patient with Buerger's disease. The patient also had superficial thrombophlebitis on the dorsum of the foot.

Aetiopathology

Buerger's disease has a wide geographical variation in incidence, and amongst those presenting with extremity arterial disease the diagnosis is up to ten times more likely in Asia and the Indian subcontinent compared to Western Europe or North America [3]. In Europe and North America the prevalence of the disease, or at the very least its diagnosis, has been in decline in recent years in contrast to Indo-Asia where it remains the leading cause of peripheral vascular disease. Prevalence rates of Buerger's disease in patients with peripheral arterial occlusive disease range from 0.5-5.6% in Western European countries, to 45-63% in India, and 16-66% in Asia and the Far East (Korea and Japan). Perhaps the best population data come from Japan where the nationwide surveys estimate there are approximately 9,000 patients with the disease representing an incidence of 5 per 100,000 of the population. Recent reports suggest it is a disease in decline, even in a previously high prevalence area like Japan [4]. Historically the incidence of Buerger's disease in women has been low (1-2%); however, in recent North American reports the incidence has been as high as 23% [2].

Buerger's disease has unknown aetiology, but is undoubtedly an inflammatory vasculitis, perhaps triggered by a hypersensitivity to constituents of tobacco. It differs from other vasculitis in that the occlusive thrombus has a high inflammatory cell infiltrate with relative sparing of the vessel wall. In particular, a prominent T-cell immune inflammatory response plays a significant role [5]. Although inherent defects in immunological response are suspected in Buerger's disease, typically serum inflammatory markers and auto-antibodies are not detected. The incidence is much higher in countries with high rates of tobacco consumption. The use of unprocessed tobacco such as Bidi smoking in Bangladesh (homemade cigarettes with raw tobacco) may be more harmful than cigarette smoking. The use of unprocessed tobacco, with high nicotine and tar content, remains common in many developing countries and this may explain the high incidence of Buerger's disease in Bangladesh, India and Java. Although a causative link has not been established, there is a definite relationship between tobacco use and exacerbation and remission of the disease. Recreational drug use has also been implicated in the development of Buerger's disease, though whilst cannabis is often combined with tobacco, links to other drugs such as cocaine are tenuous.

The fact that most smokers do not develop Buerger's disease has prompted some to look for a genetic predisposition, with tobacco being the trigger. Several authors have looked at patterns in Human Leukocyte Antigen (HLA) halotypes, albeit with considerable variability in results. In high prevalence areas such as India and Japan, there is a strong association with HLA-DRB1*1501. A statistically significantly higher frequency of HLA-DR4 and a lower frequency of the HLA-DRW6 antigen has been found in patients with Buerger's disease; however, in North America, no distinctive pattern in HLA halotypes has been found. There is an association between Buerger's disease and a mutation on the prothrombin 20210 gene. Other studies have focused on the possibility of prothrombotic genetic factors.

There is mounting evidence that alterations in auto-immune responses play a role in Buerger's disease. Recent reports suggest a link between this disease and other antiphospholipid antibody syndromes. Serum auto-antibodies have been studied in patients with Buerger's disease, but there was no evidence of several commonly tested auto-antibodies (cANCA, pANCA, antinuclear antibodies, anti-Ro, anti-cardiolipin antibodies). In patients with active disease, elevated levels of anti-endothelial cell antibodies were detected. There are altered haemorrheological factors contributing to thrombosis [6]; however, no single aetiological mechanism pertains. Buerger's disease would appear to be a combination of tobacco sensitivity with underlying genetic predisposition and abnormal immunological, endothelial, and coagulation responses.

Buerger's disease is a non-atherosclerotic inflammatory occlusive disease of the arteries and veins, with the histopathological features most pronounced in the acute phase of disease activity. Affecting the medium and small vessels it has a segmental distribution with skip areas of normal vessels between diseased ones. Involvement of large arteries is unusual and rarely occurs in the absence of small-vessel occlusive disease [7]. Although principally a disease of the arms and legs, Buerger's disease has also been reported in the medium and small vessels of the cerebral, coronary, renal, gonadal and mesenteric vessels. Specimens are most often obtained from amputated tissue (Figure 2), although, biopsy of a

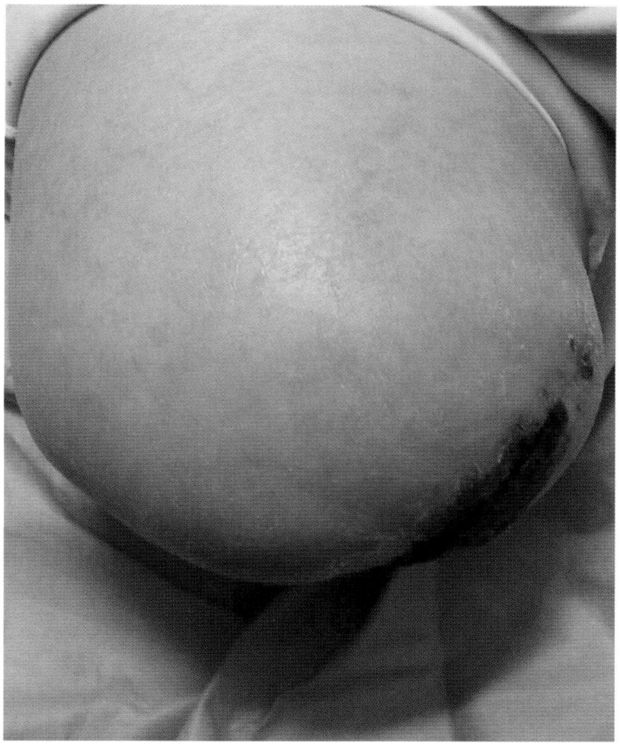

Figure 2. Above-knee amputation for intractable gangrene of the right lower leg. Persistent smoking led to the development of recurrent ischaemic necrosis of the stump.

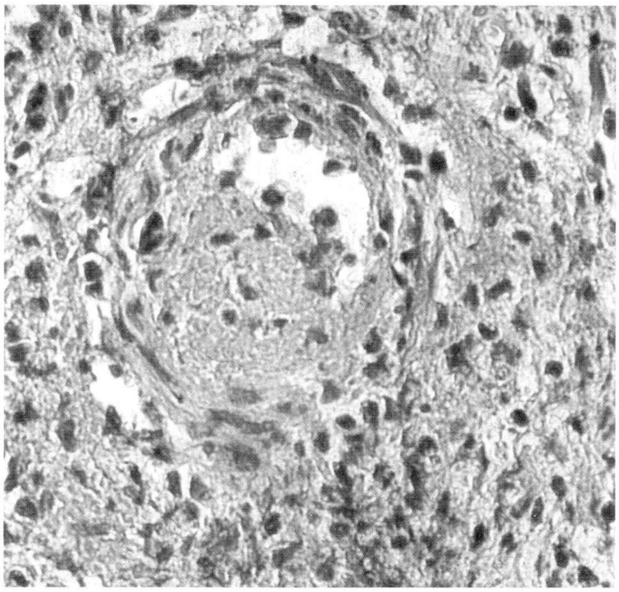

Figure 3. Histological slide of a digital artery in the intermediate stage of Buerger's disease, (H&E, X50). Note the prominent inflammatory infiltrate and early organisation of the thrombus.

superficial inflamed vein may aid diagnosis. Biopsy specimens should be avoided in ischaemic limbs due to the risk of producing a non-healing wound. Biopsy in the acute phase demonstrates acute inflammation involving all layers of the vessel wall, especially of veins, in association with occlusive thrombus (Figure 3). The thrombus has a dense inflammatory cell infiltrate which is most marked at the periphery, with polymorphonuclear leukocytes with karyorrhexis, or micro-abcesses, in which one or more multinucleate giant cells may be present. In the intermediate phase there is progressive organisation of the thrombus, and at this stage the thrombus has a more prominent inflammatory infiltrate with less inflammation seen in the vessel wall. The chronic phase shows further thrombus organisation, perhaps with recanalisation, and prominent vascularisation of the medial, adventitial and peri-adventitial layers. Interestingly, the elastic lamina is preserved unlike in other forms of vasculitis. This process leads to the formation of hypertrophied vasa-vasoral vessels with their typical corkscrew appearance on angiography. Although a distinct disease process, Buerger's disease may be found in co-existence with atherosclerosis, particularly in the older patient.

Diagnosis and investigation

The classical presentation of Buerger's disease is in a young male smoker with onset of symptoms before the age of 50 years. The distal vessels of the arms and legs are affected. The incidence in women and the elderly is increasing substantially [8]. Patients may present with claudication of the feet (typically the arch of the foot), the legs, and occasionally the arms and hands. Later, ischaemic ulceration of the extremities may supervene, and progress to distal gangrene (Figures 1 & 2). The commonest signs and symptoms in three large series are displayed in Table 1. The largest available study on 825 patients with Buerger's disease found 42 patients (5%) with arm arterial involvement only, 616 (75%) with leg involvement only, and 167 (20%) with both. The most frequently affected arteries were the anterior (41%) or posterior (40%) tibial arteries in the legs, and the ulnar artery (11.5%) in the arms [4]. In particular, a young patient presenting with early onset of advanced peripheral vascular disease and associated superficial

Table 1. Common symptoms and signs in Buerger's disease. Modified from Olin *et al* [2], Sasaki *et al* [4], and Wysokinski *et al* [8].

	Olin	Sasaki	Wysokinski
Demographics			
Number of patients	112	850	377
Mean age (years)	42	40	30
Signs and symptoms (%)			
Intermittent claudication	63	62	89
Rest pain	81	38	85
Ischaemic ulcers	76	45	-
Thrombophlebitis	38	16	62
Raynaud's phenomenon	44	-	10
Coldness/cyanosis/paraesthesia	69	-	-

Table 2. Suggested scoring system for the diagnosis of Buerger's disease. Modified from Papa *et al* [11].

A. Positive points		
Age at onset	Less than 30/30-40 years	+2/ +1
Foot claudication	Present/by history	+2/ +1
Arm involvement	Symptomatic/asymptomatic	+2/ +1
Migrating phlebitis	Present/by history only	+2/ +1
Raynaud's phenomenon	Present/by history only	+2/ +1
Angiography; biopsy	If typical, both/either	+2/ +1
B. Negative points		
Age at onset	45-50/more than 50 years	-1/ -2
Sex, smoking	Female/non-smoker	-1/ -2
Location	Single limb/leg not involved	-1/ -2
Absent pulses	Brachial/femoral	-1/ -2
ASO, DM, HT, HL	Discovered after diagnosis 5-10 years/2-5 years later	-1/ -2

Summary of points from A and B defines probability of the diagnosis of Buerger's disease

Number of points	Probability of diagnosis
0-1	Diagnosis excluded
2-3	Suspected, low probability
4-5	Probable, medium probability
6 or more	Definite, high probability

ASO=arteriosclerosis obliterans; DM=diabetes mellitus; HT=hypertension; HL=hyperlipidaemia

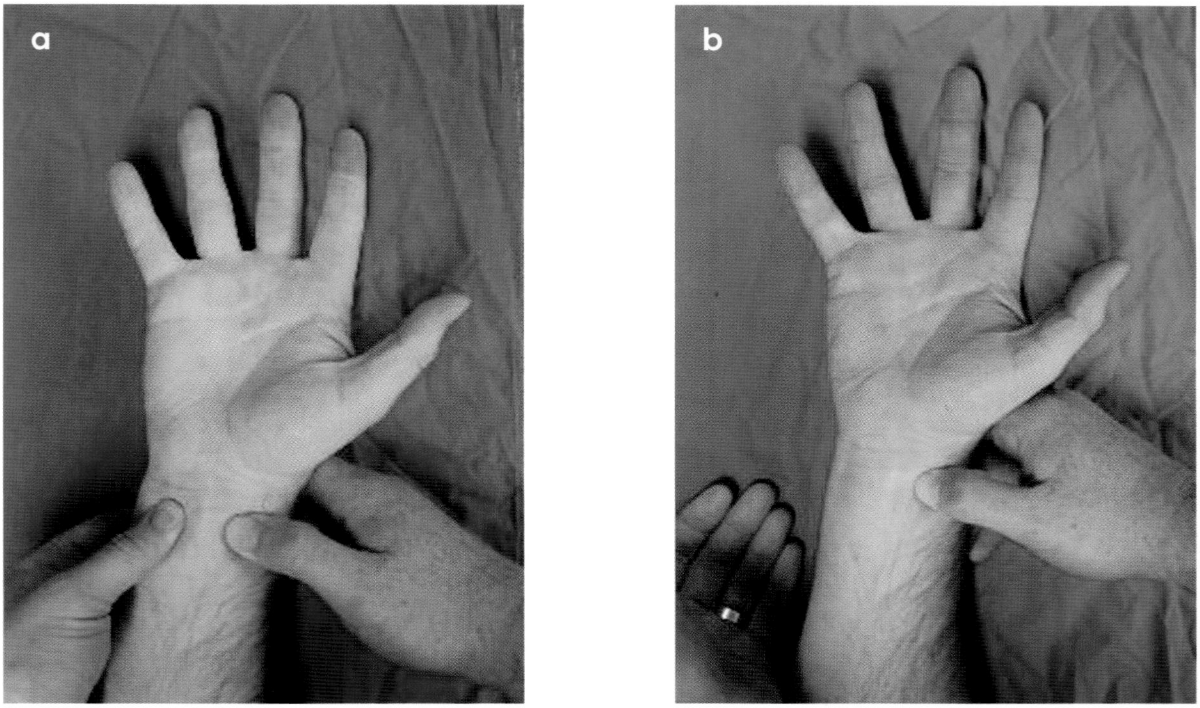

Figure 4. Allen's test is used to assess the integrity of the circulation to the hand. a) The patient makes a fist to empty blood from the hand, the clinician places thumbs over the radial and ulnar arteries, and the patient then opens the hand. b) The clinician releases the thumb pressure from one of the arteries while still compressing the other. If the hand does not fill with blood this indicates occlusion of the artery that was not compressed. However, prompt return (as in this case) indicates that the artery is not blocked. Both arteries should be assessed.

thrombophlebitis, is almost exclusive to Buerger's disease. A high index of suspicion must be exercised in any young patient with severe symptoms or signs, particularly in the absence of end-stage renal disease or diabetes.

In practice the provisional diagnosis of Buerger's disease is based on the five clinical criteria proposed by Shionoya [9]: smoking history, onset before age 50 years, infrapopliteal arterial occlusive disease, either arm involvement or thrombophlebitis migrans, and the absence of atherosclerotic risk factors other than smoking. Mills and Porter have proposed major and minor diagnostic criteria [10]. Furthermore, Papa and Adar have proposed various clinical, angiographic, and histopathological criteria and even a scoring system to aid diagnosis [11] (Table 2).

Clinical assessment should include a complete history including smoking history, use of recreational drugs and questioning about pain, particularly intermittent claudication and rest pain. A complete neurological and vascular assessment must be performed especially of the leg where the vascular system is compromised in most patients; the symptoms in the arm affect approximately half of all patients [8]. Pedal pulses are often absent whereas the proximal pulses (except the arm pulses) are present in most patients with this disease. An Allen's test of the feet and hands should be performed, as an abnormal test in a young smoker is highly suggestive of Buerger's disease (Figure 4).

Investigation

Although there are no specific diagnostic laboratory tests for Buerger's disease, exclusion of other vascular disease such as atherosclerosis, emboli, and autoimmune disease, is an important initial step. These should include the following: acute phase reactants (erythrocyte sedimentation rate and C-reactive protein), antinuclear antibody, rheumatoid factor, complement measurements, serological markers for CREST syndrome (Calcinosis, Raynaud's phenomenon, oEsophageal disease, Sclerodactyly, Telangiectasia) and scleroderma (anticentromere antibody and Scl-70), and a complete hypercoagulability screen, including antiphospholipid antibodies.

Non-invasive Doppler pulse volume and waveform analysis should confirm the diagnosis of arterial insufficiency. Furthermore, segmental pressures and waveforms demonstrate the distal vessel disease with relative sparing of proximal vessels. When two or more limbs are affected an echocardiogram is indicated to exclude a proximal embolic source. This may be supplemented by interrogation of the proximal large vessels and distal run-off using any combination of several diagnostic modalities now available, which may include digital subtraction arteriography (DSA), computerised tomography angiography (CTA) and magnetic resonance angiography (MRA).

Angiography remains the most useful to aid diagnosis, demonstrating normal non-atherosclerotic proximal arteries, with distal disease affecting the small and medium-sized vessels. Buerger's disease is characterised by segmental occlusive disease interspersed with normal-appearing vessels often with "corkscrew" collaterals bridging the gaps. Typical arteriographic features used for diagnosis have been described by Olin and colleagues [2] as follows:

- Involvement of small and medium-sized vessels such as the digital arteries in the fingers and toes and the palmar, plantar, tibial, peroneal, radial, and ulnar arteries.
- Segmental occlusive lesions with areas of diseased arteries interspersed with areas of normal-appearing arteries.
- Evidence of more severe disease distally.
- Evidence of collateralisation around areas of occlusion (corkscrew collaterals).
- Proximal arterial segments with no evidence of atherosclerosis and no arteriographic evidence of arterial emboli.

Perhaps the most characteristic feature of Buerger's disease is corkscrew-shaped vessels, representing dilated vasa vasorum of the occluded main arteries. In one recent study these were present in 39 (27%) of 144 limbs affected by Buerger's disease, whereas this appearance was seen in only two (3%) of 63 limbs in patients with atherosclerosis [12]. Another finding of this study was that corkscrew-shaped vessels that extend from the sites of the arterial occlusion to the periphery of the feet without opacification of the main pedal arteries indicated a poor prognosis. The majority of patients have three or four limbs involved, and even asymptomatic extremities usually have evidence of disease on angiography [3,7].

Histological evidence is most pathognomonic of Buerger's disease in the acute phase when tissue may be available from amputation or biopsy. However, biopsy of areas involved with active disease runs a high risk of non-healing and as such should be discouraged. Pathological specimens typically show:

- thrombus in the artery or vein, with a cellular infiltrate in the vessel wall and in the thrombus itself (usually lymphocytic or polymorphonuclear leucocyte);
- no disruption of the internal elastic lamina (fibrinoid necrosis) with involvement of all layers of the vessel wall;
- significant endothelial cell and fibroblast proliferation in the vessel wall and in the thrombus, with varying degrees of lymphocytic infiltration and occasional giant cells;
- evidence of organisation of the thrombus;
- recanalisation of the vessel, with perivascular fibrosis and vascularisation of the blood vessel wall;
- evidence of collateral and anastomotic vessels;
- focal and segmental lesions that involved the artery, the vein and sometimes the nerve.

None of the above features is pathognomonic and the diagnosis should be made on a combination of

Table 3. Case report.

A 44-year-old woman was admitted as an emergency with acute ischaemia of her left hand (Figure 5). She was a smoker with no other cardiovascular risk factors. She had a history of Raynaud's phenomenon affecting both hands, and claudication affecting both legs. No evidence of auto-immune, vasculitic or embolic disease was noted. On angiographic assessment she had normal proximal vessels, distal small and medium-vessel disease bilaterally, and segmental and distal occlusion of her radial and ulnar arteries at the left wrist (Figure 6). Catheter-directed thrombolysis was attempted for 48 hours; unfortunately, no recanalisation occurred. She underwent a 7-day treatment with intravenous iloprost resulting in stabilisation of her pain and symptoms, and limb preservation. She has stopped smoking and continues to maintain limited function of her left hand.

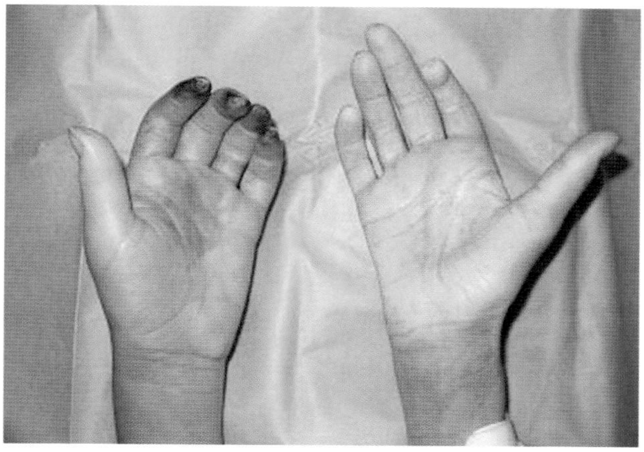

Figure 5. The hands of a patient with Buerger's disease. On the left there is finger-tip ulceration and necrosis. On the right there are chronic trophic changes and Raynaud's phenomenon.

clinical presentation, arteriography, exclusion of confounding processes and, where possible, histology (Table 3). Particular care must be taken in the older patient where atherosclerotic vessel involvement may co-exist with Buerger's disease.

Management

By far the greatest treatment priority in those diagnosed with Buerger's disease is effective smoking cessation. In a longitudinal follow-up study of 120 patients diagnosed with Buerger's disease at the Cleveland Clinic, the incidence of amputation in the patients who stopped smoking was only 6% compared to 43% in those who continued to smoke [2].

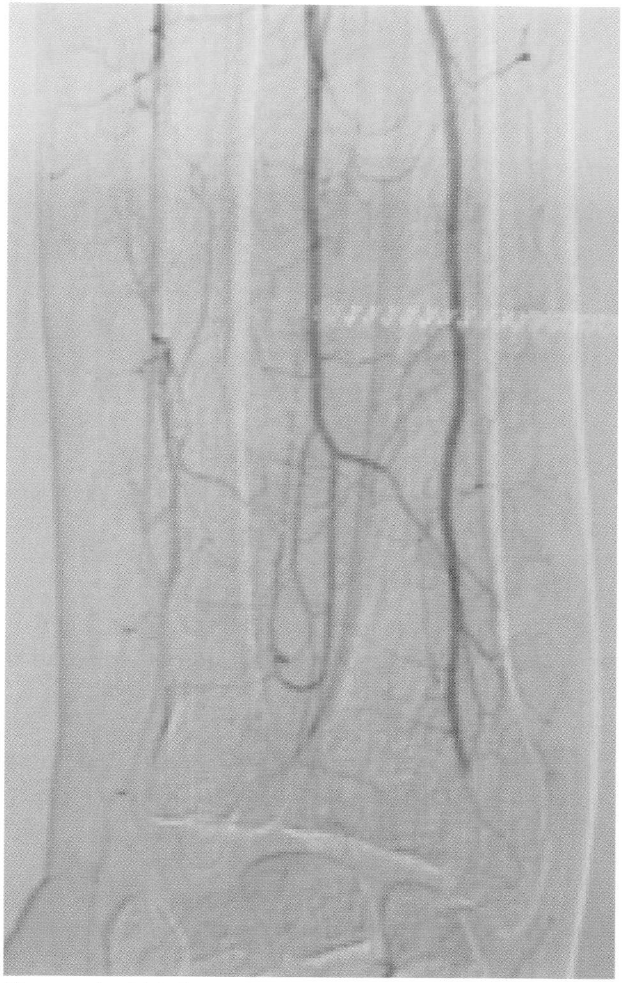

Figure 6. Distal occlusion of the radial and ulnar arteries in a patient with Buerger's disease on digital subtraction angiography.

So strong is the link that if disease activity persists after apparent smoking cessation, supporting evidence of abstinence should be sought, such as urinary nicotine and cotinine levels. Even passive smoking has been implicated in the perpetuation of this process. Patients may need help and counselling to stop smoking and even inpatient management has been suggested [7].

Local measures are important to prevent secondary complications, particularly in areas of ischaemic ulceration or necrosis. Patients should be educated on the need to protect extremities and avoid extremes of temperature. The use of correct fitting footwear is essential to prevent mechanical, thermal or chemical trauma; indeed, one study revealed that approximately 50% of amputations could be traced to a non-healing ulcer from a preventable injury or poor fitting shoes [3].

Pharmacotherapy may include anti-inflammatory agents, vasoactive drugs and prostaglandin analogues. Non-steroidal anti-inflammatory drugs are effective in the short-term relief of thrombophlebitis, but do not have a disease-modifying effect. If significant vasospasm is present, calcium channel blocking agents such as nifedipine should be considered. Similarly, other vasoactive drugs, such as pentoxifylline or cilostazol, may reasonably be tried in patients with critical ischaemia, although there is no good scientific evidence to support their use. Fiessinger and colleagues conducted a prospective randomised double-blind trial comparing intravenous iloprost (a prostaglandin analogue) to aspirin and noted a significant improvement in pain and trophic changes in the iloprost group, and a reduction in amputation rate at 6-month follow-up [13]. A recent prospective randomised trial showed a significant advantage for oral iloprost in relief of pain and freedom from amputation, though no difference in ulcer healing [14].

Analgesia is often a problem in patients with Buerger's disease and standard analgesics are often ineffective. Narcotic analgesics may be required for severe ischaemic pain and even prolonged epidural analgesia is indicated occasionally. Other novel approaches to symptom and pain control have included the use of implanted electrical spinal cord stimulation, which has an analgesic affect and improves skin microcirculation.

Surgery

Sympathectomy, either surgical or chemical, has been tried with success by many authors. There would appear to be evidence that this may at least contribute to pain control and healing of superficial ulceration. Sayin and colleagues reported on 216 patients treated for Buerger's disease of the leg and carried out lumbar sympathectomy in 183 (85%)[15]. Intra-arterial thrombolysis, in particular selective thrombolysis, has its supporters, and there are anecdotal reports of recanalisation of crural vessels using this technique. Surgical revascularisation is often unhelpful due to the distal nature of Buerger's disease and the lack of an identifiable outflow vessel. Inada and colleagues reported in 236 patients with Buerger's disease, but only 11 (4.6%) were amenable to surgical revascularisation [16]. However, in those with critical ischaemia suitable for distal bypass, autologous vein is recommended. Sasajima and colleagues recently reported their experience with 71 infra-inguinal bypasses using autologous vein for critical ischaemia, with 85% to crural vessels. They cited a very respectable primary patency rate of 49% and secondary patency rate of 62.5% at 5 years [17]. In those who stop smoking, patency and limb salvage rates are significantly higher. Omental transfer has been shown by some to achieve limb salvage and significant success in terms of pain control and ulcer healing, but is not widely practised outside Asia. The future may hold new promise with encouraging reports already from small clinical trials on the use of intramuscular gene transfer of vascular endothelial growth factor. In general the treatment of these patients requires combination of several modalities in a specialist centre.

Outcome and complications

Although good evidence on the effect of Buerger's disease on longevity is lacking, it is not generally thought to reduce life-expectancy. However, in those unable to stop smoking the amputation of one or more limbs is inevitable. These patients are also at risk of early onset atherosclerosis, the cardiovascular and cerebrovascular complications of which will certainly hasten death. In those who stop smoking their future prospects are reassuringly good [18].

Key points

- Buerger's disease is a rare non-atherosclerotic inflammatory vasculitis affecting the small and medium-sized vessels.
- Affecting primarily young men who smoke, it is an uncommon cause of peripheral arterial disease in Western Europe and North America, but remains common in Indo-Asia.
- Tobacco consumption is intimately related to disease activity, and smoking cessation remains the cornerstone of treatment.
- Prognosis is favourable in those who stop smoking, but in those who continue, amputation of one or more limbs is likely.

References

1. Buerger L. Thrombo-angiitis obliterans: a study of the vascular lesion leading to pre-senile spontaneous gangrene. *Am J Med Sci* 1908; 136: 567-80.
2. Olin JW, Young JR, Graor RA, Ruschhaupt WF, Bartholomew JR. The changing clinical spectrum of thromboangiitis obliterans (Buerger's disease). *Circulation* 1990; 82: IV3-IV8.
3. Szuba A, Cooke JP. Thromboangiitis obliterans. An update on Buerger's disease. *West J Med* 1998; 168: 255-60.
4. Sasaki S, Sakuma M, Yasuda K. Current status of thromboangiitis obliterans (Buerger's disease) in Japan. *Int J Cardiol* 2000; 75: S175-S181.
5. Lee T, Seo JW, Sumpio BE, Kim SJ. Immunobiologic analysis of arterial tissue in Buerger's disease. *Eur J Vasc Endovasc Surg* 2003; 25: 451-7.
6. Bozkurt AK, Koksal C, Ercan M. The altered hemorheologic parameters in thromboangiitis obliterans: a new insight. *Clin Appl Thromb Hemost* 2004; 10: 45-50.
7. Olin JW. Thromboangiitis obliterans (Buerger's disease). *N Engl J Med* 2000; 343: 864-9.
8. Wysokinski WE, Kwiatkowska W, Sapian-Raczkowska B, Czarnacki M, Doskocz R, Kowal-Gierczak B. Sustained classic clinical spectrum of thromboangiitis obliterans (Buerger's disease). *Angiology* 2000; 51: 141-50.
9. Shionoya S. Buerger's disease: diagnosis and management. *Cardiovasc Surg* 1993; 1: 207-14.
10. Mills JL, Porter JM. Buerger's disease: a review and update. *Semin Vasc Surg* 1993; 6: 14-23.
11. Papa MZ, Rabi I, Adar R. A point scoring system for the clinical diagnosis of Buerger's disease. *Eur J Vasc Endovasc Surg* 1996; 11: 335-9.
12. Suzuki S, Yamada I, Himeno Y. Angiographic findings in Buerger disease. *Int J Cardiol* 1996; 54: S189-S195.
13. Fiessinger JN, Schafer M. Trial of iloprost versus aspirin treatment for critical limb ischaemia of thromboangiitis obliterans. The TAO Study. *Lancet* 1990; 335: 555-7.
14. Oral iloprost in the treatment of thromboangiitis obliterans (Buerger's disease): a double-blind, randomised, placebo-controlled trial. The European TAO Study Group. *Eur J Vasc Endovasc Surg* 1998; 15: 300-7.
15. Sayin A, Bozkurt AK, Tuzun H, Vural FS, Erdog G, Ozer M. Surgical treatment of Buerger's disease: experience with 216 patients. *Cardiovasc Surg* 1993; 1: 377-80.
16. Inada K, Iwashima Y, Okada A, Matsumoto K. Nonatherosclerotic segmental arterial occlusion of the extremity. *Arch Surg* 1974; 108: 663-7.
17. Sasajima T, Kubo Y, Inaba M, Goh K, Azuma N. Role of infrainguinal bypass in Buerger's disease: an eighteen-year experience. *Eur J Vasc Endovasc Surg* 1997; 13: 186-92.
18. Ohta T, Ishioashi H, Hosaka M, Sugimoto I. Clinical and social consequences of Buerger disease. *J Vasc Surg* 2004; 39: 176-80.

Case vignette

The value of biopsy for a leg ulcer: Pyoderma gangrenosum

John F Thompson MS FRCS (Ed) FRCS, Consultant Surgeon, Royal Devon and Exeter Hospitals, Exeter, UK

A 69-year-old man was admitted with a painful leg ulcer (Figure 1). He had a history of heavy smoking, claudication and a family history of venous ulceration. Clinical examination revealed absent popliteal pulses and an ankle brachial pressure index of 0.8. He had wasting of the calf muscles, but no varicose veins.

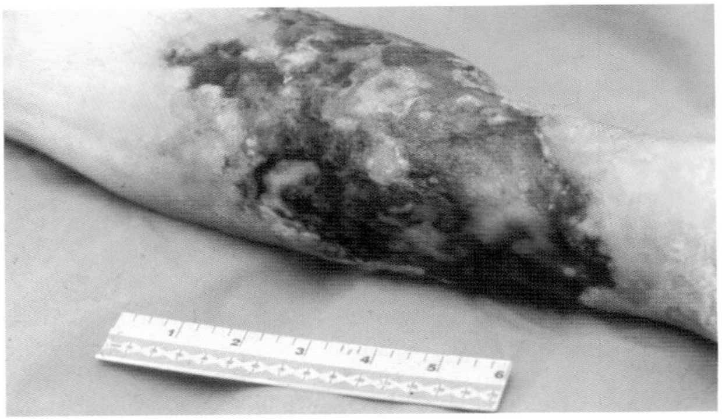

Figure 1.

The unusual distribution of the ulcer raised questions as to the aetiology. A biopsy was suggested that confirmed the diagnosis of Pyoderma gangrenosum. He was treated with a combination of intravenous antibiotics and steroids. The ulcer was excised and grafted with a meshed split skin graft (Figure 2). The graft was successful and he made a complete recovery (Figure 3).

Longstanding refractory ulcers should be treated with suspicion in view of the possibility of malignant change (Marjolin's ulcer). Ulceration in an atypical site should be biopsied; close collaboration with colleagues in the dermatology department should be a part of vascular surgical practice.

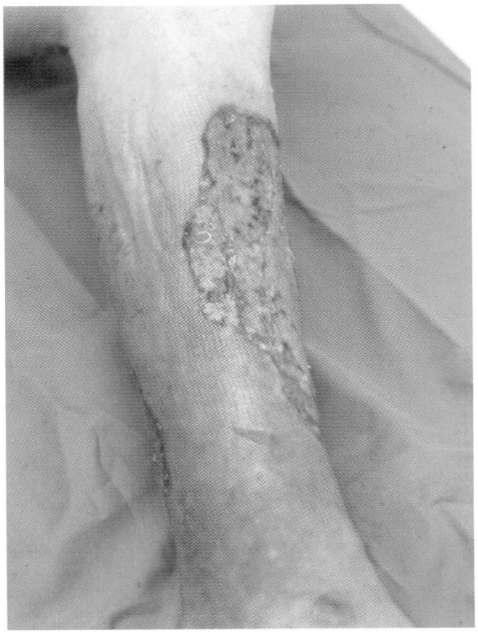

Figure 2.

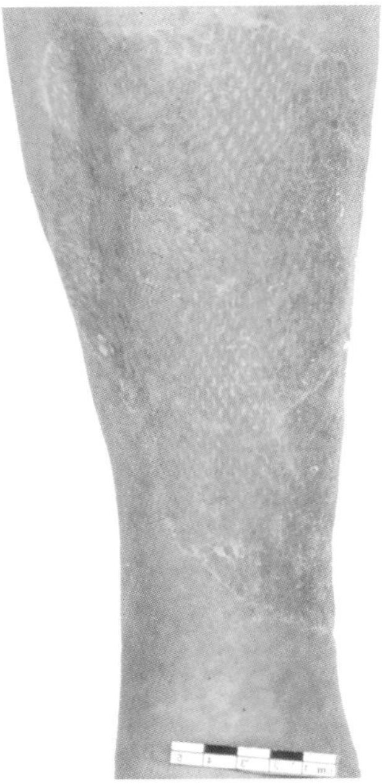

Figure 3.